Sports Supplement Review

3RD ISSUE

By Bill PHILLIPS

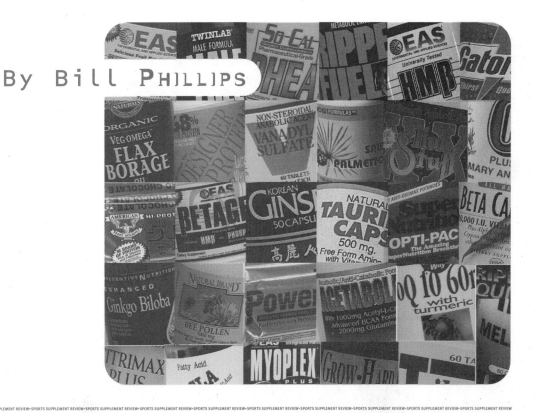

Sources CONSULTED

Literally hundreds and hundreds of athletes contributed to the information contained in this book. Other data sources included textbooks, medical journals, scientific conference abstract presentations, and reports from supplement manufacturers and distributors. To give individual credit to each and every text consulted or each person interviewed would be impossible. However, a comprehensive list of very important references does appear in the back of this book.

I would also like to specifically thank the numerous experts who made significant contributions to this book, including: Brett Hall, R.D.; Vicki Douthitt, Ph.D.; TC Luoma; Dan Duchaine; Keith Klein (Chapter 14); Will Brink (Chapter 11); Torbjorn Akerfeldt (Chapter 15); Charles Staley, Ph.D. (Chapter 17); and Charles Poliquin (Chapter 18).

I would also like to acknowledge the diligent efforts of Graphic Designers Chris Monck and Craig Korn; as well as Associate Editor, Sue Daniel; my All-Star Word Processor, Leigh Rauen; Copy Editors, Virginia Cusack and Robert Wehner; and Production Coordinator, Mike Sitzman. Without the assistance of these fine individuals, this friggin' book would have taken me twice as long, and it probably would have been only half as good.

Oh, by the way, the dude on the front cover is lifetime drug-free bodybuilder Roger Applewhite; the cover photo is the work of Kal Yee. The back cover photo is me and was taken by Dennis Lane.

Important NOTICE

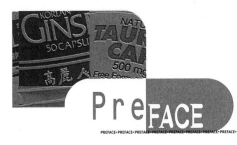

PreFACE

By Jeffrey Stout, M.P.E., Ph.D.

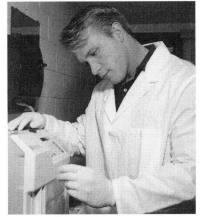

Professor of Exercise Science at Creighton University
Member of the American College of Sports Medicine
Consultant, EAS, Inc.

Being a Professor of Exercise Science as well as an avid weight-training athlete, I have an intense interest not only in human performance and muscle metabolism but also in the real-world applications of this field of science. Thus, I follow the latest findings regarding sports supplements quite closely.

Because of my "schooling," I have learned to look at the supplement industry with skepticism, if not cynicism. I've discovered there are many supplements which are promoted as performance enhancers, muscle builders, and/or fat burners that don't come close to living up to the advertising claims that are made about these products. But, I've also learned there are some products that really do work, and over the past year, I've tried several supplements that produced such remarkable results, I could hardly believe they were drug free!

There is a scientific basis for the use of some supplements—there's a logical reason why they work, but it's not always easy, even for someone with my education and experience, to determine which supplements are for real and which ones are bogus.

Fortunately, the book you're about to read, which I have thoroughly reviewed, takes this very complex issue and makes it simple and easy to understand. The *Sports Supplement Review, 3rd Issue,* is very well researched and referenced, authoritative, yet highly comprehensible. It's an excellent, straightforward source of scientific and real-world information that can benefit experts, those new to this field, as well as everyone in between.

I highly recommend the *Sports Supplement Review, 3rd Issue,* to anyone who's interested in building a lean, strong, muscular, healthy body. I've already applied the information I learned in this book to my own workouts and can definitely see and feel the difference! I'm certain your workouts and pursuit of a better body will be enhanced as well by the application of the information in this new, great book!

3

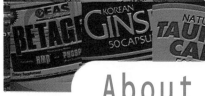

About THE AUTHOR

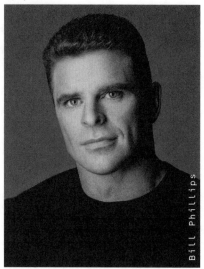

Bill Phillips

The author of this book, Bill Phillips, is probably best known as the founder and Executive Editor of *Muscle Media*, one of the nation's fastest growing strength-training magazines. Under Phillips' direction, *Muscle Media* has gained a reputation as the "tell-it-like-it-is" fitness and physique-development publication because of its straightforward, brutally honest approach to the numerous topics that pertain to bodybuilding and fitness. *Muscle Media* is distributed on over 45,000 newsstands and has a loyal and growing worldwide readership of over 350,000 weight trainers.

Phillips has also written some of the most controversial yet popular books on athletic performance enhancement and bodybuilding—over 500,000 copies of his books have been distributed in 22 countries over the past 3 years alone, making his expertise literally world renowned. Phillips has a reputation for first-rate, perceptive reporting—for sweeping aside the surface swill and plunging into the depths of bodybuilding reality.

Some experts call Phillips "bodybuilding's early warning system" because of his positively uncanny instincts and the way he consistently reveals what tomorrow's most talked about stories in fitness and physique development will be—from new trends in bodybuilding drug use to the latest scientific breakthroughs in supplements, training, and nutrition—Phillips always seems to be at least one step ahead of the game.

Phillips, a bodybuilder himself, has the introspection that allows him to closely relate to and empathize with the desires and needs of the hardcore fitness and physique enthusiast. This, combined with over a decade of interaction with leading scientists, medical doctors, and literally thousands of strength trainers from around the world, gives him a unique perspective that many other information providers in this industry lack. Phillips can evaluate the scientific rationale and basis behind various supplements as well as the potential of a supplement to produce positive effects in the *real world*.

Phillips' expertise on physique development and athletic performance are not only sought out by fitness buffs and world-champion athletes but also by numerous

"A-list" Hollywood celebrities who rely on their extraordinary physiques to maintain their thriving superstar status. Phillips has also appeared as an industry expert on national network news programs like the *CBS Evening News* and *ABC's Good Morning America* as well as being quoted in dozens of newspapers, including: the *New York Times, Rocky Mountain News,* and *Wall Street Journal,* to name a few.

Not only is Phillips committed to discovering and reporting the truth about topics such as which bodybuilding supplements work and which ones don't, his company, Experimental and Applied Sciences, Inc. (EAS), has gone to unprecedented levels to advance the science of natural performance enhancement. Last year alone, Phillips' corporation allocated over one million dollars to university studies to further the science of sports nutrition. This money funded research grants in the area of human performance and muscle metabolism at prestigious institutions such as Kent State University, Iowa State University, Creighton University, the University of Nebraska at Omaha, the University of Memphis, Witchita State University, State University of New York at Stony Brook, and Nottingham University in England.

Phillips' partnership with the scientific community and support of university clinical research underscore his commitment to provide consumers with credible information and to identify new products that may enhance muscle building, fat loss, and sports performance.

Phillips believes that the answers to safe, legal performance enhancement and muscle building lie in scientifically designed nutritional supplements used in conjunction with effective nutrition and exercise programs. Although Phillips admits the science of sports supplements has not quite caught up with that of bodybuilding drugs, he remains optimistic and cites that almost every month, new, exciting discoveries in this area of science are being made.

And, Phillips believes this all-new, completely updated *Sports Supplement Review, 3rd Issue,* will provide fitness and physique enthusiasts with the most up-to-date, practical, scientific, and real-world information on bodybuilding supplements available anywhere today!

Table OF CONTENTS

SPORTS SUPPLEMENT REVIEW, 3RD ISSUE•SPORTS SUPPLEMENT REVIEW, 3RD ISSUE•SPORTS SUPPLEMENT REVIEW, 3RD ISSUE•SPORTS SUPPLEMENT REVIEW, 3RD ISSUE•SPORTS SUPPLEMENT REVIEW, 3RD ISSUE•SPORTS

8

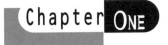

Chapter ONE

Introduction

You and I are quite likely different in many ways, but there's one thing we definitely have in common—we both want to gain more size and strength and build a lean, muscular physique. (Of course, you wouldn't be reading this book if you didn't want to build a better body—you'd be out doing whatever it is "regular" people do.)

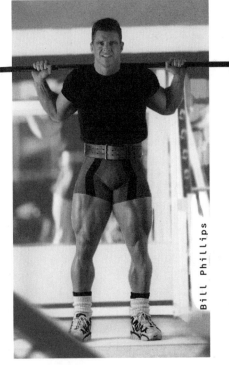

Bill Phillips

You and I—we're dedicated to being better than the "average Joe." We have discipline, drive, and we're determined to build the best body our genetics will allow!

We know it takes hard work and dedication, but we're always looking for the "extra edge." And today, more so than ever before, bodybuilders like you and me are desperately searching for *supplements* that will help us get better results faster from the time we spend working out, in part because of the health risks, legal ramifications, and lack of availability of performance-enhancing drugs like steroids.

The good news is that over the past few years, legitimate scientific research has uncovered powerful new supplements that really do work—supplements that really can boost athletic performance, accelerate gains in size and strength, and even promote fat loss! The science of supplements is moving forward at a meteoric pace—exciting new discoveries are being made literally every month!

The bad news is that not all supplements work. There are many irreputable companies and "snake-oil salesmen" that are blatantly ripping consumers off left and right. They use false advertising and other scams to make a quick buck. Unfortunately, trying to figure out what works and what doesn't can be a confusing and sometimes frustrating endeavor—there are so many supplements on the market, and they're all supposed to "perform miracles."

9

•SPORTS SUPPLEMENT REVIEW, 3RD ISSUE•SPORTS SUPPLEMENT REVIEW, 3RD ISSUE•SPORTS SUPPLEMENT REVIEW, 3RD ISSUE•SPORTS SUPPLEMENT REVIEW, 3RD ISSUE•SPORTS SUPPLEMENT REVIEW, 3RD ISSUE•SPORTS SUPPLEMENT REVIEW, 3RD ISSUE•SPORTS SUPPLEMENT

Sifting through all the B.S. and uncovering the *facts* could be a full-time job; in fact, for me, it is! For the past 16 years, I've been studying muscle-building products. I've tried virtually everything you can think of, including steroids back in the mid-'80's. I've spent literally thousands of hours gathering information on supplements, and I've worked with some of the most brilliant sports medicine doctors and scientists on the planet! I've made it my business to know what works and what doesn't, and in this new book, I'm going to share virtually everything I know with you!

In this, the *Sports Supplement Review, 3rd Issue*, not only will I give you the latest scientific and real-world information on popular supplements like creatine, HMB, ephedra, whey protein, vanadyl sulfate, and so on, but I'll also give you the complete low-down on new supplements like DHEA, CHP, androstenedione, melatonin, chrysin, *Tribulus terrestris*, and many more. And, I'll give you an idea of what's right around the corner—what the hottest supplement trends in the coming year will be.

If you've ever wondered *exactly* which supplements will really help you build muscle size and strength, boost your endurance and athletic performance, and even accelerate fat loss, this will be one of the most exciting books you'll ever read!

This easy-to-read book contains *all* the answers you're looking for—I guarantee it! For example, do you want to know which supplements will help you pack on pounds of rock-hard muscular bodyweight? If so, check out Chapter 4. You'll be amazed at how powerful and effective some of these supplements really are!

> "...**do** you want to know which supplements will help you pack on pounds of rock-hard muscular bodyweight? If so, check out Chapter 4."

Do you want to know which supplements will help you burn fat and build a lean, muscular physique? Well, you'll definitely want to read Chapter 12—I "spill my guts" on some amazing products that will help you lose fat faster than anything else you can get without a prescription! (I didn't even know about some of these supplements myself until just a few months ago.)

Do you worry about getting scammed or ripped off by supplement distributors that conveniently tell you less than "the whole truth" in their ads? Believe me, if you're not worried about getting *royally screwed* by unethical supplement distributors, you should be. I absolutely insist you read Chapter 13 before you spend another dollar on supplements. In this chapter, I expose the "inside secrets" of how supplement companies rip unsuspecting consumers off! (These rip-off artists really piss me off—they give the whole industry a "black eye.")

As you most likely know, or will learn from reading this book, there are more than a few supplements that really do work. How do you decide which ones you should be using and how to "stack" or combine them for maximum results? It's not easy to figure out—this is a very complicated subject. But, after you read my step-by-step instructions on how to determine *exactly* which supplements are best for **YOU** and precisely how to stack and cycle them, which you'll find in Chapters 12 and 16, you could catapult your gains in muscle size and strength and fat loss to almost unimaginable levels!

Hey... you wanna learn how to save up to $100 a month on the highest quality, most effective new bodybuilding supplements? Of course you do! In Chapter 13, I'll give you some vital tips on *where* and *when* to buy supplements to save big bucks on the best muscle builders and fat burners you can get. (I'll even tell you the best day of the month to buy supplements!)

And, as any bodybuilder with half a brain knows, even the best supplements won't produce maximum results if you don't train and eat properly. But, there's a lot of confusion about exercise and nutrition just like there is with supplements. Not anymore—after reading Chapters 17 and 18, you'll have your very own "Ph.D." in pumping iron. Read Chapter 15 and you'll discover how to use regular old food to kick your body's anabolic hormones into high gear so you can make gains literally year-round. I'm serious... the information in these chapters will completely revolutionize the way you train and eat!

I promise this book will give you the *real answers* to virtually every question you could possibly ask about bodybuilding supplements. And, you'll get all this information in simple, straightforward language without pages of complicated, scientific "mumbo jumbo" and irrelevant crap.

Because I am just as interested as you are in building muscle, losing fat, and gaining strength, I understand that you want the hardcore, unadulterated truth and nothing less. Well, that's exactly what you'll get in this all-new, completely updated *Sports Supplement Review, 3rd Issue.* I've got a ton of exciting, new information to share with you (some of which has never before appeared in print!), so let's stop wasting time and get to it...

SPORTS SUPPLEMENT REVIEW, 3RD ISSUE•SPORTS SUPPLEMENT REVIEW, 3RD ISSUE•SPORTS SUPPLEMENT REVIEW, 3RD ISSUE•SPORTS SUPPLEMENT REVIEW, 3RD ISSUE•SPORTS SUPPLEMENT REVIEW, 3RD ISSUE•SPORTS

12

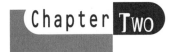

Chapter Two

What Are Supplements and How Do They Work?

The "bio-science of supplements" is a somewhat complex and confusing subject; as a matter of fact, I could write a whole book about that topic alone, but it's probably something that would be interesting to only really hardcore science types and researchers. You've got better things to do than read a 300-page book on how different molecules react with each other, how obscure compounds and chemicals are formed, and all that stuff. But it *is* important to have a basic understanding of just exactly what a "supplement" is and the primary mechanisms by which supplements work. So, in this chapter, we'll take a quick look at those two topics and then move on.

Most of us use the word "supplement" to describe a nutrient, a formulation, or some type of compound that is "drug free" or "natural." Some use terms like "sports supplement," "performance supplement," "bodybuilding supplement," etc. All these pretty much mean the same thing.

But just exactly what is a supplement, anyway? Well, according to a relatively new law called the Dietary Supplement Health and Education Act of 1994 (DSHEA), supplements or "dietary supplements," as the FDA calls them, are defined as: vitamins, minerals, herbs, or other botanicals (except tobacco), amino acids, any "dietary substance for use by man to supplement the diet by increasing the total dietary intake," and "a concentration, metabolite, constituent, extract, or combination of any of the above-listed ingredients."

This definition of dietary supplements is quite broad and has allowed a whole slew of new products to be brought to the market as "supplements"—as a matter of fact, a number of drug companies which were developing new products with the intent of bringing them to the market as pharmaceuticals are now looking to get in the dietary supplement business.

> "**...if** you're deficient in one or more nutrients, it's quite possible your body may not be able to build muscle and burn fat properly."

WHAT ARE SUPPLEMENTS AND HOW DO THEY WORK?

SUPPLEMENTS AND HOW DO THEY WORK?~WHAT ARE SUPPLEMENTS AND HOW DO THEY WORK?~WHAT ARE SUPPLEMENTS AND HOW DO THEY WORK?~WHAT ARE SUPPLEMENTS AND HOW DO THEY WORK?~WHAT ARE SUPPLEMENTS AND HOW DO THEY WORK?~WHAT ARE SUPPLEMENTS AND HOW DO THEY WORK?~WHAT ARE SUPPLEMENTS AND HOW DO THEY WORK?~WHAT ARE SUPPLEMENTS AND HOW DO THEY WORK?~WHAT ARE SUPPLEM

According to this law, dietary supplements include many of the things you would suspect, such as vitamins, antioxidants, minerals, amino acids, protein powders, and so on. But it's interesting to note that "dietary supplements" now include many things that prior to late 1994 might have been considered drugs or "unapproved food additives" by the FDA. Look at DHEA and melatonin for example. These very popular "supplements" are synthetically manufactured prohormones that exert "drug-like" effects on the body.

In the United States, the rule is you can buy anything that is classified as a dietary supplement without a prescription. Most of these products are available at health-food stores, through mail-order companies, and at big supplement chains, like General Nutrition Centers (GNC).

The United States has one of the most liberal and "open" policies in terms of supplement legislation, and the FDA isn't very happy about it. (They may try to "redo" this law in the not-too-distant future.) In Canada, many products that are considered supplements in the U.S. are available only with a prescription, or they're not available at all. In parts of Europe, it's much the same. In fact, there are some countries in Europe where you can buy steroids over the counter but can't buy supplements like vanadyl sulfate, amino acids, chromium picolinate, etc. (Crazy, huh?!)

Basically, what we'll discuss in this book are products that would likely be classified as dietary supplements by the FDA, which, by the way, does not "approve" supplements. They only have the power to get involved if a supplement is determined to be harmful or if a marketer of a supplement makes a "drug claim." An example of a drug claim would be if a company advertised or labeled a supplement as a cure for cancer or some other disease that would usually call for treatment with medicine.

> **"...despite** what some 'old-school' dietitians, doctors, or other 'experts' might tell you, there indeed is a very sound, scientific basis for supplementation."

In this book, we won't talk about things like anabolic steroids, fat-burning drugs, and other products you can legally obtain only with a prescription. The products we'll talk about are, for the most part, easy for almost anyone to get, legal, and generally considered safe.

Another thing that is important to understand before we jump into the main substance of this book is just exactly how supplements work in the first place. I basically put the effects of supplements into three general categories.

The first way a supplement might help you build muscle, lose fat, and improve your health is simply by making up for deficiencies. This has basically been what most dietitians, nutritionists, doctors, etc. have viewed supplements as—a means of protecting your body against vitamin and mineral deficiencies and so on. Vitamin supplements have been widely used for decades as a means of preventing serious, even fatal diseases, which are caused by nutrient deficiencies.

It's widely accepted that active individuals, like bodybuilders and other athletes who exercise intensely, have greater demands for a number of nutrients, which makes it even that much more likely we will suffer deficiencies without supplementation. And if you're deficient in one or more nutrients, it's quite possible your body may not be able to build muscle and burn fat properly.

For example, it is well known that the trace mineral chromium is essential for insulin to exert its anabolic effects.[180] It's also been shown that a great number of people may not consume the appropriate amount of chromium through their diets, thus leaving them in a deficient state.[197] In this case, consuming chromium supplements may help build muscle. (Makes sense, huh?)

Now, another mechanism by which supplements may exert a positive effect on your efforts to build a better body is by providing a nutrient that is "under-supplied" to cells or not normally available in "optimal" levels in the diet. In this case, a nutrient is required by an organism (like a muscle cell), and a specific concentration of this nutrient results in what I'd call "better-than-normal" cell function. For a dietary supplement to exert a positive effect under this scenario, normal consumption of the supplied nutrient must be "suboptimal."

Let's look at the very popular bodybuilding supplement creatine (which we'll review in-depth later in this book) as an example. Very few athletes have what doctors would call a "creatine deficiency," but numerous scientific studies have clearly established that the amount of creatine an athlete normally supplies through his or her diet is not the "optimal" amount.[19] Supplementing the diet with extra doses of creatine can very reliably enhance performance, improve recovery, and promote gains in lean body mass.[79]

So, even if you don't have a nutrient deficiency, it is absolutely, positively possible to benefit from using a supplement that provides optimal levels for a cell to "up-regulate" its natural function.[294]

A third mechanism by which a dietary supplement may work is when it produces a pharmacological or "drug-like" effect on cellular processes. Under this scenario, the dietary supplement can exert a positive effect on muscle metabolism and/or performance when it contains a compound which is normally not required by a cell but is capable of altering normal cell function.

Let's look at the herb guarana (remember, herbs are considered dietary supplements under the new FDA regulations). This herb contains caffeine which may alter muscle function and fat metabolism.[293] Of course, neither guarana nor caffeine

WHAT ARE SUPPLEMENTS AND HOW DO THEY WORK?

SUPPLEMENTS AND HOW DO THEY WORK?~WHAT ARE SUPPLEMENTS AND HOW DO THEY WORK?~WHAT ARE SUPPLEMENTS AND HOW DO THEY WORK?~WHAT ARE SUPPLEMENTS AND HOW DO THEY WORK?~WHAT ARE SUPPLEMENTS AND HOW DO THEY WORK?~WHAT ARE SUPPLEMENTS AND HOW DO THEY WORK?~WHAT ARE SUPPLEM

are nutrients that are required by a cell. But, they are capable of altering normal cell function.

So, despite what some "old-school" dietitians, doctors, or other "experts" might tell you, there indeed is a very sound, scientific basis for supplementation. Remember, a supplement can work through three different "modes of action": by preventing or correcting a nutrient deficiency; by providing "optimal" levels of a nutrient that a cell needs to perform at its best; and finally, a supplement may work by providing a cell with a substance that it doesn't require but which alters cell function in somewhat of a "drug-like" manner.

Oh, by the way, this is not some wacky theory I threw together. It's a concept which scientists who are up to date on this topic accept; in fact, these ideas were recently presented at a conference sponsored by the National Institutes of Health (NIH) which is a government-funded group that spends literally <u>billions</u> of (taxpayer) dollars on scientific research.[196]

"*Alright already...* which supplements should I take to build muscle and burn fat?" you ask. Hang in there, we're gettin' to that...

Hot New Supplement Trends

As I write this chapter, it's early in the year 1997. And, I'm assuming most of you who are reading this book have examined the 1996 version of my *Supplement Review*. You might also regularly read my magazine, *Muscle Media*.

My guess is you already know a thing or two about bodybuilding supplements. You probably opened up this book asking the question, "What's new and exciting in the world of bodybuilding supplements—what can Phillips tell me that I don't already know?"

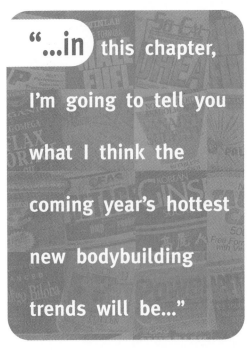

"...in this chapter, I'm going to tell you what I think the coming year's hottest new bodybuilding trends will be..."

Am I right? Is that what you're thinking? Well, if so, I've got some good news for you—this book is filled with exciting, <u>new</u> information about bodybuilding supplements! In fact, in this chapter, I'm going to tell you what I think the coming year's hottest new bodybuilding trends will be—the stuff the other industry "experts" will be talking about months from now.

WHERE I'M "COMING FROM"

Make no mistake, a lot has happened since I wrote the last version of my *Supplement Review*. There have been some amazing discoveries, which I'm anxious to tell you about. Some of this information is "red hot" to say the least. But, before we jump right in, I want to take a brief moment to tell you where I'm "coming from." In this chapter, and throughout this book, I'm going to be sharing my *opinions* with you—a whole lot of them! I'm basically going to tell you what I think is good, bad, and ugly in the world of supplements.

How do I make up my mind? I take a number of different things into consideration, such as: scientific studies, interviews with researchers and medical doctors,

HOT NEW SUPPLEMENT TRENDS

HOT NEW SUPPLEMENT TRENDS•HOT NEW SUPPLEMENT TRENDS•HOT NEW SUPPLEMENT TRENDS•HOT NEW SUPPLEMENT TRENDS•HOT NEW SUPPLEMENT TRENDS•HOT NEW SUPPLEMENT TRENDS•HOT NEW SUPPLEMENT TRENDS•HOT NEW SUPPLEMENT TRENDS•HOT NEW SUPPLEMENT TRENDS•HOT NEW SUPPLEMENT TRENDS•HOT

feedback from athletes and bodybuilders, and my own personal experiences with a product. These all play a factor in whether I think a supplement works or not.

Now, when I say something works, that doesn't necessarily mean it's a sound, scientific fact, accepted by every expert in the world. This book contains a great deal of scientifically validated and referenced information, but in some cases, the science is incomplete or inconclusive. And, once in a while, athletes are way ahead of scientists. One example of this that stands out is athletes knew anabolic steroids worked extremely well long before most doctors and scientific experts were convinced. In this instance, if you had ignored the real-world feedback and only listened to the "scientific opinion," you would have believed steroids were completely ineffective at enhancing athletic performance and muscle mass. Of course, we all know that's not the case. The point is, sometimes you have to form an opinion based on a "hunch" or sometimes limited empirical feedback.

Other times, you have to look at preliminary scientific studies or abstracts. Now, I'm aware that hardcore scientists (which I'm not) rely primarily on peer-reviewed, published studies. I'm actually a "bodybuilding theorist"—I try to piece together information, much like a detective would to solve a case. I try to come up with answers *sooner* rather than *later*.

> **"My job is to keep you on the cutting edge of bodybuilding supplement trends..."**

Unfortunately, if we waited around for every scientist, or even the majority of scientists, to agree on something before we made a move, we'd probably be waiting forever. Do you realize that many scientists don't even believe we can benefit from taking Vitamin C supplements, in spite of the fact that literally hundreds of studies show it works? I'm not trying to rip on scientists—they have their jobs to do, and I have mine. My job is to keep you on the cutting edge of bodybuilding supplement trends—to help you learn what works and what doesn't, so you can build a stronger, more muscular physique.

So, even though this book is based on a lot of scientific evidence, it's also "bridged" with my opinions and beliefs as well as *common sense*. Fortunately, I have somewhat of a unique "knack" for being right—*at least most of the time*! (Of course, no one is right 100% of the time, and I'm no exception to that rule.)

Also, as you probably know, I have a company which sells supplements—I've been in the supplement industry for seven years now. But, that does not mean the reviews you'll get in this book are not as straightforward and accurate as you'll find anywhere else. My company, Experimental and Applied Sciences (EAS), sells a relatively small line of supplements—the vast majority of products you'll read about in this book, including many that I recommend, are ones I don't even sell. (I wrote this book, first and foremost, to help you stay *informed*!) The truth is, I could sell virtually any supplement I wanted to. Every week, I get inundated with offers from different supplement companies, scientists, inventors, and so on, who all want me to promote their products. Typically, I give their products a thorough review (and occasionally try them out myself), but I rarely introduce new products to the EAS line. There's no doubt my company could make a lot more money, in the short term, if we sold supplements I just don't believe in, but that's not my style.

Now, before we jump into the exciting supplement reviews I have prepared for you, I want you to keep something else in mind—I'm not recommending that you use every one of the supplements in this book that I say might work. As we'll discuss later in this very comprehensive publication, there are various ways to determine which supplements might provide you with the most benefit, and I'll walk you through all of that. Depending on your particular goals (whether you want to build muscle size and strength, lose fat, enhance athletic performance, etc.), you'll want to use different types of supplements. Also, which supplements you use will depend on how much money you want to invest in these products. (By the way, later in this book, I'll tell you how to save hundreds of dollars on supplements!)

Throughout the majority of this guide, I'll discuss supplements using their "generic names," but in Chapter 10, I'll review specific brand names, and I'll tell you what I think of each of them.

Now, back to the material you'll find in this chapter: as I explained, in this section of my book, I'm including cutting-edge information on the latest and hottest supplement trends. Whether these supplements stand the test of time—whether we look back a year or two from now and determine that these things have been proven to work in the real world <u>and</u> in scientific studies—remains to be seen. There's a chance these trends will turn out to be bodybuilding supplement fads and nothing more. But, I think there's a chance some of the trends I'll introduce you to in this chapter will stand the test of time (otherwise I wouldn't have even put them in the book).

Okay, here's what's new in the world of bodybuilding for 1997!

TESTOSTERONE BOOSTERS THAT WORK!

Testosterone, or "T" as bodybuilding experts call it, is today, and actually always has been, the most coveted muscle-building hormone in existence. For decades, scientists and athletes alike have been mesmerized with the amazing powers of testosterone—it's literally the hormone that separates the men from the boys. It's the four-carbon ring which every anabolic steroid is derived from, and not only does it help build muscle but recent research shows it *may* elevate your mood, slow down the aging process, boost your sex drive, and perhaps even increase the odds that you'll be successful in the business world.

HOT NEW SUPPLEMENT TRENDS

HOT NEW SUPPLEMENT TRENDS•HOT NEW SUPPLEMENT TRENDS•HOT NEW SUPPLEMENT TRENDS•HOT NEW SUPPLEMENT TRENDS•HOT NEW SUPPLEMENT TRENDS•HOT NEW SUPPLEMENT TRENDS•HOT NEW SUPPLEMENT TRENDS•HOT NEW SUPPLEMENT TRENDS•HOT NEW SUPPLEMENT TRENDS•HOT NEW SUPPLEMENT TRENDS•HOT

CHAPTER 3

Any doubt that testosterone truly is "king" was erased last year when a very comprehensive study published in the July 4, 1996, issue of the *New England Journal of Medicine* revealed supraphysiological doses of synthetic testosterone allowed weight-training men to gain almost twice as much lean body mass as their non-testosterone-supplemented counterparts. This study also revealed that men who took testosterone but didn't even train with weights gained more muscle than a group of men who regularly trained with weights. Basically, taking testosterone and sitting on the couch appears to produce greater gains in muscle size and strength than working your ass off in the gym and not taking testosterone. (Those of you who are experienced bodybuilders are probably saying to yourself, "Duh!" But to the scientific community, this study was revolutionary.)

Anyway, the bottom line is, testosterone is and always has been *the* muscle-building hormone. Unfortunately, testosterone medicine and its chemical cousins, anabolic steroids, are illegal, very hard to get, and if used improperly, may have serious side effects. So, what does all this have to do with drug-free bodybuilding supplements? Shouldn't I save this information for the next edition of my *Anabolic Reference Guide*? Well, not necessarily. I now know (and you're about to learn) how we might be able to double, if not triple, our testosterone levels without using any "drugs." No, I'm not talking about the impotent "testosterone boosters" of yesteryear—crap like boron (that was shown to slightly increase testosterone in post-menopausal women but didn't do jack squat in healthy, weight-training males). No, it's not like that at all. Let me explain...

It All Started With DHEA...

About two months after I finished the 1996 version of my *Supplement Review*, the bodybuilding world went bonkers for a compound called DHEA (dehydroepiandrosterone). This trend wasn't started by any new, breakthrough studies which showed DHEA supplementation could dramatically increase gains in muscle size and strength in bodybuilders (which is how the creatine and HMB crazes got started). Rather, DHEA became popular basically because *it became available.* You see, up until a few years ago, DHEA was stuck in some type of FDA limbo—it wasn't really a drug, but it wasn't really a supplement either: that is, until the Dietary Supplement Health and Education Act (DSHEA) of 1994 was passed. This piece of legislation (which I told you about in Chapter 2) defined what a dietary supplement is, and as it turns out, this law basically made it okay for prohormones (like DHEA) to be sold as dietary supplements.

DHEA is an interesting compound, but it's *not* what I'm excited about. However, DHEA does cause an increase in testosterone for some people—mainly women and mature adults whose bodies don't produce that much DHEA naturally. Let's go through a crash course on DHEA and quickly move on to the *really* exciting part...

The Facts About DHEA

Dozens and dozens of supplement companies now sell DHEA. It's purported to do just about everything: burn fat, build muscle, cure Alzheimer's disease, prevent cancer, extend your life, to name only a few of the bold claims some marketers have made. But what does it really do? Let's take a look.

DHEA is an androgenic hormone produced by the adrenal glands. It's actually two steps up the hormonal metabolic pathway from testosterone production. Our bodies start making DHEA when we're around the age of 7, and its secretion peaks when we are about 20-24 years old. Then, DHEA levels begin to decline at a steady pace of about 20% per decade, until they hit a low of approximately 10% of peak levels by the time a person is in his/her 80's.[11]

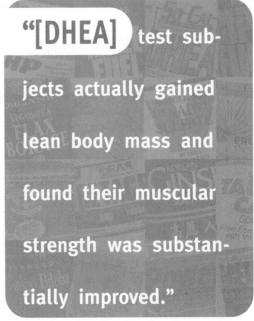

"[DHEA] test subjects actually gained lean body mass and found their muscular strength was substantially improved."

DHEA is a substrate which serves a variety of purposes. It can lend itself to everything from cellular energy production, to fat metabolism, to sexual maturation, to muscle growth, etc.

Interestingly enough, the science of oral DHEA supplementation is actually quite young. Only in the past five years have scientists begun to look at its effects on patients with various maladies, ranging from heart disease to diabetes. It has also been evaluated to some extent in healthy individuals.

One of the most interesting studies examined the effects of a 50-mg daily oral dose of DHEA in men and women over the age of 50.[105] It was found that this daily dose increased subjects' DHEA blood levels to those of young adults within two weeks. This level of DHEA persisted throughout the six-month study period. Immune function was also assessed by measuring blood levels of immune cells (including: lymphocytes, T-cells, and natural killer cells) and was found to increase by 67% in men and 84% in women. A follow-up study was conducted, also using mature adults, where participants consumed 100 mg of DHEA before sleep. This caused not only a rise in DHEA levels and the expected increase in immune function, but the test subjects actually gained lean body mass and found their muscular strength was substantially improved.[302] Men in the group also experienced a significant decrease in bodyfat over the control group.

So what's going on that allows these older subjects to become leaner and stronger? One theory, backed by some good science, is that by cranking up levels of DHEA through supplementation, mature adults are able to produce greater amounts of testosterone. More testosterone equals more lean mass, which typically increases fat burning.

HOT NEW SUPPLEMENT TRENDS

HOT NEW SUPPLEMENT TRENDS•HOT NEW SUPPLEMENT TRENDS•HOT NEW SUPPLEMENT TRENDS•HOT NEW SUPPLEMENT TRENDS•HOT NEW SUPPLEMENT TRENDS•HOT NEW SUPPLEMENT TRENDS•HOT NEW SUPPLEMENT TRENDS•HOT NEW SUPPLEMENT TRENDS•HOT NEW SUPPLEMENT TRENDS•HOT NEW SUPPLEMENT TRENDS•HOT

To test this theory on a more personal level, my father, age 53, started taking 100 mg of DHEA per day about 6 months ago. He was recovering from hip surgery, and I encouraged him to try boosting his testosterone levels to aid in his rehabilitation efforts. His pre-supplementation blood test showed DHEA levels at 254 mcg/dl and testosterone at 485 ng/dl (nanograms per deciliter). Both of these levels were within the normal range. After 2 months of DHEA supplementation, his DHEA levels shot up to 626 mcg/dl, and his testosterone soared to 1,026 ng/dl. (That's way over the high end of normal!) The day we got his blood test back, we printed up a little sign which read, "Raging Bull" and posted it on his office door. He said that just about summed up how DHEA made him feel.

So DHEA may indeed work wonders for older adults, but what about healthy young men and women? There have been a few studies performed in young adults. One, using a high dosage (1,600 mg/day!), showed some positive results—a significant loss of bodyfat (31% in 28 days) with a concurrent increase in lean body mass.[189] But, other studies show little or no results.

Does DHEA Really "Work"?

There's no way to say whether DHEA flat out works or doesn't work for bodybuilders. As I've explained, there is evidence to suggest the older you are, the more you'll benefit from using a DHEA supplement. Typically, young men (especially under the age of 25) already make all the DHEA their bodies need to maintain optimal testosterone production. However, to the best of my knowledge, no studies have ever been conducted which evaluate the effects of DHEA supplementation on weight-training athletes/bodybuilders. And I'm certain no studies have been done with DHEA supplementation on bodybuilders who have used steroids (who may have artificially suppressed their natural testosterone production with the use of these drugs). It's possible that young bodybuilders may experience some benefit from using DHEA, as intense exercise (especially overtraining) can suppress testosterone production. It's also possible that DHEA supplementation may help former steroid users increase their natural testosterone production, but this is mere speculation at best.

> "It's possible that young bodybuilders may experience some benefit from using DHEA..."

Is It Safe?

Because DHEA is relatively powerful stuff, certain people should flat out not use it, and others should use the supplement with caution. For example, any man with prostate hypertrophy or any other medical condition, such as high blood pressure, etc., should consult with a physician before using the compound. I've also discovered that women, and some men, may experience problems with acne while using DHEA.

How Much Do You Take?

In terms of dosages, I suggest 100-200 mg/day for men, taken in 2 evenly divided doses—one in the morning and another before going to bed. I don't think women need any more than 25 mg/day, and some notice a positive effect with as little as 5 mg. (It may relieve symptoms of PMS, according to a researcher I interviewed from Louisiana State University.) I've received feedback from a lot of bodybuilders who have tried mega-dosing (taking 1,000 mg of DHEA or more per day), but from what I can discern, this doesn't necessarily produce fantastic results. The optimal dosage of DHEA is widely debated, but my *opinion* is, if you use 200 mg/day and don't "feel it," you ain't gonna—at any dosage.

All in all, DHEA is great stuff for folks over 40, and it *might* work for some younger lifters. But, keep reading, and I'll tell you about something new, which I think is better than DHEA, and it's definitely "hot"!

Androstenedione—The East German "Secret Weapon"

When it comes to "drug free" testosterone boosters, the first-place trophy goes to the adrenal hormone *androstenedione* (pronounced, "an-dro-sten-de-own"). It's the next step up from DHEA and is the *direct* precursor to testosterone—only one step away. It's naturally made in both men and women. And, guess what else? Amazingly enough, it's also found in the pollen of Scotch pine trees. So, lo and behold, it's now a "dietary supplement"! Guess what else? In reasonable amounts, and taken orally, the liver will convert it to testosterone! *Yippee*!! Androstenedione could be the most controversial supplement of the decade—word of it is spreading like wildfire through gyms across America!

Background Information

Androstenedione was first isolated in 1935, but it wasn't looked into until the late '50's when scientists determined androstenedione is converted in the body to testosterone.[243] There are two different pathways in the body that can create androstenedione: either from DHEA (dehydroepiandrosterone) or from a hormone called "17 alpha-hydroxyprogesterone." Scientists found androstenedione can be converted to testosterone (and vice versa).

In 1962, the first significant study was done with *orally* administered androstenedione on a small group of women.[164] One group of women used 100 mg

23

HOT NEW SUPPLEMENT TRENDS

CHAPTER 3

HOT NEW SUPPLEMENT TRENDS•HOT NEW SUPPLEMENT TRENDS•HOT NEW SUPPLEMENT TRENDS•HOT NEW SUPPLEMENT TRENDS•HOT NEW SUPPLEMENT TRENDS•HOT NEW SUPPLEMENT TRENDS•HOT NEW SUPPLEMENT TRENDS•HOT NEW SUPPLEMENT TRENDS•HOT NEW SUPPLEMENT TRENDS•HOT NEW SUPPLEMENT TRENDS•HOT

of DHEA; another used 100 mg of androstenedione. (In women, a normal serum testosterone level is under 100 ng/dl; the normal range of serum testosterone for a man is between 300 and 1,000 ng/dl.) Here are the results:

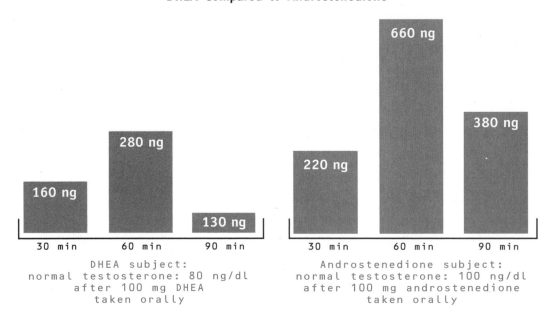

Testosterone Levels After Administration of DHEA Compared to Androstenedione

	DHEA subject			Androstenedione subject		
	30 min	60 min	90 min	30 min	60 min	90 min
	160 ng	280 ng	130 ng	220 ng	660 ng	380 ng

DHEA subject:
normal testosterone: 80 ng/dl
after 100 mg DHEA
taken orally

Androstenedione subject:
normal testosterone: 100 ng/dl
after 100 mg androstenedione
taken orally

Source: V.B. Mahesh and R. B. Greenblatt, "The In Vivo Conversion of Dehydroepiandrosterone and Androstenedione to Testosterone in the Human," *Acta Endocrinologica* 41 (1962) : 400-406.

As you can see, at the same dosage, the androstenedione subject achieved much higher testosterone levels compared to the DHEA subject. For many years, this research was overlooked, but a few decades later, it was "rediscovered."

The East German Secret

To the best of my knowledge, androstenedione was first used as a performance-enhancing substance by the East Germans. Secret documents, which were discovered after the unification of East and West Germany, showed that a team of biologists, physiologists, and physicians, who were put in charge of coming up with novel programs to improve athletic performance in East German Olympic athletes, experimented extensively with androstenedione.

A dude named Michael Oettel (a pharmacologist working at the East German FKS [Research Institute for Body Culture and Sport] in Leipzig), must have been aware of that 1962 study, because in 1980 and 1981, he detailed a way of using androstenedione nasal spray and oral versions to elevate testosterone in GDR (German Democratic Republic) Olympic athletes.[24] I don't have full translations of all the androstenedione research, but I do have this significant tidbit: "By nasal intake of androstenedione, the testosterone/epitestosterone ratio increases and returns to normal within one day. [This ratio is the parameter used to detect 'cheaters' in drug testing.] However, even though the ratio returns to normal, the serum testosterone level remains elevated." (Basically, the GDR athletes could be "juiced" but not "tagged"! [Follow me?])

Oettel performed seven different experiments with androstenedione on performance athletes. In two experiments, the androstenedione was given in *oral* form; the rest were done with nasal spray. He concentrated on the nasal spray because there was a consistently rapid conversion to testosterone (15 minutes), while the activity of the oral versions could be influenced by the subject's state of digestion. What struck me about these experiments was that, in all cases, the dosage was given only once or twice a day, yet serum testosterone remained elevated for a few days after the end of treatment.

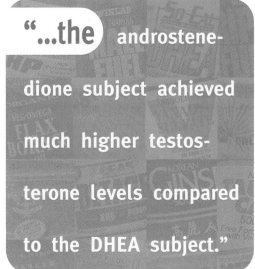

"...the androstenedione subject achieved much higher testosterone levels compared to the DHEA subject."

So how did the androstenedione nasal spray work? Well, according to Raik Hannemann, a promising young GDR swimmer, it was, "...like a volcanic eruption." According to Hannemann, it was mandatory for any athlete who wanted to participate in the 1988 Seoul Olympics, but he also stated, "It tore up my nasal membranes." (Androstenedione nasal spray was pretty harsh!)

The androstenedione "supplements" which are becoming popular among bodybuilders are not nasal sprays—they're tablets and capsules. How effective are the "orals" compared to the nasal spray? Well, the East Germans felt the absorption process with tablets and capsules was much slower—that's why they took it nasally. (Remember, their goal was get results *fast*, then get it out of the system to beat drug tests.) However, one study, quoted in a German patent application (German Patent number DE 42 14 953 A1), stated that oral doses of androstenedione, given to men at levels of 50 mg and 100 mg, raised testosterone levels from 140% to 183% and 211% to 237%, respectively.

Although there is some research showing it causes a significant surge of serum testosterone as well as sustained levels, we don't have studies documenting increases in muscle mass. The East German scientist, Oettel, felt his twice-a-day "pulses" of testosterone increased the performance of his athletes. He focused on the positive effect of androgens on the central nervous system and how enhanced neuron firing improves athletic performance.

There might be another indication that once-a-day testosterone surges are effective. In a 1989 study, researchers compared two groups of laboratory animals.[273] One group got a large dose of testosterone each day; the other received the same

HOT NEW SUPPLEMENT TRENDS

CHAPTER 3

HOT NEW SUPPLEMENT TRENDS•HOT NEW SUPPLEMENT TRENDS•HOT NEW SUPPLEMENT TRENDS•HOT NEW SUPPLEMENT TRENDS•HOT NEW SUPPLEMENT TRENDS•HOT NEW SUPPLEMENT TRENDS•HOT NEW SUPPLEMENT TRENDS•HOT NEW SUPPLEMENT TRENDS•HOT NEW SUPPLEMENT TRENDS•HOT NEW SUPPLEMENT TRENDS•HOT

milligram total, spread throughout the day in smaller doses. The single dose increased muscle mass <u>more</u> than the smaller, frequent dose schedule!

Many testosterone delivery systems, like the daily skin patch or weekly injection, release testosterone into the blood slowly and gradually. Administering testosterone in a single pulse, once a day, is a new idea. There may be fewer side effects with this single delivery.[230] It's possible that by spiking your natural testosterone levels only once or twice a day, you may keep the body from lowering its natural production of testosterone—a problem that occurs with the use of anabolic steroid drugs.

Is It Cheating?

With the exception of pro football, androstenedione has not been banned in any of the drug-tested sports. The International Olympic Committee has added DHEA, but not androstenedione, to its prohibited-substance list. Even though the testosterone/epitestosterone ratio may rise to 14:1 during the day of androstenedione use, it could fall below 6:1 (within the passing range) the day after stopping its use. In one previous instance, an athlete tested positive for testosterone on his random drug test and justified his 13:1 testosterone/epitestosterone ratio by showing the sports authorities a bottle of androstenedione. Since the substance was not banned, his positive result was thrown out. Was the athlete using androstenedione, or had he used an injectable testosterone? From a urine test, there is no way of telling.

But, is using androstenedione cheating? *By itself*, androstenedione is not a muscle builder. It, like DHEA, only works when/if it is converted to testosterone in the body. You might say this supplement "upgrades" your body's *natural* production of testosterone.

"Androstenedione...

has created a buzz and

high expectations in the

hardcore community."

Is It Just Expensive DHEA?

There is currently only one androstenedione product on the American market: it's called Androstene 50, and it's sold by a company called Osmo. I had it tested—it's real. It costs about $50 for sixty 50-mg capsules. (Other companies will undoubtedly be coming out with androstenedione supplements soon.) If you multiplied the figures in the 1962 androstenedione study, you might assume that using 3 times the amount of DHEA (300 mg) would produce roughly the same testosterone elevation as 100 mg of oral androstenedione. But the conversion of DHEA to testosterone is more complex than the single step required of androstenedione. There may be a limitation on the extent of DHEA conversion because of insufficient levels of enzymes.[164] Likewise, there may be limitations on the conversion of androstenedione to testosterone.

What's the Best Dosage of Androstenedione?

We haven't seen blood test results for dosages higher than 100 mg of androstenedione taken orally. If a 100-mg dose can produce a threefold increase of serum testosterone, can a 200-mg dose produce a sixfold increase? Or would the available liver conversion enzymes be limiting? No one knows. There is possibly a big market for androstenedione as a libido booster at the modest 100-mg dosage, since the testosterone elevation is likely superior to many of the libido products currently available. And, as I'll explain later in this chapter, some bodybuilders are stacking DHEA, androstenedione, and a compound called *Tribulus terrestris* and are reporting stunning results!

Should androstenedione be used one, two, or three times a day? And, what's the best dosage? We don't know. My best guess is that 50-100 mg, taken first thing in the morning and perhaps another 50-100 mg in the evening would work well (to enhance the anabolic drive). For a strength boost, a dose 60 minutes before training could produce favorable results. (After an oral dose, testosterone levels peak at about 60 minutes.) Absorption may be better on an empty stomach, but we aren't sure.

Side Effects?

Since androstenedione seems to cause a brief burst of testosterone, it may or may not cause any of the usual testosterone side effects: acne, prostate hypertrophy, and a decrease in HDL (good) cholesterol. It should not be used by anyone with any known health problems without first consulting a physician. Because of its potency, I would <u>not</u> recommend this supplement to women as it may cause acne, facial hair growth, and lowering of the voice. It is not a drug; thus, it does not pose all the health risks of anabolic steroid use, such as liver toxicity, kidney stress, etc.

What's Next?

Unlike the popular bodybuilding supplements, HMB and creatine, androstenedione has virtually no research studies on its effect on muscle mass. But some athletes still seek more "drug-like" bodybuilding supplements. Androstenedione, without published research, has created a buzz and high expectations in the hardcore community. In bodybuilding, testosterone is almost a magic word. Androstenedione, being only one step away, might develop a little magic of its own. But, more research is needed before it could be called a "sure thing."

This <u>is</u> a hot new trend for certain and one I will follow and keep you posted on through *Muscle Media*.

Tribulus Terrestris—Could It Boost the Effects of DHEA and/or Androstenedione?

When I wrote the *1996 Supplement Review*, I was somewhat equivocal (unde-cided) about the herbal supplement *Tribulus terrestris*. Over the last year, I have learned more about it, and I have received quite a bit of feedback from people who have tried this product. I have had the opportunity to discuss the compound at length with some experts who have studied it for years. One of them is Dr. James Wright, who introduced some of the potential benefits of *Tribulus terrestris* supple-mentation through an article in the September 1996 issue of *Muscle & Fitness*. Dr. Wright is very well versed in bodybuilding—as a matter of fact, he has written numerous books about steroids and other bodybuilding compounds, which I have often referred to. Also, another expert whom I hold in very high regard, Strength Coach Charles Poliquin, has confirmed that numerous European Olympic athletes use *Tribulus terrestris*. I would hardly rate *Tribulus terrestris* as a "sure thing," but I think it will be one of the most talked about bodybuilding supplements of 1997.

What Is This Stuff?

Tribulus terrestris (a.k.a. "puncture vine") is a plant which grows in some moderate climates and many tropical areas of the world. It has played an important role in folk medicine for centuries. The ancient Greeks used it as a diuretic (it actu-ally does work for this—this is an added benefit) and a general mood-enhancing tonic. In India, it has been used as a diuretic, antiseptic, and anti-inflammatory, while in China, the herb has been a frequent component of therapies for a variety of dis-eases affecting the liver, kidneys, and cardiovascular system.

This compound is extremely rich in substances of potential biological signif-icance, including: saponins, flavonoids, alkaloids, and other nutrients. The presence and quantities of the pharmacologically important metabolites depend on the parts of the plant used, but generally, the above-ground parts have the highest concen-trations (leaves, fruits, and, to a lesser extent, shoots). And where the plant is grown is also important, as are the conditions of growth, cultivation, and harvesting.

Interestingly, in Bulgaria and the Balkan countries, *Tribulus terrestris* is used primarily as a compound to treat infertility and a lack of libido. It has been exten-sively studied by scientists at the Chemical Pharmaceutical Research Institute in Sofia, Bulgaria. Their studies on this compound, going back two decades, offer the most compelling data available. I have not been able to find any evidence that it's been researched at any universities in the United States.

Until the publication of the *Handbook of Chinese Herbs and Formulas* (Vol. 1) by Dr. Him-che Yeung in 1983 and the *Chemical Constituents of Oriental Herbs* by Hsu, Chen, and Hong in 1985, little was known about this plant in America, other than by a small group of scientists, herbalists, and doctors trained in Oriental and Ayurvedic (Indian herbal medicine) traditions. It is just now starting to catch on in bodybuilding, as a result of its use by eastern European Olympic and world-champion strength athletes.

How Does It Work?

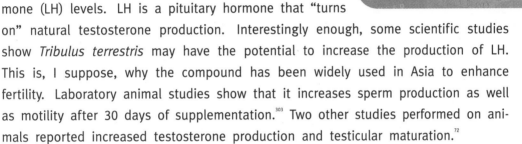

"Like DHEA and androstenedione, *Tribulus terrestris* is being promoted as a testosterone enhancer..."

Like DHEA and androstenedione, *Tribulus terrestris* is being promoted as a testosterone enhancer, but it does not work by the same mechanism—both DHEA and androstenedione provide the raw material for testosterone formation; *Tribulus terrestris* is purported to enhance testosterone levels by increasing luteinizing hormone (LH) levels. LH is a pituitary hormone that "turns on" natural testosterone production. Interestingly enough, some scientific studies show *Tribulus terrestris* may have the potential to increase the production of LH. This is, I suppose, why the compound has been widely used in Asia to enhance fertility. Laboratory animal studies show that it increases sperm production as well as motility after 30 days of supplementation.[303] Two other studies performed on animals reported increased testosterone production and testicular maturation.[72]

Another study examined the effects of *Tribulus terrestris* on boars experiencing an absence of libido (sex drive). (Why they would be studying this, I have no F-in' idea. Hey... what do you call a boar that can't "get it up?" A boring boar! [Okay... so I'm not a comedian.]) Anyway, these animals, after ten days of supplementation, were reportedly jumping each other like rabid bunnies.

Now, to more substantial stuff—a study involving healthy individuals taking 750 mg/day of *Tribulus terrestris* evaluated hormonal responses and revealed LH *increased* in males from 14.38 ml/U/ml to 24.75 ml/U/ml (that's a 72% increase). The *free* testosterone in males went from 60 ng/dl to 84.5 ng/dl (an increase of 41%).[181] To avoid becoming confused by these numbers, keep in mind that free testosterone is only a portion (the biologically active portion) of total serum testosterone. Normal blood levels of <u>total</u> testosterone are between 300 and 1,000 ng/dl.[131]

Another study including over 200 male subjects suffering from impotence (often caused by low testosterone levels) showed that many (but not all) of the men experienced an increase in LH and testosterone as well as sperm production and motility.[303]

Now, there are no clinical studies to my knowledge (and I looked everywhere) that offer any evidence this increase in LH, testosterone, or sex drive directly relates to any type of enhanced athletic performance or muscle building. (Although I definitely believe *Tribulus terrestris* can significantly "lift" performance in the bedroom.)

HOT NEW SUPPLEMENT TRENDS

HOT NEW SUPPLEMENT TRENDS•HOT NEW SUPPLEMENT TRENDS•HOT NEW SUPPLEMENT TRENDS•HOT NEW SUPPLEMENT TRENDS•HOT NEW SUPPLEMENT TRENDS•HOT NEW SUPPLEMENT TRENDS•HOT NEW SUPPLEMENT TRENDS•HOT NEW SUPPLEMENT TRENDS•HOT NEW SUPPLEMENT TRENDS•HOT NEW SUPPLEMENT TRENDS•HOT NEW SUPPLEMENT TRENDS•HOT

As far as I can tell, only one study was done on healthy subjects—all others were performed on subjects with impaired testosterone function or the absence of libido.

But, you'd be surprised at how many bodybuilders who have experimented with steroids have crippled their natural LH and testosterone production. Thus, *Tribulus terrestris,* by itself, may help some bodybuilders—especially those who have used steroids or are coming off the drugs.

Some marketers of *Tribulus terrestris* make some pretty wild claims about what this compound can do—they allege it can cure at least two dozen diseases, lower blood pressure and cholesterol, enhance mood, etc. I'm really not buying into all that hype—it just seems a little too hard to believe. As a matter of fact, I don't think using *Tribulus terrestris* by itself has the potential to significantly boost gains in muscle size and strength. HOWEVER, if you were to use it in conjunction with androstenedione and/or DHEA, it could hit hard! You see, DHEA and androstenedione provide your body with the raw materials (precursors) for testosterone. But, this does not necessarily mean these compounds will be converted to testosterone by your body. I just reviewed a blood test yesterday from a 32-year-old athlete I train, and despite the fact that he had *above normal* DHEA levels, his testosterone was *below normal*—so was his LH. My guess is that despite the fact that there was plenty of "raw material" for testosterone production, his pituitary (the body's hormone "control center") was not signaling testosterone production. If supplementing *Tribulus terrestris* increased LH, in the presence of high DHEA or androstenedione levels... look out! Dare I say, a "steroid-like" effect might be seen?!

I've only talked to four bodybuilders who've tried this stack (*hardly* a significant number), but something "big" seems to be happening. To start with, the occurrence and "intensity" of erections have increased so much it sounds like it's almost embarrassing. I don't know what's causing this effect—whether it's really the increase in hormone levels or if something else is going on (despite what some contend, there are compounds which increase potency and libido that are not directly attributable to increases in testosterone; yohimbine is one such agent). Whatever the case, something very conspicuous and "noticeable" is going on. These same athletes report the strength and intensity of their weight-training sessions is improved. I may try this stack myself, and I am going to fund research to investigate what's going on—to determine if LH and testosterone levels are indeed going up significantly. If there is an effect on those hormones, the research will go to a second phase where test subjects' body composition (muscle and fat) will be analyzed. Basically, we'll try to determine if this stack helps you pack on muscle and lose fat, and if so, at what dosage? The research will also collect safety data.

> "If supplementing *Tribulus terrestris* increased LH... look out!"

As you might imagine, these studies will take several months, but as soon as I know more, I'll pass the information along to you in *Muscle Media*.

Is It Safe?

I should warn that some people get an upset stomach from using *Tribulus terrestris* (about one or two out of ten as far as I can tell). This may be minimized by taking it with food. Also, I would have a hard time believing that *Tribulus terrestris* would produce a dramatic effect for a long period of time. I recommend using it on a cycle of no more than six weeks in the manner I describe in Chapter 12. I'm convinced that any compound, be it a supplement, herb, or drug, that alters some hormonal axis of the body, will be overridden as the body adjusts its feedback mechanisms. Thus, if you decide to use *Tribulus terrestris* and/or DHEA and/or androstenedione, try cycling it six weeks on and four to six weeks off.

At this time, *Tribulus terrestris* is not widely available, but it can be found as a component of some supplements like Tribestan and another called Tribestrone. I suspect many more *Tribulus terrestris*-containing supplements will come out on the market this year.

No significant adverse effects have been noted in any of the clinical trials or human research studies. Toxicity is extremely low in both acute and long-term animal studies. No negative effects are presently known to exist when *Tribulus terrestris* is used as a nutritional supplement (it's a dietary supplement because it's an herb). However, I would not recommend that women who are pregnant or lactating use this product. I think it has the potential to alter hormonal chemistry significantly. Also, I would not recommend it to individuals with enlarged prostates or any other medical conditions without first consulting a physician.

It seems that experimenting with a dosage of 750-1,250 mg/day, in divided doses with meals, and stacking it with DHEA (about 100 mg/day) and androstenedione (around 100 mg/day) may work well. But, I must reiterate, there is no conclusive data available regarding the bodybuilding effects of this supplement. For now, it's merely a <u>trend</u>, not a sure thing.

Chrysin (a.k.a. Flavone X)—Another Possible Testosterone Booster

So far in this chapter we've talked about possible testosterone boosters, such as DHEA and androstenedione, which supply the raw materials from which testosterone is made. We also discussed *Tribulus terrestris*, an interesting herb that might stimulate the body to make more LH, which gives the signal for testosterone production. Now, we come to yet another "dietary supplement" which might boost testosterone, but this one, hypothetically, works through yet another mechanism. In this case, the compound is called chrysin (those of you who read *Muscle Media* might recognize this as a supplement Dan Duchaine wrote about last year—he called it "Flavone X").

HOT NEW SUPPLEMENT TRENDS

HOT NEW SUPPLEMENT TRENDS•HOT NEW SUPPLEMENT TRENDS•HOT NEW SUPPLEMENT TRENDS•HOT NEW SUPPLEMENT TRENDS•HOT NEW SUPPLEMENT TRENDS•HOT NEW SUPPLEMENT TRENDS•HOT NEW SUPPLEMENT TRENDS•HOT NEW SUPPLEMENT TRENDS•HOT NEW SUPPLEMENT TRENDS•HOT NEW SUPPLEMENT TRENDS•HOT

Anyway, some studies suggest chrysin may enhance testosterone production by minimizing the conversion of testosterone to estrogen, a process which occurs naturally in our bodies and accelerates as testosterone levels go up. A compound with this type of activity is called an "anti-aromatase." You see, the process by which the body converts testosterone to estrogen is called aromatization; thus, something that works against this conversion is called an anti-aromatase. Got that? Good.

What Is Chrysin?

Chrysin is the chemical name for a particular "isoflavone," which is a naturally occurring chemical extracted from a plant called *Passiflora coerulea*.[300] Small amounts are also found in honeycomb. Flavones are *not* the same thing as sterols. Scientific evidence shows that flavones may indeed be biologically active and exert powerful effects.

How Does Chrysin Work?

Well, scientific studies from Europe (where the product has been patented for 2 years) show that it has the potential to increase natural production and blood serum levels of testosterone by over 30%. Exactly how this works is a bit complicated, but I'll try to keep it simple. First, let's talk about two of the "major" steroid hormones in your body—testosterone and estrogen. I'm sure you have a pretty good idea of what testosterone is—it's the *manly hormone*. Estrogen, on the other hand, is a hormone that is dominant in females. But, men's bodies also produce estrogen, and the level of estrogen in your blood may signal the pituitary to turn testosterone production off or on. You see, the more estrogen your pituitary "senses," the less testosterone it allows the body to create. If our bodies begin to produce more testosterone than normal (perhaps as a result of using DHEA, androstenedione, and/or *Tribulus terrestris*), or if someone takes a testosterone-based drug/anabolic steroid, the body converts a greater amount of this androgenic hormone to estrogen through this aromatizing process. (This is what causes "bitch tits" in guys who use a lot of steroids.)

Experts believe if you can minimize the conversion of testosterone to estrogen, testosterone levels in the blood could increase without an excessive amount of estrogen being produced; thus, the pituitary gland would not shut down natural testosterone manufacturing.

There are currently several prescription drugs that work as "anti-aromatase" agents. Teslac (delta 1-testolactone) and Cytadren (aminoglutethimide) have been shown to help increase testosterone levels when taken orally.[74, 244, 284] In-vitro studies comparing the aromatase-inhibitory effects of chrysin, head to head with Cytadren, show almost identical activity![44, 127] (That's powerful stuff, baby!)

When I first read about chrysin, I was skeptical, but over the past few months, I've talked to several experts from the United Kingdom who have offered some compelling evidence and anecdotes about chrysin's effects. (So now I'm "less skeptical.") One of my "chrysin contacts" has trained a number of the UK's top Olympic athletes and powerlifters. He thinks the stuff works. (Hypothetically, if chrysin were stacked with other testosterone-enhancing supplements, the effects could be synergistic—hopefully this is something future studies will reveal.)

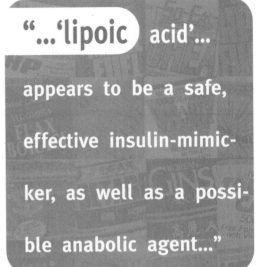

"...'lipoic acid'... appears to be a safe, effective insulin-mimicker, as well as a possible anabolic agent..."

Chrysin is not readily available on the market because so few people are aware of it, and it's extremely expensive. However, there is a chance someone will figure out how to produce it at a reasonable cost, and you will see it on the market within the next six months. Chrysin appears to be safe—human studies have been done on the compound in Europe, but further research is definitely needed, and from what I understand, it's being planned.

Drawing from the dosages recommended in existing foreign patents, and going by the feedback I've received from the handful of professionals who've experimented with it, an effective dose *might* be between one and three grams per day, divided into two or three separate doses. Possibly, the right time to take chrysin would be in the morning, an hour before working out and then before going to sleep.

I'll try to keep you posted on anything new I learn about chrysin in future issues of *Muscle Media* and in updates to this book. As I stated in the introduction of this chapter, this is one of those trends that may or may not pan out, but as I explained, I'm giving you the no-holds-barred "inside scoop"—I'm letting you in on some of the best-kept secrets... the stuff that's going on behind the scenes in drug-free bodybuilding.

LIPOIC ACID—A NEW INSULIN MIMICKER WITH BIG POTENTIAL

As *Muscle Media* reported several years ago, one of the most intriguing new frontiers in bodybuilding is tapping into the anabolic effects of insulin. As you may or may not know, insulin is your body's primary "nutrient-storage" hormone. It escorts amino acids, glucose, and other nutrients into muscle cells—these nutrients literally can't get in without insulin "unlocking the door" first.

Over the years, we've seen some interesting insulin-mimicking supplements hit the bodybuilding market. Some of them have a great "gym reputation," including vanadyl sulfate, which has been shown in some studies to mimic the action of insulin, thereby possibly allowing more glucose and amino acids to be taken up by muscle cells.[111]

HOT NEW SUPPLEMENT TRENDS

HOT NEW SUPPLEMENT TRENDS•HOT NEW SUPPLEMENT TRENDS•HOT NEW SUPPLEMENT TRENDS•HOT NEW SUPPLEMENT TRENDS•HOT NEW SUPPLEMENT TRENDS•HOT NEW SUPPLEMENT TRENDS•HOT NEW SUPPLEMENT TRENDS•HOT NEW SUPPLEMENT TRENDS•HOT NEW SUPPLEMENT TRENDS•HOT NEW SUPPLEMENT TRENDS•HOT

CHAPTER 3

Chromium supplements are thought to work in a similar manner—by improving the action of insulin, chromium can help some (but definitely not all) bodybuilders get better results faster from their workouts.[7, 191]

A lot of "extreme" bodybuilders have actually been using insulin medications intended for diabetics. These potent drugs reportedly produce dramatic results when combined with intense weight-training and an appropriate nutrition program (they're also stacking it with growth hormone, steroids, and IGF-1). This is among the most dangerous trends, so far as drug use goes, in bodybuilding. If you screw up with this stuff, it could kill you—not 40 years from now, not 10, not even next week. If you're using insulin today and you take too much of it, you could be dead in a matter of hours. Needless to say, any strategies that could be employed to optimize the anabolic effects of insulin which do not include extreme, radical measures, like those I described above, would be of interest to bodybuilders.

Recently, I've had the opportunity to review a great deal of information about a very interesting compound called "lipoic acid," which not only appears to be a safe, effective insulin-mimicker, as well as a possible anabolic agent, but it's also a powerful antioxidant.[217] And, it appears to have a variety of health-enhancing effects. Here's the story...

> "...lipoic acid supplementation may help speed recovery, increase endurance, and give you fuller, more 'pumpable' muscles."

Lipoic Acid—The Basics

Known by different names—lipoic acid, lipoate, alpha-lipoic acid, and thioctic acid—this compound acts as a coenzyme for several reactions in the body, one of which is a process called "glycolysis"—the process responsible for converting blood sugar to energy. Lipoic acid exerts this effect by supporting the activity of the mitochondria, which are small structures found in every muscle cell that act as "powerhouses."

Lipoic acid is a nutrient the body can make and is therefore not considered "essential"; however, there have been studies showing the addition of lipoic acid to the diet of type II diabetics (those with insulin insensitivity not requiring insulin therapy) significantly increases the body's utilization of blood sugar.[217] Because muscle represents the primary "disposal" site of blood sugar, it is likely that lipoic acid is aiding in muscular uptake of blood sugar—possibly leading to greater glycogen synthesis. In one study, using 1 gram of intravenous lipoic acid per day, diabetics increased their metabolic clearance rate of glucose by 50%.[132]

This compound has been used in Germany for years as a treatment for diabetes, much like insulin is used in the U.S. today. A group of doctors from

Munich, headed by a doctor named Hans Tritschler, reported at an international conference on diabetes that lipoic acid may not only increase glucose uptake by muscle cells but may actually *decrease glucose uptake by fat cells* at the same time.[277] The result of this action may well be more energy production in the muscles and less fat stored in the body.

Lipoic acid is also thought to be a very powerful antioxidant. Two studies looking at this effect showed that lipoic acid helps protect red blood cells and fatty acids from both oxidative damage (the type usually experienced from intense training) and UVA damage from intense exposure to sunlight.[59, 170]

No tests have been performed on healthy, exercising subjects, *yet*. But it is well established that a large and ever-growing percentage of the American population suffers some degree of insulin insensitivity, especially individuals carrying a substantial amount of excess bodyfat or those who have diets high in saturated fats (which means most of the population), even though they may not be overweight. If insulin insensitivity is a problem for you and you're trying to build muscle and lose fat, lipoic acid supplementation may help speed recovery, increase endurance, and give you fuller, more "pumpable" muscles.

So far, clinical studies show that lipoic acid is quite safe—no toxicity has been observed; however, any time you're experimenting with a supplement that may act as an insulin mimicker, you should proceed very cautiously. As a matter of fact, lipoic acid has a reputation for being a rather potent agent, and if you take too much of it all at once, you could experience low blood sugar levels, which include symptoms such as fatigue, anxiety, jitteriness, confusion, frustration, etc. If you decide to try lipoic acid, start with a small dosage—approximately 100-200 mg with a meal. Eventually, working up to a dose of 400-600 mg/day, taken in divided doses with meals (for example, 200 mg with 3 separate meals), could produce very nice results. I don't think bodybuilders would need to take more than 600 mg/day. Studies appear to show that there is no added benefit to larger doses.[217] Apparently an effective dose of lipoic acid for its antioxidant purposes could be as low as 200-300 mg/day.[210]

As far as I can tell, lipoic acid looks like the most potent natural insulin-mimicking compound on the market—better than even vanadyl sulfate and chromium. All in all, lipoic acid looks like an exciting new supplement that may help enhance the anabolic effects of insulin and may help protect the body against damage from free radicals by working as an antioxidant. Lipoic acid supplements have been on the market for over a year now and are being carried by such companies as Jarrow, Solgar, and Ethical Nutrients. However, because the science is so young in this area, lipoic acid has not yet taken off. Also, the raw material needed to make this stuff is mega-expensive! But, manufacturers in Europe have told me they're confident they can get the price of this product down.

HOT NEW SUPPLEMENT TRENDS

HOT NEW SUPPLEMENT TRENDS•HOT NEW SUPPLEMENT TRENDS•HOT NEW SUPPLEMENT TRENDS•HOT NEW SUPPLEMENT TRENDS•HOT NEW SUPPLEMENT TRENDS•HOT NEW SUPPLEMENT TRENDS•HOT NEW SUPPLEMENT TRENDS•HOT NEW SUPPLEMENT TRENDS•HOT NEW SUPPLEMENT TRENDS•HOT NEW SUPPLEMENT TRENDS•HOT

EAS researchers are designing studies to examine the effects of lipoic acid and its bodybuilding applications. I'll admit—this is a compound EAS *may* release as a part of our bodybuilding supplement line, *if* we can demonstrate, through clinical studies, that it offers positive effects for bodybuilders. (Geez... could I make it any easier for these "knock-off artists"—the ones who make a living trying to copy-cat EAS products—to know what to do next?)

TIMED-RELEASE SUPPLEMENTS

One of the "trends" in bodybuilding supplementation, taking place "behind the scenes," which I think has a great deal of potential does not revolve around the discovery of any unique, new compound. This trend, which I think could double, if not triple, the effectiveness of numerous supplements on the market right now, has to do with how the ingredients in dietary supplement formulas are delivered to the body.

The Problem

One of the reasons some weight trainers don't get the results they're looking for from using various supplements has to do with the fact that consuming these products in a manner which facilitates their maximum effectiveness can be complex. As a matter of fact, it can be a royal pain in the ass. I often forget to take my supplements exactly when I'm supposed to, even though I am well aware of the importance of the proper timing and patterning of supplement intake throughout the day to optimize effectiveness.

You see, most dietary supplements (unlike a lot of drugs) have a very short "half-life"—they're in and out of the system in a matter of hours. Thus, it's important to take multiple doses throughout the day in order to maintain an elevated level of these vital nutrients.

Unfortunately, you can't take your entire daily dose of most supplements in one serving—this would most likely lead to poor intestinal absorption, only short-term elevations in blood levels of these key substrates, and in some cases, a stomachache.

The Solution

One possible solution to this problem may be on the horizon. I have been following the progress of a few very astute researchers who have been attempting to "borrow" some of the sophisticated, "timed-release" delivery systems developed by the pharmaceutical industry and adopt them to allow us to take merely one dose of a supplement each day and have it slowly release into the bloodstream for a long period of time. Not only would this make using supplements more convenient for busy people like you and me but the consistent release of key nutrients into the blood, over an extended period of time, could enhance the positive effects of many supplements, including: water-soluble vitamins, minerals, amino acids, prohormones, etc.

Here's something else exciting—as many of you know, when we go to sleep, our bodies typically go through a period of anabolism (the building up of tissue) during the first few hours, but then our bodies shift into a stage of protein breakdown. This occurs, in part, because of a shift in certain hormone levels and also because of the simple fact that levels of key anti-catabolic factors fall during a prolonged period of fasting, which occurs during sleep. If you were able to take a supplement at night, before you went to sleep, that slowly released certain amino acids and anti-catabolic factors, like HMB, into the bloodstream throughout this fasting state, you may experience a shift in overall protein balance in favor of muscle growth. Also, it's not impossible that before the end of the year we'll see timed-release pro-hormone formulas that contain compounds, such as androstenedione and DHEA.

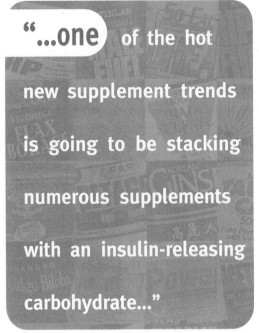

"**...one** of the hot new supplement trends is going to be stacking numerous supplements with an insulin-releasing carbohydrate..."

Hypothetically, releasing these compounds into the bloodstream several hours after you go to sleep could cause an elevation in testosterone that could "turn on" the protein-synthetic machinery at a time when it typically "turns off." And, it's not impossible this same technology could be used with growth-hormone-releasing formulas to provide a long-term increase in growth-hormone levels, instead of the quick "burst" you get from consuming supplements like arginine and ornithine.

I'll keep you posted on any new developments regarding this exciting technology through *Muscle Media* and in updates to this book. I must admit, this is one of the most exciting new trends in bodybuilding supplementation that I can think of— if you're a regular user of supplements and are up to date on the science of supplements, I'm sure you can understand the huge ramifications of this technology.

LOADING SUPPLEMENTS WITH INSULIN-RELEASING CARBOHYDRATES

As you'll learn in the next chapter (and as you may already know), scientists have conclusively determined that consuming the blockbuster-supplement creatine monohydrate with a carbohydrate source such as dextrose (which causes a dramatic release by the pancreas of the potent anabolic hormone insulin) enhances the effects of creatine—driving more of this vital nutrient into muscle cells where it can work its magic.

You might be saying to yourself, "That's fine and dandy—I've been consuming my creatine with fruit juice, or I've been using a premixed formula like

HOT NEW SUPPLEMENT TRENDS

HOT NEW SUPPLEMENT TRENDS~HOT NEW SUPPLEMENT TRENDS~HOT NEW SUPPLEMENT TRENDS~HOT NEW SUPPLEMENT TRENDS~HOT NEW SUPPLEMENT TRENDS~HOT NEW SUPPLEMENT TRENDS~HOT NEW SUPPLEMENT TRENDS~HOT NEW SUPPLEMENT TRENDS~HOT NEW SUPPLEMENT TRENDS~HOT NEW SUPPLEMENT TRENDS~HOT

Phosphagen HP... what's new about that?" Well, think about it... why would creatine be the only key supplement that is affected in this way? (Tip—*it's not!*)

Insulin transports numerous important nutrients into muscle cells, including: virtually all amino acids, glucose, and other key substrates such as creatine, which I just mentioned.[226, 227]

I'm predicting that in 1997, one of the hot new supplement trends is going to be stacking numerous supplements with an insulin-releasing carbohydrate to enhance their effects. This will include key cell-volumizing amino acids like glutamine, taurine, alanine, as well as branched-chain amino acid supplements and others, such as HMB.

Let's "Load" Everything!

Let's look at something else we've learned from the numerous scientific studies performed on creatine monohydrate. Research clearly shows that doing a "loading phase" (taking a large amount of the supplement for approximately one week) significantly enhances uptake of creatine. I believe the loading phase with creatine (something else we'll discuss in the next chapter in detail) helps saturate muscle cells with creatine, not just because it's filling up the muscle reserves but also because the enzyme systems that help shuttle creatine into muscle cells are highly active during the first few days of supplementation and are very efficient in transporting or storing this nutrient in muscle tissue.

I suspect creatine is <u>not</u> the only supplement that you could benefit from "loading up" on. In fact, my fellow prognosticator Dan Duchaine recently explained that loading up on glutamine and using it along with an insulin-releasing carbohydrate drink, especially right after your workout (when your body is primed for maximum nutrient uptake) could produce fantastic results. We'll talk more about the particulars of glutamine loading in Chapter 4, but suffice it to say, Duchaine and several other experts, including me, are convinced glutamine loading, concurrent with spiking insulin levels with a high-glycemic carbohydrate, could produce phenomenal results.

Because of all the things we've learned about creatine and how to maximize its effects through loading (taking a high dose for a short period of time) and stacking it with an insulin-releasing carb, I think we'll be able to extend this knowledge to other supplements, especially those which act directly at the muscle cell site, and get much better results from some of the most popular supplements on the market.

> **"...glutamine** loading, concurrent with spiking insulin levels with a high-glycemic carbohydrate, could produce phenomenal results."

Of course, scientific studies are needed to validate this theory, and my company, EAS, has already provided the funds for research grants at two separate universities to evaluate the effects of an insulin-releasing carbohydrate and the effects of consuming a loading dose of supplements like HMB. As the results come in, I'll be sure to keep you posted.

PEOPLE TRYING TO MAKE MONEY OFF THE SUPPLEMENT "PYRUVATE"

Please reread the subheading above... Notice I *didn't* say this hot trend will be "athletes experiencing great results using pyruvate." The trend here is people *trying* to make money off pyruvate. Let me explain...

When I wrote about the dietary supplement pyruvate in the 1996 version of my *Supplement Review*, it was really the first time anyone in the sports supplement business had discussed this novel compound and its applications. It captured the interest of many supplement users.

Coincidentally, when I wrote about pyruvate and created an interest in this supplement in the marketplace, I inadvertently set off a vicious (but almost hilarious) fury of posturing, gamesmanship, and legal battling over the legal rights to pyruvate.

You see, a doctor named Ronald Stanko, along with Abbott Laboratories (a huge drug company), as well as the University of Pittsburgh, all shared (or claimed to share) ownership rights to various use patents regarding pyruvate.

Then, along came a company called Med-Pro Industries which acquired patent rights to several uses for pyruvate (this stuff is patented for virtually everything you can think of—fat loss, weight loss, enhanced performance, antioxidant activity, as well as for a variety of medical and surgical applications). Med-Pro proceeded to grant certain rights to various companies and individuals. In the meantime, Dr. Stanko was busy setting up several more companies and selling various individuals stock. I'm not an expert in math, and to be honest, I'm not really even an expert in business, but as far as I can tell, between Med-Pro and Stanko, approximately eight different people or companies think they own the rights to pyruvate, and they're suing each other.

The last time I checked, there were 16 attorneys involved in the pyruvate deal—Abbott is fighting for its share of the potential profits, Dr. Stanko is looking for his cut, Med-Pro Industries is certain they're sitting on a pot of gold, and the University of Pittsburgh is looking for its fair share. To make a long (boring) story short, it's a very complicated business "situation."

So What?!

So you say you don't give a frog's fat ass about who has the rights to pyruvate—you just want to try the stuff to see whether it works for you. Well, then

HOT NEW SUPPLEMENT TRENDS

HOT NEW SUPPLEMENT TRENDS•HOT NEW SUPPLEMENT TRENDS•HOT NEW SUPPLEMENT TRENDS•HOT NEW SUPPLEMENT TRENDS•HOT NEW SUPPLEMENT TRENDS•HOT NEW SUPPLEMENT TRENDS•HOT NEW SUPPLEMENT TRENDS•HOT NEW SUPPLEMENT TRENDS•HOT NEW SUPPLEMENT TRENDS•HOT NEW SUPPLEMENT TRENDS•HOT

here's *your* problem—those involved with all this pyruvate business are so busy fighting about the legal rights to the supplement that I have to question whether an appropriate amount of money or time is being put into answering the lingering questions about the best dosage, not to mention how to manufacture it. A few months ago, I had a couple batches of pyruvate that are on the market tested, and they didn't look so good. One contained a mere 33% of the claimed calcium pyruvate content, while another had concentrations of three foreign chemicals that the analytical lab couldn't even distinguish. (Not good.)

What Is Pyruvate Anyway, and What Does It Do?

For those of you who are not familiar with pyruvate, let me give you the "crash course." Pyruvate is a compound that occurs naturally in the body and is the end product of the metabolism of sugar and starch. It's the gateway compound to the Krebs (or citric acid) cycle. This is an energy cycle of chemical and enzyme actions that produce ATP or its direct precursors. Many compounds are involved in the Krebs cycle, all starting with pyruvate.

Exactly how pyruvate exerts its powerful effects is not known, but from what I can discern, in a nutshell, it works by increasing "cellular respiration" or the amount of energy the mitochondria (the cell's metabolic furnace) uses as well as inhibiting fat production in the body.[258] Some studies using high dosages have even shown pyruvate reduces fat without exercise.[259]

Originally, the compound was being developed as a fat-loss drug by Abbott Laboratories, but when the DSHEA was passed in 1994, Abbott apparently abandoned its development of this compound as a drug because it could be sold over the counter as a dietary supplement.

Quality pyruvate does work—it really does seem to accelerate fat loss and enhance performance, but the unanswered question is, AT WHAT DOSAGE?

How Much?

As I mentioned in my last *Supplement Review*, the scientific studies pertaining to pyruvate supplementation—the ones which show it enhances fat loss in obese women up to 48%—have been done using huge dosages (36 grams/day).[259] Despite the claims by Dr. Stanko that pyruvate is effective in much lower dosages, as little as two to five grams a day, I'm not convinced reliable substantiation for this claim exists, and I'm positive it can't be found in the public domain (in published scientific studies).

The fact is, double-blind, placebo-controlled university studies (performed by competent experts) need to be conducted on athletes using reasonable dosages of pyruvate in order to evaluate whether this supplement actually produces an effect at a dose that is economically feasible and doesn't make you sick to your stomach. Consuming

30 grams of pyruvate, especially versions bound to calcium or sodium, could make you feel pretty bad.

Because I want to know whether pyruvate works for bodybuilders (and if so, at what dosage) as much as anyone, my company, EAS, is funding a series of university research programs to evaluate the effects of various dosages of pyruvate on athletic performance. In fact, the first study was just recently completed at Creighton University. It evaluated the effects of sodium pyruvate on critical power, which is a good indicator of both aerobic metabolic processes and anaerobic work capacity. In this study, scientists supplemented one group of exercising test subjects with eight grams of sodium pyruvate and another group with eight grams of

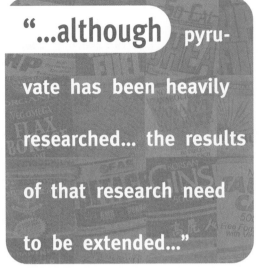

"...although pyruvate has been heavily researched... the results of that research need to be extended..."

a placebo. Both men and women with an average age of 21 years participated in the study. After 14 days of supplementation, preliminary data showed no "significant" effect, but there was what scientists call a "trend" towards an increase in both anaerobic and aerobic performance. What's interesting is that the differences between subjects *within* groups were quite extreme. As it turns out, the women in the study showed more of a "trend" for improvement than the men. Remember, the test subjects used eight grams of pyruvate a day. Since the women weighed a lot less than the men in this study, it's possible the reason the guys didn't show a trend for greater performance is because they didn't take enough. The dose per pound of bodyweight was obviously higher in the gals than the guys. Maybe I'm wrong, but my *guess* is that pyruvate works wonders at a dose of one gram per ten pounds of bodyweight. (I weigh about 200 lbs, so I think I would need 20 grams/day. Get it? No? Alright, here's the math, bro: 200 lbs ÷ 10 = 20. Duh.)

The point I cannot emphasize strongly enough is that although pyruvate has been heavily researched (*quality research* by Dr. Stanko), the results of that research need to be extended—we need to continue to look at the effects of various dosages of pyruvate on young, healthy, non-obese, weight-training men and women to see what the effects are. And, even though EAS is not one of the companies trying to cash in big on pyruvate—we do recognize that we have a legitimate obligation to the bodybuilding supplement community, which is why we are awarding these research grants to universities in an effort to evaluate what this stuff does.

I would not call pyruvate a scam or a product based on no science, but more research needs to be done to determine which type of pyruvate is most effective—either the sodium or the calcium form (the only two forms available). At this point, companies that make bold claims for pyruvate—based on studies that used different types of pyruvate and completely different dosages—are doing customers a disser-

41

HOT NEW SUPPLEMENT TRENDS

CHAPTER 3

HOT NEW SUPPLEMENT TRENDS•HOT NEW SUPPLEMENT TRENDS•HOT NEW SUPPLEMENT TRENDS•HOT NEW SUPPLEMENT TRENDS•HOT NEW SUPPLEMENT TRENDS•HOT NEW SUPPLEMENT TRENDS•HOT NEW SUPPLEMENT TRENDS•HOT NEW SUPPLEMENT TRENDS•HOT NEW SUPPLEMENT TRENDS•HOT NEW SUPPLEMENT TRENDS•HOT NEW SUPPLEMENT TRENDS•HOT

vice. For example, several companies (ProLab Nutrition, a multilevel distribution company called New-Vision International, Inzer, CytoCharge, Pinnacle, OMW, and Med-Pro) are making claims such as, "Increase fat loss by 48%... accelerate weight loss by 36%," etc. And the recommended daily dosage of the supplement they're selling is two grams per day! Depending on which study you refer to, this is anywhere between 1/9 and 1/15 of the dosage shown to be effective in clinical studies. (I wouldn't want to have to explain this to the FTC. They do not condone this type of thing.)

Here's what I would suggest to the pyruvate parties—stop spending money on attorneys, and start investing in *scientific research*.

If these individuals focused on these areas, we would soon know how much pyruvate is needed to produce the optimal effect and if that amount is realistic—if it were something you could afford. (Right now, consuming 20 grams of pyruvate a day could cost you anywhere from $10 to $18, which, even for the most devout supplement users, is quite expensive.) We'd also know if it were possible to consume this amount without getting your mineral and electrolyte balances all screwed up or without making you sick to your stomach.

Of course, I'll keep you posted on any new developments—especially the results of the clinical studies EAS is funding regarding the effectiveness of pyruvate—in future issues of *Muscle Media*.

> **"...'Anabolic Burst Cycling' is a hot new trend that will take the bodybuilding world by storm in 1997."**

CALORIE AND SUPPLEMENT CYCLING WILL BE IN VOGUE

Another new and exciting trend which is already catching on like wildfire is calorie and supplement cycling. As you may have read in my magazine, *Muscle Media*, and which you will learn even more about in Chapters 15 and 16 of this book, it appears acute calorie cycling (consuming a high-calorie diet for 2 weeks followed by a low-calorie diet for 2 weeks, and then repeating this pattern over and over again) could offer significant advantages to bodybuilders seeking enhanced muscle growth without the increases in bodyfat which occur with most long-term, high-calorie nutritional programs. I learned about this revolutionary concept from a Swedish researcher named Torbjorn Akerfeldt.

Mark my words, "Anabolic Burst Cycling" is a hot new trend that will take the bodybuilding world by storm in 1997.

In concert with calorie cycling comes the concept of acute supplement cycling—using certain supplements in relatively high doses for two weeks and then switching to other supplements. This theory is also being promoted by Torbjorn

Akerfeldt. He believes the body's adaptive mechanisms are so efficient that the down-regulation of enzymes, receptors, and hormones occurs so rapidly that it is necessary to constantly attempt to "trick" or "manipulate" these systems through frequently changing your diet, training, and even your supplement program.

The exciting thing about calorie and supplement cycling is that even though the concept is truly revolutionary, it is far from complicated and very "doable." In fact, it's downright easy!

If you want to be on the leading edge of one of the most exciting body-building trends, perhaps the most exciting of 1997, be sure to thoroughly review Chapters 15 and 16. Mark my words—calorie and supplement cycling could revolutionize natural bodybuilding!

PRO BODYBUILDERS GETTING OFF STEROIDS

What if I told you 1997 would be the year many top-level amateurs and pro bodybuilders would get off steroids and start using more sophisticated nutrition and supplementation programs? What's that? You say you'd encourage me to undergo a thorough psychological evaluation? Well, you *might* be right. But, I can *feel* that something is getting ready to change—in a big way!

Hey... anabolic steroids work; in fact, they work so damn well, especially when they're combined with growth hormone, insulin, IGF-1, and anti-catabolic drugs like Cytadren, they're literally destroying the physiques (not to mention the health!) of top bodybuilders. I mean, give me a break—open up an issue of *Flex* magazine (that publication has the "best" photos of pro bodybuilders you'll find anywhere), and look at the bodies of these "superstars." What the hell is going on here? What happened to physiques like Frank Zane's, or even bodies like Arnold's? Arnold didn't have a huge, bloated, distended abdomen that looked like he just swallowed a pumpkin nor a protruding forehead or a huge jaw (not to mention a moonface, which some of these guys have, even when their bodyfat is two percent). Make no mistake, bodybuilding drugs are ruining physiques left and right, and I think the bodybuilding world has recognized this.

Things *are* going to change. Not all at once, but the seeds for a dramatic transformation are being planted at this time. In fact, just last week, I met, in my office, for five hours, with a guy who is arguably the world's greatest professional bodybuilder (I'm not talking about Dorian Yates, even though he's the current Mr. Olympia). Guess what? This top dog agreed with me—steroids are on the way out. And, to set a positive example, this guy is getting off all the juice—even if it means getting his ass kicked at the Mr. Olympia. This year, he is going to go into the show completely bodybuilding drug free. Suffice it to say, he will not be as cut up, nor as big, as he was at last year's show, but given time, I think he could build an even better physique using the training, nutrition, and

HOT NEW SUPPLEMENT TRENDS

HOT NEW SUPPLEMENT TRENDS•HOT NEW SUPPLEMENT TRENDS•HOT NEW SUPPLEMENT TRENDS•HOT NEW SUPPLEMENT TRENDS•HOT NEW SUPPLEMENT TRENDS•HOT NEW SUPPLEMENT TRENDS•HOT NEW SUPPLEMENT TRENDS•HOT NEW SUPPLEMENT TRENDS•HOT NEW SUPPLEMENT TRENDS•HOT NEW SUPPLEMENT TRENDS•HOT NEW SUPPLEMENT TRENDS•HOT

supplementation programs I outline in this very book. In fact, after I told him about some of the exciting new supplement concepts that are on the horizon (things you'll read about in this book), he became extremely excited and even more confident about his potential to build the "perfect physique," drug free! In fact, at the time this book is being published, this bodybuilding champion has already been off steroids for 13 weeks and is starting a supplement program I've designed for him.

Of course, as every long-term steroid user will find out the hard way, when you go off these drugs—especially after being "on" for years—the body will go through quite a shock. It takes some time before the hormonal system gets "up and running" again, but eventually it will "kick in."

You know what else I've discovered? Even though a lot of pro bodybuilders use supplements—they'll throw down a few protein-powder drinks a day and maybe take some creatine—the majority of these men and women have a very low level of understanding of how much can be done with proper nutrition and supplementation. It's not that they're stupid, not by any stretch of the imagination—and it's not that they lack determination and discipline (even with bodybuilding drugs, you've got to have so much discipline to work so damn hard to build a championship physique). I think it's just a matter of focusing so much on drugs that they don't have the time nor are they in the state of mind to thoroughly investigate the potential of various supplement stacks and cycles. I mean, think about it—if your livelihood depends on making sure your competitors don't get some type of "chemical advantage" over you, you've got to work very hard just to stay up to date on all of the latest trends in the drug world. This takes up a lot of these athletes' time and energy.

I predict the type of physiques that are built with huge amounts of bodybuilding drugs are going to be out of vogue in the not-too-distant future, and a new breed of lean, symmetrical, muscular (but not grotesquely huge) physique stars will rule the competitive-bodybuilding world. And, the "champions" who don't go with this new trend will find themselves on the sidelines—with no possibilities for endorsement contracts, low placings at pro-bodybuilding shows, and fewer appearances and seminars (where these guys make the majority of their money).

Hey... my crystal ball might not be working perfectly, but this is the "vibe" I'm getting. In a year, let's look back and see if this trend hasn't become a reality. It's a trend that really needs to take place because, let's face it, the use of muscle-building drugs in the sport/art of bodybuilding is out of control. It doesn't have to be that way—since steroids became very popular in bodybuilding in the late '70's, there have been a number of *scientifically validated* advancements in bodybuilding supplementation that can offer a real advantage to drug-free weight trainers.

SUMMARY

All in all, I believe 1997 is going to be a very exciting year in bodybuilding! The new trends I described in this chapter, which include the use of powerful testosterone-releasing supplement stacks; the development of timed-release supplement technology; implementing strategies such as loading supplements and using insulin-releasing carbohydrates to shuttle more nutrients into the muscle cells; and the concept of cycling calories and supplements, may very well offer serious bodybuilders like you and me new ways to build more muscular, stronger bodies without the use of drugs. *Oh, man... things really are starting to heat up!*

Hey... if you found this chapter interesting, please read the rest of this book very carefully because I have so much important information to share with you—information which I'm certain will help you build a better body!

Onward and upward...

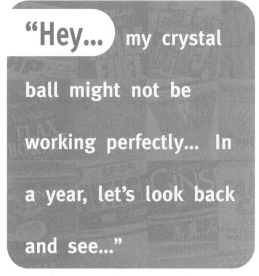

"**Hey...** my crystal ball might not be working perfectly... In a year, let's look back and see..."

SPORTS SUPPLEMENT REVIEW, 3RD ISSUE•SPORTS SUPPLEMENT REVIEW, 3RD ISSUE•SPORTS SUPPLEMENT REVIEW, 3RD ISSUE•SPORTS SUPPLEMENT REVIEW, 3RD ISSUE•SPORTS SUPPLEMENT REVIEW, 3RD ISSUE•SPORTS

46

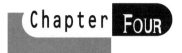
Tried and True:
Bodybuilding's Top Ten Supplements

Now that we've talked about some new, exciting supplement trends which will be the subject of heated debates in coming months, let's examine some supplements that seem to be standing the test of time, both in the scientific setting and in the real world. In this chapter, I'm going to review what I think the top ten bodybuilding supplements on the market are. As with the last chapter, I'll discuss these supplements primarily using their "generic names." Some of these supplements are available in multinutrient products, where various supplements are combined for added value and convenience. This is something I'll go over in Chapter 10, where I review various supplements by their brand names.

So, what do I think the <u>best</u> supplements in bodybuilding are—the ones that are backed by scientific data (<u>real</u> science that shows these supplements actually do something!) and the ones which are popular in gyms across America? Just keep readin', and you'll find out!

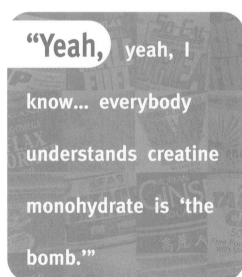

"**Yeah,** yeah, I know... everybody understands creatine monohydrate is 'the bomb.'"

CREATINE MONOHYDRATE PLUS CARBS IS THE BEST

Yeah, yeah, I know... everybody understands creatine monohydrate is "the bomb." It's *the one that works*—it's probably helped more bodybuilders gain more size and strength, faster, than anything else in history, with the sole exception of anabolic steroids. This might sound like hype, but those of you who've tried creatine monohydrate and who know anything at all about bodybuilding understand creatine packs a wallop—it works *big time!* But, I'm not going to waste your time reviewing the same old information about creatine. Nope, I'm going to bring you up to date on some fascinating things I've learned over the past year (from the top scientific experts in the world) about how to maximize the effects of creatine monohydrate. For example, notice that I have rated creatine

TRIED AND TRUE: BODYBUILDING'S TOP TEN SUPPLEMENTS

CHAPTER 4

SUPPLEMENTS~TRIED AND TRUE: BODYBUILDING'S TOP TEN SUPPLEMENTS~TRIED AND TRUE: BODYBUILDING'S TOP TEN SUPPLEMENTS~TRIED AND TRUE: BODYBUILDING'S TOP TEN SUPPLEMENTS~TRIED AND TRUE: BODYBUILDING'S TOP TEN SUPPLEMENTS~TRIED AND TRUE: BODYBUILDING'S TOP TEN SUPPLEMENTS~TRIED AND TRUE: BODYBUILDING'S TOP TEN SUPPLEMENTS~TRIED AND TRUE:

monohydrate **plus carbs** as the best bodybuilding supplement on the market. That's because solid scientific research now points to the fact that creatine works better when it's consumed along with a potent insulin-releasing carbohydrate source like dextrose (also known as glucose). A whole lot better! In fact, according to Dr. Paul Greenhaff, quite likely the world's leading expert on creatine supplementation, it works up to 60% better![102, 103, 104]

And, according to two recent studies performed at Creighton University, creatine monohydrate *plus* carbs (specifically, Phosphagen HP) does indeed seem to work better than regular creatine. In fact, in a recent study, athletes who used Phosphagen HP gained more lean mass, ran faster, jumped higher, and gained more strength than athletes who used regular creatine.[265] Another study revealed athletes who used creatine plus carbs (Phosphagen HP) boosted their anaerobic performance 30% more than athletes who used regular creatine.[264] That's some amazing stuff, folks, especially when you consider how potent regular ole creatine is! I'll review this groundbreaking new research in more detail in a moment, but first, let's take a look at what creatine is, what it does, and why it has so rapidly become the most popular sports supplement in America.

The Creatine Story

If, a couple years ago, you were to tell me there was a supplement (<u>not</u> an anabolic steroid or some other bodybuilding drug) that would help bodybuilders pack on as much as 10 rock-hard pounds of muscular bodyweight in less than 2 weeks; increase their bench press by 25 lbs in a mere 10 days; get a pump like they were loaded up on Dianabol (a pump that lasts for hours and hours); and, all the while, help them run faster, jump higher, and recover from exercise more quickly, I would have said that you were *full of it!*

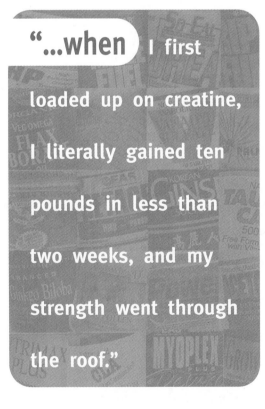

"...when I first loaded up on creatine, I literally gained ten pounds in less than two weeks, and my strength went through the roof."

But, when I first started using creatine monohydrate back in the summer of 1994, every last speck of doubt I had about this compound's effects was erased in a matter of days. That's because when I first loaded up on creatine, I literally gained ten pounds in less than two weeks, and my strength went through the roof. (Although my results were extraordinary—different people get different results—stories like mine are <u>not</u> rare. Bodybuilders everywhere are experiencing phenomenal gains with this stuff!)

Now, creatine is the most popular supplement in bodybuilding, and it's catching on like wildfire in all kinds of sports. One source recently reported that three out of four medal winners at the 1996 Summer Olympic Games were using creatine. (It's not banned because it occurs naturally, in relatively high concentrations, in certain foods. It would be impossible for the International Olympic Committee to ban this substance, even though it puts those who are *not* using the compound at an extreme *dis*advantage.) Soon, it will be difficult for athletes who don't use creatine supplements properly to compete against those who do use this powerful, natural supplement.

Over the last couple of years, I have reviewed over 100 articles in the applicable scientific literature on creatine and muscle function, and I have worked closely with some of the leading creatine researchers in the world: specifically, Anthony Almada and Dr. Paul Greenhaff. If there is one supplement that I know more about than any other, it's creatine monohydrate. In fact, my brain is almost filled to capacity with creatine facts, both relevant and irrelevant. For example, did you know creatine was discovered in meat extracts way back in 1832 by a French scientist named Chevreul, who named it after the Greek word for flesh? Did you know that in 1923, scientists discovered the average human body contains over 100 grams of creatine and that over 95% of that is stored in muscle tissue? Here are some more borderline irrelevant creatine facts—a pound of beef contains two grams of creatine—so does a pound of salmon. A pound of tuna contains 1.8 grams, and herring is the king of creatine-providing foods, supplying a whopping 3 grams of creatine per pound. Interesting, huh? Well, maybe not, but suffice it to say, if I ever get on the game show *Jeopardy* and they have a "creatine category," I'm home free!

So What Is Creatine?

Creatine is a compound that's naturally made in our bodies to supply energy to our muscles. Chemically, it is called "methylguanido-acetic acid." Creatine is formed from the amino acids arginine, methionine, and glycine through a chemical process which is not worth explaining.

Creatine is manufactured in the liver and may also be produced in the pancreas and kidneys. It is transported in the blood and taken up by muscle cells, where it is converted to creatine phosphate (CP), also called "phosphocreatine." This reaction involves the enzyme creatine kinase which helps bond creatine to a high-energy phosphate group.

Typically, the average person metabolizes about two grams of creatine per day, and that same amount is normally synthesized by the body; thus, you generally maintain a creatine balance. Once creatine is bound to a phosphate group, it is *permanently stored* in a cell as phosphocreatine *until* it is used to produce chemical energy called adenosine triphosphate (ATP). When this takes place, creatine can be

TRIED AND TRUE: BODYBUILDING'S TOP TEN SUPPLEMENTS

SUPPLEMENTS•TRIED AND TRUE: BODYBUILDING'S TOP TEN SUPPLEMENTS•TRIED AND TRUE: BODYBUILDING'S TOP TEN SUPPLEMENTS•TRIED AND TRUE: BODYBUILDING'S TOP TEN SUPPLEMENTS•TRIED AND TRUE: BODYBUILDING'S TOP TEN SUPPLEMENTS•TRIED AND TRUE: BODYBUILDING'S TOP TEN SUPPLEMENTS•TRIED AND TRUE:

released to spontaneously form creat*in*ine, which is then removed from the blood via the kidneys and excreted in the urine. Creat*in*ine is routinely checked in blood tests, serving as a crude, suggestive marker of how well the kidneys are filtering the blood. Although creatine supplementation can raise blood creat*in*ine, it has never been shown to be toxic or harmful to the kidneys.

The richest source of creatine in food is in animal muscle, such as meats and fish. But, to increase athletic performance and boost lean body mass, creatine must be taken in concentrations which are not reasonably obtained from a whole-food diet. For example, you would have to consume ten pounds of raw steak a day for five days to load your body with creatine. (Vegetarians usually have a very low intake of creatine, by the way.)

The Use of Creatine by Athletes

It is rumored that athletes in the former USSR and Bulgaria may have been using creatine to enhance athletic performance since the early 1970's. While this may be true, the first documented use of creatine supplementation by athletes was with British track and field competitors who competed in the 1992 Olympics in Barcelona. Creatine was given credit for powering several of the British athletes who won gold medals. The *London Times* reported (August 7, 1992) that Linford Christie, the 100-meter gold medalist, supplemented with creatine before the 1992 Olympics, and a European magazine called *Bodybuilding Monthly* reported that Sally Gunnele, the 400-meter gold medalist, also used creatine. The *London Times* also reported that Colin Jackson, the champion British 110-meter hurdler, used creatine before the Olympics.

Shortly thereafter, U.S. champion athletes began using creatine. Since then, scientists have elucidated more secrets on how to best utilize creatine for optimal benefit. Now, champion athletes and bodybuilders around the world swear by creatine's effects.

Low-potency creatine supplements were available in Britain, but creatine supplements especially designed for strength enhancement were not commercially available until March of 1993, when the research scientists at EAS introduced the compound to the sports nutrition market under the name **Phosphagen**™.

The Science of Creatine

The first scientific study that I could find which indicates creatine may have "bodybuilding effects" was published in *The Journal of Biological Chemistry* 67 (1926) : 29-41. That's right—*over 70 years ago*, researchers already had some indication that creatine promoted weight gain and improved nitrogen balance, which is often associated with muscle growth. (Think about it—if it took us almost seven decades from the time scientists first found evidence to suggest creatine might enhance muscle building and athletic performance to the time we found out how to use it, how many other naturally occurring compounds are out there that might help bodybuilders gain muscle size and strength? It's inevitable that there are others just waiting to be "discovered.")

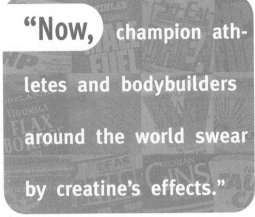

"Now, champion athletes and bodybuilders around the world swear by creatine's effects."

In 1981, an article published in the *New England Journal of Medicine* by Dr. I. Sipila and colleagues reported that supplementation with creatine in a group of patients suffering from a condition called "gyrate atrophy" (a genetic ailment of the eyes caused by a metabolic inability to efficiently metabolize ornithine and synthesize creatine) improved the test subjects' strength, increased their bodyweight by ten percent, and partially reversed the Type II muscle fiber atrophy associated with this disease.[252] One athlete in this group of test subjects improved his best time in the 100-meter sprint by two seconds.

Later that decade, Dr. Eric Hultman and his colleagues (including Dr. Paul Greenhaff), working in the Department of Clinical Chemistry at the Karolinska Institute in Sweden, "invented" the practice of creatine loading. (Dr. Eric Hultman is the scientist who developed the concept of carbohydrate loading, which literally millions of endurance athletes and even bodybuilders practice.) However, it was not until 1992 that Hultman's discoveries were peer reviewed and published in the journal *Clinical Science*.[113] (It's too bad for Dr. Hultman that he did not patent the use of creatine for enhancing athletic performance—he would be a multi-multi-millionaire today!)

The idea of loading and then using a maintenance dose was pioneered by Dr. Paul Greenhaff at the University of Nottingham in 1993 and 1994; these results were published in collaboration with Dr. Hultman.[126] Dr. Greenhaff and his colleagues performed biopsies on muscles to study the effects of creatine loading. They discovered that consuming at least 20 grams of creatine a day in divided doses for one week led to an average increase in muscle creatine concentration of about 25%. Greenhaff's study showed that supraphysiological (higher than normal) muscle creatine levels can be maintained after the loading phase by ingesting a maintenance dose of as little as 2 grams/day (although most bodybuilders I know maintain at a dose of 5-15 grams/day).

In 1993, a study peer reviewed and published in *Scandinavian Journal of Medicine, Science and Sports*[17] demonstrated that creatine supplementation can significantly increase body mass (in only one week) and that it was responsible for improved performance in high-intensity intermittent exercise.

In 1994, Anthony Almada and colleagues performed a study at Texas Women's University which was the first to demonstrate that the increase in bodyweight seen with creatine supplementation was, in fact, lean body mass (fat-free mass) and that test subjects who used creatine experienced an increase in strength (as measured on the bench press). This study was peer reviewed and published in the journal *Acta Physiologica Scandinavica*.[79]

Over the past 4 years, at least 20 separate, double-blind, placebo-controlled, university studies have demonstrated that creatine monohydrate supplementation increases athletic performance; strength; recuperation; speed in the 100-, 200-, and 400-meter sprints; and *possibly accelerates fat loss*. Basically, a boatload of scientific data shows creatine monohydrate works—it produces fast and significant results even in the most rigorous trials.[18, 47, 79, 106, 107, 153, 264] Just ask around—your gym buddies will confirm creatine has a great reputation for producing dramatic results in the real world as well!

How Creatine Enhances Muscle Size and Strength Gains

The goal of the bodybuilder is to use progressive resistance exercise to force the muscles to adapt and grow. This increased workload or progressive resistance can be achieved in several ways: by increasing the force of contraction through increased resistance such as when lifting a heavier weight, by increasing the duration of time that the muscle is under tension or contracted, and by increasing the frequency of exercise.

Creatine helps in all three ways: it helps build lean body mass, which allows still greater force to be used; provides energy so duration of exercise or work can be lengthened; and speeds recovery so exercise frequency can be increased.

"**Basically,** a boatload of scientific data shows creatine monohydrate works..."

Muscle "Cell-Volumizing" May Assist Muscle Growth

Animal-cell studies suggest that creatine may promote muscle growth by stimulating protein synthesis. There are two possible actions involved—the first is simply due to the increased work which your muscles can produce due to their increased energy content and the delay in muscle fatigue. The second way is a "bonus" that comes from the increased amount of creatine absorbed in the muscle tissue. As creatine is taken up into the muscle cells, it can also associate with water. As more creatine is stored, more water may be brought into the muscle cell. This gives muscles a full, or "pumped," feel and look. It may also increase the volume of the muscle cell. Scientific studies show that when a muscle cell is volumized, or "super-hydrated," it may trigger protein synthesis and minimize protein breakdown (it may also increase glycogen synthesis).[115, 118] This could equate to enhanced muscle growth—the muscle fibers could become larger and stronger. This is a concept that was pioneered by EAS researchers Anthony

Almada and Ed Byrd and is one that is now widely accepted in the sports nutrition industry.

Here's an analogy I often offer to explain cell volumizing: think of your muscle cells as individual water balloons (muscles are made up of at least 70% water). If you can get more water inside of them, they get bigger and firmer—if you let water out, they get smaller and softer... get the picture? When muscles start to "swell" with creatine and water and then you train with weights, the pumps you get are unbelievable! (A creatine pump is the closest thing I've ever experienced to a steroid pump!) Anyway, this cell-volumizing effect may explain why many creatine monohydrate users gain solid, muscular weight rapidly when they start using this supplement.

It seems you get most of the size and strength gains from creatine monohydrate within the first month of use. After a month of taking creatine monohydrate, I think your muscle cells are pretty much saturated with this stuff. And, I believe the initial weight gained from using creatine monohydrate is mostly water—from the cell-volumizing effect. However, this is not simply "water retention." Cell-volumizing means more water *inside* muscle cells; water retention (which can make you look smooth) happens outside the cells—there's a BIG difference!

I believe that after the first couple of weeks of creatine use, you actually start gaining more muscle tissue—not just water. This may occur because the strength increases experienced while supplementing with creatine allow you to train heavier and/or more intensely, thus triggering signals for new muscle growth. And I believe the cellular hydration caused by creatine monohydrate use also creates a more favorable environment for muscle growth.

Now, I don't have rock-hard, scientific facts to back this up. But I do have some evidence. In two relatively recent studies performed on weight trainers who consumed the creatine-rich supplement, Phosphagain®, those using the supplement gained significantly more lean body mass than nonusers who followed the same workout program.[152, 153] But, when the researchers measured the test subjects' total body water, it wasn't any different than before the study. This suggests the mass increase was somehow attributable to actual muscle tissue.

Some Evidence Exists that Creatine Is a Lactic-Acid Buffer

So we know that creatine enhances the energy reserve for muscle cells and that it may very well enhance cell volume. Now, new evidence suggests that it may work as a lactic-acid buffer as well. In a new study performed by Dr. Michael Prevost of Louisiana State University, evidence (which supports previous studies by Dr. Hultman's group in Sweden) indicates creatine may buffer lactic acid and improve exercise recovery time in short-duration, maximal-intensity exercise (like weight training). The results from this study are being reviewed by a major exercise physiology journal at this time and will most likely be published later this year.

TRIED AND TRUE: BODYBUILDING'S TOP TEN SUPPLEMENTS

SUPPLEMENTS•TRIED AND TRUE: BODYBUILDING'S TOP TEN SUPPLEMENTS•TRIED AND TRUE: BODYBUILDING'S TOP TEN SUPPLEMENTS•TRIED AND TRUE: BODYBUILDING'S TOP TEN SUPPLEMENTS•TRIED AND TRUE: BODYBUILDING'S TOP TEN SUPPLEMENTS•TRIED AND TRUE: BODYBUILDING'S TOP TEN SUPPLEMENTS•TRIED AND TRUE:

CHAPTER 4

54

Remember, when muscles use the anaerobic energy system to contract during intense exercise, they produce lactic acid—it's the stuff that's partially responsible for that "burning" feeling which occurs as the muscle becomes fatigued. This results in "burnout," which decreases exercise frequency and duration. When you can't exercise any longer because your muscles burn and won't contract, it is probably due to either running out of energy or to excessive lactic-acid buildup. I don't want to get into this issue in too much detail, but in a nutshell, a lactic-acid buffer works by absorbing hydrogen ions released during the energy-producing reactions. Creatine may absorb hydrogen ions in the process of creatine phosphate transferring a high-energy phosphate group to ADP to form ATP.

Further scientific research is necessary to verify this, but even if creatine does not buffer lactic acid, it can extend the exercise or work period by virtue of increased energy stored in the muscles. In other words, you can train or perform longer and harder because you have more muscle energy available.

What About Creatine Phosphate or Creatine Citrate?

The most popular form of creatine on the market is creatine *monohydrate*. All of the recently published scientific studies have been conducted with this form. It is virtually tasteless and is an adequately soluble compound in water. Creatine monohydrate contains more creatine per weight of material than any other form of creatine. It's simply a molecule of creatine with a molecule of water attached to it so it's more stable. When creatine monohydrate dissolves in water, the molecule of water that was attached to it is released, as is the creatine. Creatine monohydrate contains about 880 mg of "free" creatine in every gram. In this form, creatine can be purified and stabilized.

Creatine *phosphate* is not the best form to use as a supplement to shuttle creatine into the muscles. None of the scientific studies have used creatine phosphate as a <u>dietary</u> source of creatine, as it has never been shown to have an ergogenic or anabolic effect when taken orally. (There are injectable forms of creatine phosphate available in Europe for the treatment of certain cardiac muscle ailments. Two studies with injectable phosphocreatine have shown an ergogenic effect.)

A molecule of creatine phosphate is actually one molecule of creatine bound to one phosphate group. A gram of creatine phosphate contains 623 mg of "free" creatine. Since the phosphate group weighs more than a molecule of water, a molecule of creatine phosphate weighs more than a molecule of creatine monohydrate. This means a gram of creatine monohydrate contains 41% more creatine than a gram of creatine phosphate. Real creatine phosphate is also very, very expensive.

Yet another form of this supplement, called creatine *citrate*, is also being hyped as a superior supplement in this category. Creatine citrate does dissolve a little better in water than creatine monohydrate, but creatine citrate is a less concentrated form. It contains approximately 400-500 mg of "free" creatine per gram. Like I said, in a glass of water, creatine citrate may dissolve better than creatine monohydrate, but keep in mind that creatine monohydrate contains almost twice the "free" creatine as creatine citrate. Dr. Paul Greenhaff has studied creatine citrate versus creatine monohydrate in laboratory experiments (unpublished data). These show there is no advantage to using creatine citrate over monohydrate. As a matter of fact, it was necessary to supply test subjects with much more creatine citrate than creatine monohydrate in order to attain the same level of muscle saturation. And, I can tell you from my own personal experience, creatine citrate tastes like battery acid, and it's more expensive.

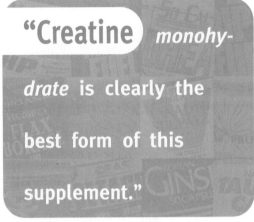

"*Creatine* monohydrate is clearly the best form of this supplement."

Creatine *monohydrate* is clearly the best form of this supplement.

Is Creatine Monohydrate Use Safe?

More good news about creatine—it appears to be very safe, even when used in relatively large quantities by athletes. There have been no adverse effects reported in any of the studies, other than the usual gastric upset or intolerance that a lot of compounds are known to cause in a few people. Although very long-term safety studies have not been conducted with people taking large amounts of creatine over many years, there are no mechanisms known that would suggest to researchers that such studies would show any different effects.

One study conducted with a group of men and women, 32-70 years of age, found that creatine loading at 20 grams/day for 5 days, followed by a 10-gram/day maintenance dose for 51 days, produced no adverse effects. However, this regimen did produce some very important benefits other than performance enhancement. There was a 22% decrease in VLDL cholesterol and a 23% decrease in blood triglycerides.[78] The VLDL cholesterol and triglycerides are complementary risk factors in heart disease and adult-onset diabetes. The men in this study also found a decrease in the concentration of blood sugar after an overnight fast, suggesting that creatine may improve insulin action. Earlier studies point to creatine reducing blood sugar in diabetic patients, but this is something that needs further research in order to make any definitive statement.

Is It Legal?

Creatine is not a steroid nor a drug. It's made in our bodies naturally and is normally present in many foods in relatively high quantities (although it would be extremely impractical, if not impossible, to regularly take in the amount

55

TRIED AND TRUE: BODYBUILDING'S TOP TEN SUPPLEMENTS

SUPPLEMENTS•TRIED AND TRUE: BODYBUILDING'S TOP TEN SUPPLEMENTS•TRIED AND TRUE: BODYBUILDING'S TOP TEN SUPPLEMENTS•TRIED AND TRUE: BODYBUILDING'S TOP TEN SUPPLEMENTS•TRIED AND TRUE: BODYBUILDING'S TOP TEN SUPPLEMENTS•TRIED AND TRUE: BODYBUILDING'S TOP TEN SUPPLEMENTS•TRIED AND TRUE:

CHAPTER 4

of creatine necessary for enhanced performance through a diet consisting of whole foods alone—that's why creatine supplements are so popular). Creatine is legal and is allowed in all types of competition. It has not been banned by any sports association nor any government agency.

Taking Creatine Supplementation to the Next Level

Okay, what we've discussed so far about creatine is certainly interesting, but we knew almost all of this last year. Now let's look at what's new in the world of creatine! Well, for starters there's some *very good news*—over the past year, five university studies have offered evidence that the effectiveness of creatine monohydrate can be boosted to an even higher level—*a much higher level!* Here's the story...

Dr. Paul Greenhaff, one of the pioneers of creatine supplementation for enhanced athletic performance and unquestionably the most "active" creatine researcher in the world, discovered certain individuals could be classified as "non-responders" to creatine supplementation. His research showed that although most athletes respond very well to creatine supplementation, about two people out of ten don't. Dr. Greenhaff's research led him to believe the anabolic hormone insulin was a potent "up-regulator" of muscle creatine intake.[103, 104] EAS researcher Anthony Almada also believed insulin had a role in creatine uptake, based on animal studies done in the '70's.[290] He hypothesized that by combining creatine with just the right amount of insulin-releasing carbohydrates and other nutrients, he could create a "high-performance" creatine supplement.

> **"...a simple carbohydrate called dextrose would be the ideal insulin-releasing agent to combine with creatine."**

Almada then carefully examined Dr. Paul Greenhaff's work and met with him in England to learn more about it. Then he analyzed the insulin-potentiating effects produced by different types of carbohydrates. He theorized that a simple carbohydrate called dextrose would be the ideal insulin-releasing agent to combine with creatine. Then he spent weeks evaluating what the appropriate dosage of dextrose might be. His goal was to produce a formula that would cause a substantial increase in insulin—enough to effectively transport more creatine into muscle cells—yet he didn't want to create a formula that was too high in carbohydrates, one that contributed excess and unnecessary calories to the diet.

Almada's research led him to hypothesize that a formula containing 35 grams of dextrose, combined with 5 grams of creatine monohydrate, may produce a powerful effect. For good measure, Almada also included one gram of taurine, an amino acid that may act as an insulin mimicker and further potentiate the uptake of creatine into muscle cells. And, to help ensure optimal function of the creatine transport systems in the body, Almada included disodium phosphate (sodium is an essential cofactor for creatine transport across the gut and muscle cells), magnesium phosphate, and potassium phosphate. (All of these nutrients may play an important role in the formation of phosphocreatine.)

Almada called this new formula Phosphagen HP™—High Performance Creatine Transport System™. This product was developed by piecing together scientific data, not by throwing out some wild theories that were more marketing hype than scientific reality, which is what many other companies do.

Putting It to the Test

Almada proceeded to evaluate whether Phosphagen HP really was more effective than creatine monohydrate. He sought the assistance of a researcher named David Noonan, a member of the exercise science team at the University of Nebraska at Omaha. (Neither Noonan nor his colleagues have any financial interest in EAS or any supplements.)

Noonan's assignment was to test creatine vs. Phosphagen HP, so he selected 30 subjects and randomly divided them into 3 groups of 10. One group received a placebo (35 grams of carbohydrates), another group used a supplement containing 5 grams of creatine monohydrate, and another used Phosphagen HP. All the subjects had a minimum of three years of weight-training experience, and all were college football players.

Before the study, Noonan and his research team measured the test subjects' body composition by DEXA analysis (a highly accurate method for evaluating fat-free mass and bodyfat). They also measured the test subjects' maximum strength in the bench press, their top speed in a 100-meter sprint, and their best vertical jump. During the study, all test subjects were instructed to follow the same nutrition and exercise program they were using before the study and were told to take four servings of their supplement a day for five days, followed by two servings a day thereafter.

Now, it's important to point out that this was a "double-blind" study. This means that none of the test subjects, nor the researchers, knew who was getting what. All three groups consumed a supplement that came in a blank packet, and all the supplements looked and tasted like fruit-punch Kool-Aid (which is how Phosphagen HP tastes).

During this study, and virtually all the studies that EAS provides funding for, no representatives from EAS were involved in the data collection or analysis. All the testing and monitoring of the subjects was done by researchers at the university. At the end of the study, researchers once again evaluated the test subjects' "lean" and fat mass (by DEXA), as well as their maximum strength, speed,

REVIEW•SPORTS SUPPLEMENT REVIEW, 3RD ISSUE•SPORTS SUPPLEMENT REVIEW, 3RD ISSUE•SPORTS SUPPLEMENT REVIEW, 3RD ISSUE•SPORTS SUPPLEMENT

•SPORTS SUPPLEMENT REVIEW, 3RD ISSUE•SPORTS SUPPLEMENT REVIEW, 3RD ISSUE•SPORTS SUPPLEMENT REVIEW, 3RD ISSUE•SPORTS SUPPLEMENT REVIEW, 3RD ISSUE•SPORTS SUPPLEMENT REVIEW, 3RD ISSUE•SPORTS SUPPLEMENT REVIEW, 3RD ISSUE•SPORTS SUPPLEMENT REVIEW, 3RD ISSUE•SPORTS SUPPLEMENT

TRIED AND TRUE: BODYBUILDING'S TOP TEN SUPPLEMENTS

SUPPLEMENTS•TRIED AND TRUE: BODYBUILDING'S TOP TEN SUPPLEMENTS•TRIED AND TRUE: BODYBUILDING'S TOP TEN SUPPLEMENTS•TRIED AND TRUE: BODYBUILDING'S TOP TEN SUPPLEMENTS•TRIED AND TRUE: BODYBUILDING'S TOP TEN SUPPLEMENTS•TRIED AND TRUE: BODYBUILDING'S TOP TEN SUPPLEMENTS•TRIED AND TRUE:

CHAPTER 4

and vertical jump. The preliminary study results are very interesting, to say the least! Just look at the charts below!

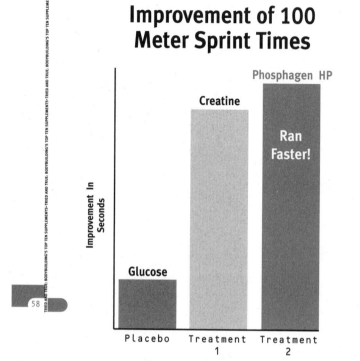

Improvement of 100 Meter Sprint Times

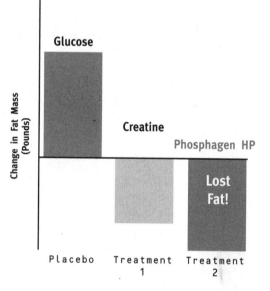

Enhanced Loss of Bodyfat Mass

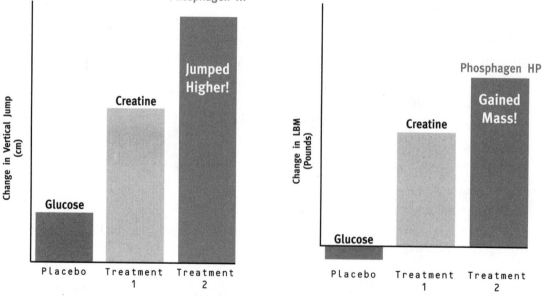

Enhanced Explosive Muscular Force

Enhanced Gains in Lean Body Mass

Source: J. Stout, et al., "The Effects of a Supplement Designed to Augment Creatine Uptake on Exercise Performance and Fat-Free Mass in Football Players." To be presented at the 1997 ACSM National Conference.

These data clearly indicate that in this study, Phosphagen HP outperformed creatine in all areas! Phosphagen HP users gained more mass (in just four weeks!), showed a trend for fat loss, jumped higher, and ran faster than those who used creatine or the placebo!

More New Studies Show Creatine *Plus Carbs* Works

Since this ground-breaking study showing the powerful effects of combining precise amounts of carbohydrates with creatine was revealed, several other studies have confirmed and extended these findings. For example, a second study from Creighton University documented the effects of creatine monohydrate plus carbohydrates (Phosphagen HP again) on "anaerobic work capacity." This study revealed Phosphagen HP produced a 30% greater increase in performance than regular creatine![264]

Another interesting study conducted by Dr. Green, and others, at the University of Nottingham in England, shows that when test subjects take creatine with insulin-releasing carbs, it not only increases the uptake of creatine by muscle cells more than 50% (as previously shown by Dr. Greenhaff) but may also increase muscle glycogen formation by over 200%. (Perhaps this is why my muscles get so "pumped" when I take this stuff!) And, this study showed even athletes who don't respond to creatine get results when they use it along with a carbohydrate that causes a rapid release of insulin.[102] Make no mistake, strong scientific evidence suggests creatine *plus carbs* really is greater than creatine supplementation alone.

Is using a supplement like Phosphagen HP better than simply taking creatine and mixing it with grape juice or another type of fruit juice? (Fruit juice elevates insulin release, too.) I think so. Keep in mind that an 8-oz glass of grape juice contains roughly 35 grams of carbohydrates (about the same amount as in a serving of Phosphagen HP). However, the carbohydrates from grape juice are roughly 50% fructose and 50% glucose. But, consuming fructose doesn't produce anywhere near the insulin release of consuming straight glucose or dextrose.[179] I'd bet good money that the carbohydrate source in Phosphagen HP produces a greater insulin-releasing effect than consuming an equal amount of grape juice. That greater insulin-releasing effect could equal greater creatine uptake.

What about the cost of Phosphagen HP versus plain creatine monohydrate and juice? I went to the grocery store and took a look at the price of grape juice, and even though it varies from brand to brand, the average price at my grocery store was $.65 for an 8-oz serving. Add that to the price of five grams of creatine monohydrate, and then compare it to a serving of Phosphagen HP, and you'll find that Phosphagen HP is *less* expensive (and more convenient!) than mixing creatine monohydrate with grape juice (at least according to my analysis). And with grape juice, you don't get the sodium, phosphates, nor the taurine—ingredients Almada

TRIED AND TRUE: BODYBUILDING'S TOP TEN SUPPLEMENTS

SUPPLEMENTS-TRIED AND TRUE: BODYBUILDING'S TOP TEN SUPPLEMENTS-TRIED AND TRUE: BODYBUILDING'S TOP TEN SUPPLEMENTS-TRIED AND TRUE: BODYBUILDING'S TOP TEN SUPPLEMENTS-TRIED AND TRUE: BODYBUILDING'S TOP TEN SUPPLEMENTS-TRIED AND TRUE:

thinks may play a role in making Phosphagen HP even more effective. I don't think you can go wrong with Phosphagen HP—it's been shown to be effective in several university studies, it's convenient and economical, and it works in the real world. I think it is *the best* sports supplement on the market, and I challenge anyone to prove otherwise.

Does Creatine Need to be Cycled?

The concept of "cycling" supplements is a holdover from the use of anabolic steroids. Cycling means to use a product for a while and then discontinue its use and keep repeating this "cycle." Steroid-using athletes often cycle steroids to minimize side effects and to keep the body from down-regulating its receptors to these drugs.

According to Dr. Paul Greenhaff, there is no scientific proof cycling creatine offers any strong advantage. Even though, as he explains, taking creatine does shut down the natural production of creatine by the body. But, he explains this also occurs when you're eating large amounts of meat which, of course, contain creatine—it's a natural feedback mechanism. But, Dr. Greenhaff explains, once you stop using creatine, your body begins to synthesize the compound naturally again.

Anecdotal reports from athletes who have tried cycling creatine offer inconclusive evidence—some contend that by taking a few weeks off from creatine supplementation and then coming back with another loading phase, they are able to enhance their gains in size and strength; others believe they get better results by continuing to use the supplement. One thing I do regularly, which I think works well, is to use a high dosage of creatine, approximately 30 grams/day for a week, and then cut back to 5-10 grams/day for 4 or 5 weeks; then go back and reload with 30 grams/day. During these intermittent reloading phases, it seems like I get an extra boost. I think it's worth a try.

Another novel strategy which EAS researcher Anthony Almada thinks might be effective, especially for athletes competing in a bodybuilding contest or some other sporting event where they need to "peak" is to discontinue creatine supplementation two or three weeks before the competition and allow creatine reserves to decline. According to Dr. Greenhaff's study, it takes around four weeks for the "excess" creatine to diffuse out of the muscle. Even if it takes longer, the muscle creatine level will still not go below previous baseline levels. Almada suggests that 1 week to 10 days before competition, begin creatine loading again, using 20 to 30 grams/day in divided doses with dextrose. (The best time to take a serving of creatine is right after you work out because of the metabolic environment created by strenuous exercise.) Remember, the "extra" creatine loaded into your muscles has not yet had time to fully diffuse (empty). At this time, there should be enough creatine transporter proteins to pack more creatine into the muscles even though they still contain more than a baseline amount of creatine. The net result may be a renewed super-loading of creatine. This is another idea I think might be worth trying.

Summary

In the ever-growing, confusing world of bodybuilding supplements, this is one area where you just can't go wrong—use a creatine supplement along with a high-glycemic carbohydrate source to load your muscles. Use 20-30 grams of creatine a day for a week and then cut back to 5-15 grams/day for a maintenance dose. If you're like most people (myself included), you'll notice a dramatic increase in size and strength. You'll get better pumps in the gym; your muscles will be noticeably stronger and "fuller." It's the closest thing to an anabolic steroid effect that I've ever felt from any natural supplement.

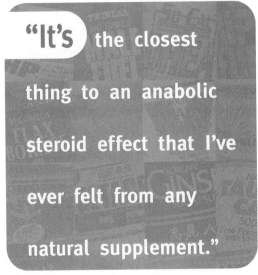

"It's the closest thing to an anabolic steroid effect that I've ever felt from any natural supplement."

WHEY PROTEIN—A BODYBUILDING ALL-STAR

Every bodybuilder understands, or *should* understand, the importance of protein supplementation. Weight-training athletes require more protein (a lot more!) than sedentary folks. Without protein (which the body breaks down into amino acids), you can't build muscle—it's as simple as that. As far as I'm concerned, no matter what kind of diet you follow—whether it's low or high in complex carbohydrates or fats—and despite the number of calories you take in, your diet *must* be rich with protein.

This belief has long been held by bodybuilders—going back some four decades—yet only in recent years has it become accepted by the scientific community. Studies with both strength and endurance athletes have clearly indicated that exercise increases the need for protein and amino acids.[90, 158] Studies have also shown that the anabolic effects of intense training are increased by a high-protein diet.[82, 101, 289]

I'm convinced that the harder and more intensely you train, the more important dietary protein becomes to maximizing the muscle-building process. For serious bodybuilders, I recommend a protein intake of 1-1.5 grams of quality protein per pound of bodyweight per day. For example, I weigh around 200 lbs; therefore, I try to consume 200-300 grams of protein a day, in 5 or 6 divided doses. I know some bodybuilders who consume as much as 500 grams of protein a day, but I have a hard time believing that much is necessary. One of the concerns I have with these *extremely* high-protein diets is that the body is very adaptive—if you constantly bombard it with huge amounts of protein, far above and beyond what's needed to promote anabolic drive, your system could become so "expert" at breaking down protein tissue that in spite of the higher protein intake, your liver could

TRIED AND TRUE: BODYBUILDING'S TOP TEN SUPPLEMENTS

CHAPTER 4

SUPPLEMENTS•TRIED AND TRUE: BODYBUILDING'S TOP TEN SUPPLEMENTS•TRIED AND TRUE: BODYBUILDING'S TOP TEN SUPPLEMENTS•TRIED AND TRUE: BODYBUILDING'S TOP TEN SUPPLEMENTS•TRIED AND TRUE: BODYBUILDING'S TOP TEN SUPPLEMENTS•TRIED AND TRUE: BODYBUILDING'S TOP TEN SUPPLEMENTS•TRIED AND TRUE:

be disassembling amino acids as fast as you could consume them. (I intend to examine this paradox in a future issue of *Muscle Media*.)

In addition to providing your muscles with the vitally important amino acids it needs to grow, protein also has a nice effect on insulin stability and energy levels, especially during a diet. By consuming protein with each meal, there's a greater chance your blood sugar levels will fluctuate less. This can help you control your appetite and provide a consistent environment for greater fat loss. If you consume a diet that's too high in carbohydrates, your blood sugar levels fluctuate all day—one minute you feel great; the next you feel tired and wiped out (as you'll learn later in this book, part of this has to do with the fact that there are certain amino acids in protein and carbohydrate foods that act as "mood-altering" neurotransmitters—specifically tryptophan and tyrosine).

What Type of Protein Is Best?

There are many different types of protein sources available to you. Quality protein can be found in whole foods like eggs, milk, cottage cheese, beef, fish, poultry, etc. And, there are also a variety of protein supplements on the market: milk and egg protein, soy, beef, even vegetable protein. Out of all these different protein supplements, I'm absolutely convinced that whey protein is the best. Not only does it have a superior biological value (which means it may "yield" more usable grams of amino acids than other protein supplements), it's also very low in lactose (that nasty milk sugar that upsets many people's stomachs). Whey protein—ion-exchanged, microfiltered whey protein/peptides—is extremely high quality and very easy to use, which is another thing that is terrific about it.

> **"In the old days... protein powders were a necessary evil—they tasted like chalk and mixed like oil and water."**

In the old days (and I'm not talking about that long ago!), protein powders were a necessary evil—they tasted like chalk and mixed like oil and water. When I express how much I like products like Designer Protein™ by Next Nutrition and other whey-protein-containing supplements such as Myoplex Plus™, part of that is based on the fact that the protein is such good quality, and part of it simply has to do with the fact that these supplements taste great, they mix up easily, and they're easy on the gut. Those of you who've been bodybuilding for a number of years can appreciate these properties in a product! (It wasn't always this easy, folks!)

Another one of the great things about whey protein is that it has an especially high concentration of essential amino acids (up to 50%), half of which are muscle-preserving branched-chain aminos, and most quality whey-protein supplements are also fortified with glutamine—an amino acid which I believe is important to bodybuilders.

Whey protein also seems to support the immune system which is "taxed" by intense exercise. A scientist named Dr. Bounous and his colleagues at McGill University (in Canada) completed a series of studies which demonstrated whey protein was superior to egg albumin, soy, beef, and fish (to name a few) with regard to enhancement of both cellular and hormonal responses. Careful analysis revealed that the immunostimulating action of whey was due to the overall amino acid makeup—whey contains just the right amino acids in the right concentration. Whey protein has also been found to increase levels of glutathione (arguably the most important water-soluble antioxidant). [34, 35, 36]

I could go on and on, but suffice it to say, a great deal of evidence supports my conclusion that whey is the best protein for bodybuilders. It has the highest biological value, it's rich in the branched-chain amino acids, it may support the immune system, and it may also work as an antioxidant. Quality milk proteins, especially modern-day caseinate- and milk-protein isolates, are also good protein products. These particular proteins are naturally high in glutamine, which is a very, very important amino acid for bodybuilders. But I think whey is the all-star.

When and How to Use Whey Protein

What I try to do is consume around 100 grams of protein from quality whole-food sources, like chicken, fish, or beef, each day, and then I try to take in another 150 grams of protein from supplements, like Myoplex Plus or Designer Protein.

Of course, how much protein *you* need to supplement (and I'm convinced virtually every bodybuilder should be using a protein supplement) depends on how much quality protein you consume from regular food.

I find it extremely impractical to consume large quantities of protein from whole-food sources because I spend so much time away from my home. (I'm always at work or on the road.) To consume 300 grams of whole-food protein a day, I'd have to be eating meat every time I turned around, and day after day and week after week of high meat consumption makes me sick to my stomach. I don't have time to shop for and prepare that many whole-food meals. And, on a gram-per-gram basis, protein powders can be less expensive than meat anyway.

Here are a few tips on when to consume a quality protein supplement to help maximize your bodybuilding potential: first, and most importantly, have a protein-rich supplement (preferably with carbohydrates) right after a workout. This is when your body's protein synthetic machinery is getting ready to kick into high gear, and not having an abundant supply of all the important amino acids

TRIED AND TRUE: BODYBUILDING'S TOP TEN SUPPLEMENTS

CHAPTER 4

SUPPLEMENTS•TRIED AND TRUE: BODYBUILDING'S TOP TEN SUPPLEMENTS•TRIED AND TRUE: BODYBUILDING'S TOP TEN SUPPLEMENTS•TRIED AND TRUE: BODYBUILDING'S TOP TEN SUPPLEMENTS•TRIED AND TRUE: BODYBUILDING'S TOP TEN SUPPLEMENTS•TRIED AND TRUE:

during the post-workout recovery period could cripple your body's ability to recover and grow.

Next, try consuming a protein supplement first thing in the morning to put an immediate halt to the catabolic tailspin you go through during the latter half of your sleep cycle. Going to sleep means not eating, and not eating means your body "runs out" of protein and slows its production of insulin (remember, insulin helps escort amino acids into muscle tissue) halfway through the night, so you, in effect, stop synthesizing muscle protein needed for growth and repair. The sooner you consume a protein supplement in the morning, the better, especially if your goal is to gain muscle size and strength. One of the advantages of using a supplement for this first a.m. protein dose is that supplements are usually digested much quicker than whole-food proteins (the amino acids will get into your system much faster than if you were to eat ten egg whites, for example).

Another good time to have a protein supplement is late in the evening—I often have a protein drink an hour or so before I go to sleep—this helps ensure that I don't go any longer than necessary without consuming protein; in fact, sometimes when I wake up in the middle of the night (to use the bathroom or whatever), I'll mix up a serving of Designer Protein and drink it before I go back to sleep. Now, I probably wouldn't wake myself up on purpose to do this, but most nights, I wake up sometime during the early, early morning anyway, and slamming down a quick protein drink could help improve protein metabolism and prevent the protein breakdown that occurs naturally every night while we're sleeping. As a matter of fact, scientific evidence seems to indicate that maintaining high levels of branched-chain amino acids (like those found in whey protein) in the bloodstream can actually prevent a large percentage of this typical overnight protein breakdown. The cycle of feeding (during the daytime) and fasting (at night while we sleep) results in gains and loses of body protein. For most people, this is just fine—it's all part of homeostasis (the body's effort to *stay the same*)—but for bodybuilders, this natural building up and breaking down process is not "okay." We need to do whatever we can to try to shift this cycle in favor of the buildup of muscle tissue, and as I just described, consuming protein before you go to sleep, as soon as you wake up, and perhaps even in the middle of the night, could have a positive effect.

Other than that, while you're awake, you should make a diligent effort to consume some type of protein every few hours throughout the day. Not all of these "protein feedings" need to be supplements—as I already explained, I try to get a mixture of quality whole-food proteins and protein supplements.

As you can see, protein supplementation is simple. Just be sure to do it day in and day out. The more consistent your protein intake is, the more consistent your muscle growth will be.

HMB—Proving Itself in the Laboratory and the Real World

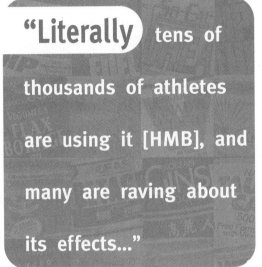

"**Literally** tens of thousands of athletes are using it [HMB], and many are raving about its effects..."

In the 1996 version of my *Supplement Review*, I introduced you to a supplement called beta-hydroxy beta-methylbutyrate (HMB), and at that time, I predicted it would be one of the most popular bodybuilding supplements on the market—right up there with creatine monohydrate. Well, HMB has been out on the market for about a year and a half now, and lo and behold—my prediction was dead right—along with creatine monohydrate, whey protein, and meal-replacement powders, HMB is one of the most popular supplements in bodybuilding today. Literally tens of thousands of athletes are using it, and many are raving about its effects, including drug-free bodybuilding champions like Bill Davey and Dan Gwartney, M.D. (both claim HMB helps them retain muscle mass while cutting up). Numerous professional athletes use it, too, including five-time Pro Bowl tight-end for the Denver Broncos, Shannon Sharpe—widely known as the NFL's most muscular man. (This guy is lifetime drug free and can bench press 470 lbs! And he's still fast enough to outrun some of the top defensive backs in the game!) Shannon Sharpe has been using HMB for about a year now and raves about its effects. (He stacks it with Phosphagen HP.) HMB was also one of the supplements used by numerous medal-winning Olympic athletes in the 1996 Olympic Games in Atlanta.

Since I first broke the HMB story, it has been featured in over 400 newspaper stories and on over 120 television news programs as an exciting, new discovery that could significantly enhance the muscle-building and fat-burning effects of exercise. It was even featured on the *CBS Evening News* in a story that was nationally televised to literally millions of viewers.

In a story last year on the television news program *Dateline*, it was stated, flat out, that creatine and HMB are two products in the sports nutrition market that are backed by science. What's so amazing about this is that the story, overall, was negative—it basically said the same thing about the bodybuilding supplement industry that I've been ranting about for the past seven years, which is that the majority of products sold as muscle builders or performance enhancers aren't backed by science!

Make no mistake, HMB is one of those exciting, new bodybuilding supplement discoveries that comes along only every once in a while. As was the case with creatine monohydrate, over the past year, a number of new and exciting scientific

REVIEW•SPORTS SUPPLEMENT REVIEW, 3RD ISSUE•SPORTS SUPPLEMENT REVIEW, 3RD ISSUE•SPORTS SUPPLEMENT REVIEW, 3RD ISSUE•SPORTS SUPPLEMENT

•SPORTS SUPPLEMENT REVIEW, 3RD ISSUE•SPORTS SUPPLEMENT REVIEW, 3RD ISSUE•SPORTS SUPPLEMENT REVIEW, 3RD ISSUE•SPORTS SUPPLEMENT REVIEW, 3RD ISSUE•SPORTS SUPPLEMENT REVIEW, 3RD ISSUE•SPORTS SUPPLEMENT REVIEW, 3RD ISSUE•SPORTS SUPPLEMENT REVIEW, 3RD ISSUE•SPORTS SUPPLEMENT

TRIED AND TRUE: BODYBUILDING'S TOP TEN SUPPLEMENTS

CHAPTER 4

SUPPLEMENTS•TRIED AND TRUE: BODYBUILDING'S TOP TEN SUPPLEMENTS•TRIED AND TRUE: BODYBUILDING'S TOP TEN SUPPLEMENTS•TRIED AND TRUE: BODYBUILDING'S TOP TEN SUPPLEMENTS•TRIED AND TRUE: BODYBUILDING'S TOP TEN SUPPLEMENTS•TRIED AND TRUE: BODYBUILDING'S TOP TEN SUPPLEMENTS•TRIED AND TRUE:

discoveries have been made regarding HMB—discoveries that reveal the powerful effects of this supplement and offer insight into how it should be used. We'll get to that in a minute, but for starters, let me give you a crash course on what exactly HMB is, how it was discovered, and how it might boost your bodybuilding progress.

What Is HMB?

HMB is an acronym for a compound called "beta-hydroxy beta-methylbutyrate." It's a metabolite of the essential amino acid leucine. In addition to what's made in our bodies, we derive HMB from food—it's present in small quantities in both plant and animal foods, including: grapefruit and catfish. HMB is not a steroid nor a drug; in fact, HMB is a natural component of mothers' milk. It's classified as a dietary supplement.

What Does HMB Do?

Most interesting to bodybuilders is that HMB appears to up-regulate our ability to build muscle and burn fat in response to intense exercise. In fact, in one study recently published in the prestigious *Journal of Applied Physiology*, it was revealed that athletes who supplemented their diets with three grams of HMB a day, for just three weeks, gained three times as much lean body mass and experienced an increase in strength two and a half times greater than test subjects who followed the same workout program but used a placebo.[205]

HMB has been extensively studied and has been found to have a very consistent, positive effect on protein metabolism. Animal studies have shown that HMB appears to be very safe and nontoxic. Human studies have documented only positive effects on health and human metabolism with HMB supplementation.

> "...HMB appears to up-regulate our ability to build muscle and burn fat in response to intense exercise."

What Do the Scientific Studies Show?

Several studies performed with animals have found that HMB may help decrease stress-induced muscle protein breakdown, and studies with humans have found that HMB may enhance increases in both muscle size and strength when combined with resistance training. Let's examine a couple of these studies "up close." The two which I think reveal a great deal about HMB's bodybuilding effects are those published in the prestigious *Journal of Applied Physiology* in November 1996.

In the first study, Dr. Nissen (a professor at Iowa State University and President of Metabolic Technologies, Inc.) got together a group of 41 guys who volunteered to participate in the study. They were between the ages of 19 and 29 and were randomly divided into 1 of 3 groups receiving varying amounts of HMB—0, 1.5, or 3 grams/day. Additionally, subjects ingested 1 of 2 different amounts of protein: either a "moderate" level of 117 grams/day or a higher level of 175 grams/day. The participants also lifted weights for an hour and a half, three days a week.

After just three weeks, the test subjects in this study who used HMB experienced some amazing things! Here are the results:

Subjects gained lean body mass in a dose-responsive manner: 0.88 lbs for the group receiving no HMB, 1.76 lbs for the group ingesting 1.5 grams of HMB, and 2.64 lbs in the group taking 3 grams of HMB per day! (The lifters using HMB gained a lot more lean mass!)

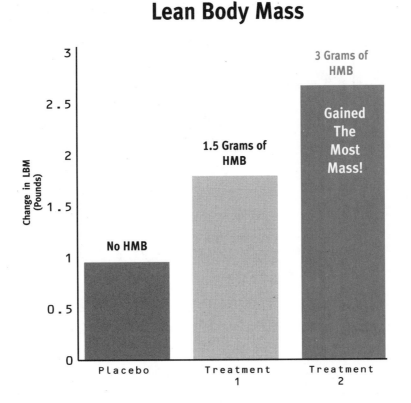

Enhanced Gains in Lean Body Mass

Source: S. Nissen, et al., "The Effect of the Leucine Metabolite β-Hydroxy β-Methylbutyrate on Muscle Metabolism During Resistance-Exercise Training," *J. Appl. Physiol.* 81 (1996) : 2095-2104.

TRIED AND TRUE: BODYBUILDING'S TOP TEN SUPPLEMENTS

SUPPLEMENTS~TRIED AND TRUE: BODYBUILDING'S TOP TEN SUPPLEMENTS~TRIED AND TRUE: BODYBUILDING'S TOP TEN SUPPLEMENTS~TRIED AND TRUE: BODYBUILDING'S TOP TEN SUPPLEMENTS~TRIED AND TRUE: BODYBUILDING'S TOP TEN SUPPLEMENTS~TRIED AND TRUE:

Researchers also found that HMB-supplemented subjects got stronger—total strength (combining increases for upper- and lower-body exercises) increased 8% in unsupplemented subjects, 13% in the 1.5-gram-HMB group, and 18.4% in the 3-gram-HMB group.

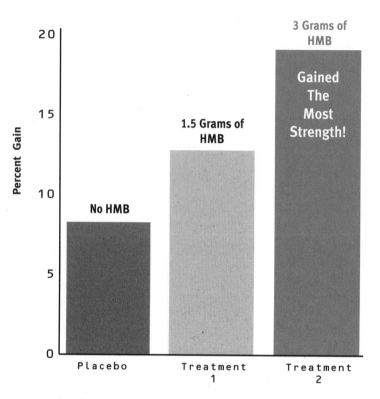

Enhanced Strength Gains

Source: S. Nissen, et al., "The Effect of the Leucine Metabolite β-Hydroxy β-Methylbutyrate on Muscle Metabolism During Resistance-Exercise Training," *J. Appl. Physiol.* 81 (1996) : 2095-2104.

In the second study, 32 guys (ages 19-22) were divided into 2 groups—1 received a placebo (no HMB); the other group got 3 grams of HMB per day. They all trained like madmen for seven weeks. The early measurements in the study indicated that the subjects who received HMB developed significantly more fat-free mass than those who lifted weights but didn't take HMB.

Bench-press strength increases were almost three times greater in the group receiving HMB, and strength increases for the squat, although not statistically significant, were also greater.

The results of these two studies are particularly impressive since the evidence of HMB's effectiveness was found in both biochemical tests (3-methylhistidine and creatine kinase—measurements designed to quantify muscle protein breakdown) and in more practical measurements (subjects gained fat-free mass and got stronger).

These benefits occurred with HMB independent of the level of protein intake in these subjects. However, it's important to note that the group consuming the least amount of protein was still ingesting about twice the RDA level suggested for maintaining nitrogen balance. So it could be that a protein intake considered normal by non-bodybuilding standards would limit the benefits of HMB. (I believe HMB works best when you use it in conjunction with a high-protein diet.)

Over the last year, five new scientific studies have been completed which confirm the bodybuilding benefits of this popular supplement. Here's a rundown: a study at Wichita State University, directed by researcher Matthew Vukovich, Ph.D., demonstrated that HMB might not only enhance the muscle-building and fat-burning effects of exercise, it may also *boost endurance*. In this study, experienced cyclists who supplemented their diets for two weeks with three grams of HMB a day (in divided doses), experienced a significant increase in VO_2max (a technical term for maximum aerobic performance). In concert with this was a reduction in blood lactate levels (a sign of muscle fatigue—lactic-acid buildup is that burning you get when you're training, which is one of the causes of muscular failure—if you can postpone this buildup of lactate, you could hypothetically do more reps, get in more muscle work, and enhance your endurance). In this study, the test subjects experienced a significant effect with HMB supplementation but did not respond to a placebo (an inert compound or a "fake" supplement, so to speak), nor from supplementation with three grams of leucine.[287] These findings will be presented at the American College of Sports Medicine conference in Denver, in May of 1997.

Another recent study demonstrated that women who train with weights and supplement their diets with HMB experience enhanced strength, an increase in lean body mass, and accelerated fat loss. This study, conducted by Dr. Nissen and his colleagues at Iowa State University, offers evidence that HMB produces similar results in both men and women, possibly indicating that the compound does not depend on any specific androgenic hormones, such as testosterone, to exert its effects. The results of this study were presented to the scientific community at the Experimental Biology meetings recently in New Orleans.[206]

In yet another recent university study, HMB was shown to enhance gains in lean body mass and strength in older individuals (between the ages of 65 and 80!)

"**Over** the last year, five new scientific studies have been completed which confirm the bodybuilding benefits of this popular supplement [HMB]."

69

TRIED AND TRUE: BODYBUILDING'S TOP TEN SUPPLEMENTS

CHAPTER 4

SUPPLEMENTS•TRIED AND TRUE: BODYBUILDING'S TOP TEN SUPPLEMENTS•TRIED AND TRUE: BODYBUILDING'S TOP TEN SUPPLEMENTS•TRIED AND TRUE: BODYBUILDING'S TOP TEN SUPPLEMENTS•TRIED AND TRUE: BODYBUILDING'S TOP TEN SUPPLEMENTS•TRIED AND TRUE:

when used in conjunction with an exercise program.[288] (Yep... old folks get results with HMB, too, which makes sense; people respond to anabolic steroid therapy at all ages.) The results of this interesting study were also recently presented to the scientific community at the Experimental Biology meetings.

Yet another scientific study, this time one that was conducted in order to try to determine the "mechanisms of action" (how HMB works) was carried out at State University of New York at Stony Brook, by Dr. Nada Abumrad and her colleague Dr. Cheng. Their *in-vitro* (in a test tube) studies showed HMB may very well increase the metabolism of fats. In this study, HMB was shown to increase fatty acid oxidation in muscle cells.[2] This confirms what many HMB users have discovered, which is that the compound may not only help build lean mass but may support fat loss. Exactly how this occurs will be the focus of continued research by Drs. Abumrad and Cheng and other researchers. The findings of this study were also recently presented to the scientific community at the Experimental Biology conference in New Orleans.

HMB even seems to improve performance in horses! Results from another scientific study, conducted by Drs. Miller, Sandberg, and Fuller at Iowa State University revealed that when horses were fed ten grams of HMB a day, they had improved oxidative metabolism and less muscle damage, which resulted in greater endurance and a more speedy recovery.[183] This first-of-a-kind study with HMB and exercising horses was also unveiled to scientists recently at the Experimental Biology meetings.

Make no mistake, study after study after study is showing that HMB works—that, *when combined with exercise*, it somehow helps up-regulate the body's endurance and seems to accelerate the rate at which you can gain muscle and burn fat.

HMB in the Real World...

We have seen that HMB works in the laboratory—it produces results that can be measured very reliably by scientists—but does it work in the real world? Well, the feedback I'm getting (and I get *a lot* of feedback from the readers of my magazine), is that HMB works. Does it produce "steroid-like" results—magically packing on pounds of muscle with little or no effort? No. Will it turn an average Joe into a superstar athlete overnight? Hardly. In fact, compared to bodybuilding's *ultimate* drug-free supplement, creatine monohydrate, HMB doesn't produce results nearly as dramatic. Those of you who have experienced

"...**weight** trainers who have plateaued... might gain an extra two to three pounds of muscle a month after incorporating HMB..."

the "power" of creatine know what I'm talking about—creatine works so well and so fast, it has spoiled a lot of bodybuilding supplement users. We're always looking for that next creatine—that next "instant gratification," fast-acting supplement. Unfortunately, HMB doesn't quite work that way. It, along with many other quality supplements, suffers from what I call "creatine envy."

There's no question in my mind that HMB works, but it's not the same type of supplement as creatine—HMB seems to shift the balance of protein metabolism in favor of new muscle growth, and it also appears to minimize the breakdown of muscle tissue (an anti-catabolic effect). In doing so, HMB can help support a consistent increase in muscle-tissue growth—according to scientific studies, it appears that HMB supplementation may double the muscle-building and fat-burning effects of exercise.

When I'm asked exactly what someone might expect from using HMB, my guess is that experienced weight trainers who have plateaued—who, in spite of their best efforts and hard workouts, aren't experiencing an increase in muscle size and strength—might gain an extra two to three pounds of muscle a month after incorporating HMB into their bodybuilding programs. Now, this might not seem like much—especially when some lifters gain as much as ten pounds during the first ten days they start loading up on creatine monohydrate, but even if you were to gain only a pound or two of new muscle tissue a month while supplementing with HMB, over a period of a year, that would be 12-24 lbs of rock-hard muscle, which, as anyone who's followed the iron game for some time knows, is an *enormous* increase in mass.

Also, keep in mind that the initial gains with creatine monohydrate are primarily due to a cell-volumizing phenomenon—an increase in fluid inside the muscle cell, which, aside from making you bigger and stronger, may also help improve protein metabolism. I don't have any evidence to suggest that HMB promotes cell volumizing—I believe the change in lean body mass with HMB consists entirely of contractile muscle tissue. Future studies, using sophisticated muscle biopsy procedures, could confirm this.

How Does HMB Work?

Dr. Nissen's research, which resulted in the discovery of HMB, actually came about after over a decade of examining the role a branched-chain amino acid called leucine plays in protein synthesis and anti-catabolism. Animal studies showed that leucine, and its metabolite KIC, were nitrogen sparing.[209] Although leucine and KIC were known to increase muscle-cell and immune-cell production, most studies were done in animals experiencing extreme stress, such as starvation or trauma. It wasn't until Dr. Nissen and his colleagues examined the downstream metabolic pathway from KIC that they discovered the powerful effects of HMB.

TRIED AND TRUE: BODYBUILDING'S TOP TEN SUPPLEMENTS

SUPPLEMENTS•TRIED AND TRUE: BODYBUILDING'S TOP TEN SUPPLEMENTS•TRIED AND TRUE: BODYBUILDING'S TOP TEN SUPPLEMENTS•TRIED AND TRUE: BODYBUILDING'S TOP TEN SUPPLEMENTS•TRIED AND TRUE: BODYBUILDING'S TOP TEN SUPPLEMENTS•TRIED AND TRUE: BODYBUILDING'S TOP TEN SUPPLEMENTS•TRIED AND TRUE:

The data suggest it takes a 60-gram dose of leucine or a 20-gram dose of KIC to produce the positive effects on muscle metabolism that are seen with a 3-gram dose of HMB. Unfortunately, consuming 60 grams of leucine or 20 grams of KIC is not only impractical and very expensive but can also cause very nasty stomach problems. Basically, it's impractical to get the positive muscle-building effects of HMB by consuming leucine and/or KIC.

Although no one is exactly sure how HMB works, Dr. Nissen's latest working hypothesis (his best guess) is that HMB may supply a precursor to muscle and to the immune system that supports maximal cellular repair. Thus, the muscle membrane is more rapidly repaired after exercise-induced damage, and muscle growth is supported by having an adequate supply of this substrate in the muscle for membrane expansion. The result is a more rapid return to positive protein synthesis.

Another hypothesis is that HMB supports a decrease in protein turnover or muscle damage. In turn, this decrease in muscle breakdown could result in more rapid neural recruitment by the muscle fibers and may act as a catalyst to faster strength increases. This could explain why in scientific studies, test subjects using HMB noticed a dramatic increase in strength after using the supplement for only a week or two.

(Fortunately, it's not vitally important to understand exactly how HMB works in order to benefit from using it!)

HMB Is Safe

HMB is a normal product of human metabolism—it's naturally present in mothers' milk and is found (albeit in small quantities) in the foods we eat. HMB also appears to be an essential part of the tissue growth process. In addition, it's a water-soluble compound (kind of like water-soluble vitamins) which is excreted in the urine in proportion to dietary intake. Thus, based on the chemistry of HMB, it would be predicted that HMB is a safe compound.

In fact, researchers have studied HMB extensively to evaluate its safety—according to Dr. Nissen, every human study that has been conducted regarding HMB included an extensive safety profile which screened for adverse reactions and organ function. They've even given psychological profiles and physical exams in each study. In none of these studies has there been any indication of a safety issue related to HMB. The only changes in blood chemistry related to a decrease in total and low-density lipoprotein (LDL) cholesterol levels.

There have also been extensive animal studies in which high levels of HMB have been administered, with no adverse effects—no toxicity at any level has been measured. I feel very safe about the use of HMB.

How Do You Use HMB?

Virtually all of the studies performed with exercising subjects used three grams of HMB in divided doses. This has been the case whether the test subject was a 165-lb, 74-year-old man; a 120-lb, 35-year-old woman; or a 215-lb, 21-year-old football player. So far, only one study to date has examined the effects of larger doses on young, weight-training men, and that study was just recently wrapped up by Dr. Richard Kreider at the University of Memphis. The very preliminary results of this study seem to indicate there is a *trend* for greater results in athletes using more than three grams of HMB a day.

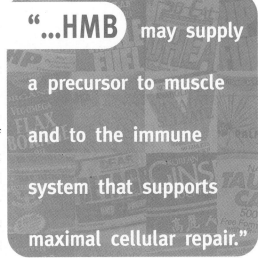

"...HMB may supply a precursor to muscle and to the immune system that supports maximal cellular repair."

Here's the way I look at it—if a 175-lb, weight-training male gets good results with HMB at a dosage of 3 grams a day, a 120-lb woman might experience significant results at 2 grams a day, and bodybuilders who weigh more than 175 lbs (like many of those who will read this book) might need a bit more of this supplement to produce maximum results.

In one study recently published in the *Journal of Applied Physiology*, Dr. Nissen and his colleagues evaluated the effects of 1.5 grams of HMB a day versus 3 grams. The test subjects who used only 1.5 grams of HMB a day made significant gains in lean body mass over subjects using no HMB, but those who used 3 grams/day experienced even greater results.

Dr. Nissen, unquestionably the world's leading expert on HMB, has speculated that three grams a day would provide the optimal effect for most individuals, but keep in mind, the majority of Dr. Nissen's work has been done using "regular" college athletes. (Those of us who follow this industry know bodybuilders often have more muscle mass than most college athletes.)

What I'm getting at is that I believe it's possible that in experienced, relatively muscular bodybuilders, the effects of HMB may not be optimal with a dosage of three grams a day—it may take four, five, or even six grams a day to achieve maximum results. This is consistent with some of the feedback I've received—athletes who have experimented with more seem to be getting better results.

Unfortunately, HMB is very expensive to manufacture (there are only two or three labs in the world that can even make it). Thus, consuming five or six grams a day could be cost prohibitive, but as you probably read about in Chapter 3, I'm "hot" on the concept of loading up on supplements, like creatine, glutamine, *and* HMB. I believe an ideal dosage pattern would be one gram, three times a day, with meals,

TRIED AND TRUE: BODYBUILDING'S TOP TEN SUPPLEMENTS

SUPPLEMENTS•TRIED AND TRUE: BODYBUILDING'S TOP TEN SUPPLEMENTS•TRIED AND TRUE: BODYBUILDING'S TOP TEN SUPPLEMENTS•TRIED AND TRUE: BODYBUILDING'S TOP TEN SUPPLEMENTS•TRIED AND TRUE: BODYBUILDING'S TOP TEN SUPPLEMENTS•TRIED AND TRUE: BODYBUILDING'S TOP TEN SUPPLEMENTS•TRIED AND TRUE: BODYBUILDING'S TOP TEN SUPPLEMENTS•TRIED AND TRUE:

CHAPTER 4

TRIED AND TRUE: BODYBUILDING'S TOP TEN SUPPLEMENTS•TRIED AND TRUE: BODYBUILDING'S TOP TEN SUPPLEMENTS•TRIED AND TRUE: BODYBUILDING'S TOP TEN

74

in addition to *two to three grams consumed with a high-glycemic carbohydrate source* (perhaps mixed with a serving of Phosphagen HP or a serving of Myoplex Plus Deluxe) *immediately following your weight-training workouts.* It is my belief that since HMB probably acts at the site of the muscle cell, insulin might help carry more HMB into the muscle cell and significantly enhance the results. (Here's another tip—try consuming a gram of HMB with a gram of Vitamin C one hour before exercise—you wouldn't believe the way this can minimize muscle soreness and improve recovery!)

After a week at this "loading dose," cutting back to three or four grams a day, in divided doses, may produce great results, and repeating this loading dose every six weeks or so may further enhance the benefits. But hey, it's just a theory—my best guess.

Another thing which I think might be a good idea is to cycle HMB—using it for four to six weeks, then taking a couple weeks off, as continued use may down-regulate some of HMB's effects. Of course, this is not the type of thing that has been substantiated with rock-hard science—it's merely another theory.

If you plan on cycling HMB, I would definitely use it for the first few weeks when changing training programs. When you alter the way you're training, or you come back after a layoff, your workouts inflict so much damage on muscle tissue that proper recovery is often difficult. I believe that when you intensify your training routine and use a powerful anti-catabolic supplement, you might be able to significantly enhance gains.

I also believe that during periods of intense dieting or "cutting," HMB may work wonders in terms of helping you maintain muscle mass while you strip off bodyfat. (By the way, an example of how I'm cycling HMB is illustrated in Chapter 16.)

What Kind of HMB Is Best?

As far as I'm concerned, the best HMB supplement on the market right now is EAS' BetaGen™ formula—each serving of this supplement contains one gram of HMB, along with two grams of creatine monohydrate, as well as an extra dose of the vitally important amino acids glutamine and taurine. Not only is BetaGen a great value, it's very convenient because it's a powdered orange drink mix. The problem I was having with HMB before, especially when I took my dosage up to six grams a day, is that I had to take 24 capsules a day. I can add BetaGen to a serving of Phosphagen HP or to a protein drink; I can mix it with yogurt, or I can just put it in a small cup of water or juice and drink it—it tastes great, and it's easy to use. Of course, the capsules work, too—that's what they've used in most of the HMB studies.

> **"As** far as I'm concerned, the best HMB supplement on the market right now is EAS' BetaGen™..."

Watch Out for Fake HMB

Okay—before I wrap it up, let me warn you about something you need to watch out for if you're shopping for HMB—there are a lot of fake versions of HMB on the market. You see, HMB is not easy to get—the patent rights are owned by the Iowa State University Research Foundation (ISURF), and they have been licensed to Metabolic Technologies, Inc. (MTI) under U.S. Patent 5,348,979. MTI has licensed several companies to sell HMB, including EAS. There are several other legitimate brands of HMB on the market. Watch for the patent number on the label—this is usually a sign that it's the real deal.

Over the past year, a number of fake HMB supplements have hit the market. Examples of these bogus versions of this popular supplement include "HMM!" by Power Star, "HMB/K+" by Dews Research, "HMB" by Proforma, and "HMB" by Nature's Resources. These knock offs were tested and shown to contain no HMB at all! This continues to be a problem as HMB gets more and more popular, and supplement companies continue to be deceptive, unscrupulous, and motivated by greed and a "make-a-buck-no-matter-how-you've-got-to-do-it" philosophy.

So there you have it—everything you could possibly need to know about HMB. As you can see, HMB sure looks like a winner; thus, I call it tried and true, even though it's relatively new. Few supplements, even ones that have been around for many years, are backed by as much solid science as HMB. No wonder it's creating so much excitement! Of course, as future studies reveal new insights as to how to use HMB to get better results faster from your exercise, I'll be sure to pass it along in my magazine, *Muscle Media*.

CAFFEINE/EPHEDRINE/ASPIRIN (OR THEIR HERBAL EQUIVALENTS)—THE FAT-BURNING STACK

As bodybuilders, one thing we all have in common is that we want *more muscle:* in essence, that's what it's all about—building your body—building a bigger, stronger physique. Thus, a true "bodybuilding supplement" is one that helps you get bigger and stronger—something like creatine or HMB. But, something else that is also unique to the bodybuilder—something that separates us from other athletes is the desire—no, make that the compulsive, *insatiable drive*—to have low bodyfat levels. After all, what's the sense of having more muscle if it's all covered up by fat—if you can't see the beautiful, heroic proportion, shape, and definition of the abdominal muscles, the intercostals; the separation in the quadriceps; the striations in your pecs? *That's* what it's all about... building a *lean*, muscular body, not just "bulking up." Thus, at one time or another, we look for supplements that help boost fat loss. And, make no mistake, there are many marketers of supplements and drugs that would like us to believe they've got the answer—that they have discovered a "miracle" for quick and easy fat loss.

TRIED AND TRUE: BODYBUILDING'S TOP TEN SUPPLEMENTS

SUPPLEMENTS·TRIED AND TRUE: BODYBUILDING'S TOP TEN SUPPLEMENTS·TRIED AND TRUE: BODYBUILDING'S TOP TEN SUPPLEMENTS·TRIED AND TRUE: BODYBUILDING'S TOP TEN SUPPLEMENTS·TRIED AND TRUE: BODYBUILDING'S TOP TEN SUPPLEMENTS·TRIED AND TRUE:

I don't think I'm going to be bursting your bubble when I tell you there is no "magic pill" which makes fat loss "simple and easy." The truth is, unless you are one of those very few genetically gifted, super-lean individuals (and I hate each and every one of you!), getting cut—taking your bodyfat down to 5%, 6%, or even 7% *is a bitch!* However, losing fat is absolutely, positively "doable." I haven't met a person on the planet who couldn't lose fat—who wasn't able to get "cut-up" once he/she had the important components of his/her program in order. Getting lean takes a ton of discipline, but it is so rewarding. It's so exciting to see those muscles in the mirror that we've worked so hard to develop—the vascularity, the striations, the definition.

Start with Diet and Exercise

Of course, any successful fat-loss program has to be centered around decreasing calorie intake and/or increasing calorie expenditure. How do we do this? Well, it's really not that complicated. To increase calorie expenditure, you need to exercise more, and to decrease energy intake, you simply need to eat less. To burn fat, you've got to create what's called an "energy deficit," which means the fuel your body needs is pulled from existing storage compartments—principally bodyfat.

(Okay... so this is very basic stuff—I just wanted to make sure we were all on the same page before we dove into a discussion about fat-burning compounds.)

The Fat Burners

I'm aware that it's very "in vogue" to use weight-loss drugs, like Redux (dexfenfluramine) and fen/phen (a combination of the drugs phentermine and fenfluramine). In fact, literally tens of thousands of prescriptions are written for these compounds every week. I tried Redux and fen/phen just to see what it felt like, and I can't say I was all that thrilled with either of them. They both gave me a brutal headache when they started to wear off (late in the afternoon/early evening), and they do some weird stuff—it's like your mouth isn't hungry, but your stomach roars. I've never had worse hunger pains in my life than when I was taking these compounds. They make my brain feel like a sponge, too—I can't think clearly when I'm on them. Plus, from what I understand (from what I've read in the scientific journals), these drugs are not without serious side effects; in fact, there have been numerous deaths from a disease called "pulmonary hypertension" blamed on these compounds. (Man... that would suck!)

Anyway, where was I... Oh, I was getting ready to explain which supplements help with fat loss. There are several compounds I think may help accelerate fat loss when they're used as part of an effective bodybuilding program, including: HMB, CLA, and even pyruvate (in a dosage of 15-25 grams/day, *I suspect*), but the "granddaddy" of all fat burners is a combination of the over-the-counter drugs caffeine, ephedrine, and aspirin, or their herbal equivalents: guarana, ephedra, and willow bark.

This "stack" has been shown effective in numerous scientific studies.[13, 14, 38, 275] In fact, some studies offer evidence this stack is up to 29% more effective than Redux (the #1 selling weight-loss pharmaceutical in America). This stack is cheap, effective, and relatively safe.

Caution: This Is Powerful Stuff

Before I go any further, I need to warn you that a person with any type of heart disease, high blood pressure, thyroid disease, diabetes, enlarged prostate, or anyone taking MAO-inhibitor drugs for depression or appetite suppression should stay away from any ephedrine or ephedra-containing compounds. And I want to warn that you should never exceed the recommended dose of these products. I would also suggest that those of you who may have problems with peptic ulcers avoid this stack, as the aspirin and caffeine both can aggravate that condition. The reason some people experience serious side effects from using these compounds is, near as I can tell, because they overdose on them—they take much more than the recommended dose and then wonder why they end up in trouble. These compounds are strong and should be used with caution!

How Does the Stack Work?

The most powerful component in this stack is ephedrine/ephedra. It's a "beta-adrenergic agonist." It's long been regarded as a fairly potent thermogenic compound, but it was found to be even more effective when combined with caffeine and aspirin. It's true that caffeine is also a fairly good thermogenic compound, but it hardly measures up to ephedrine. When the two are combined haphazardly (in random amounts), their thermogenic qualities are additive: one plus one equals two. However, when the 2 are combined in fairly specific ratios—200 mg caffeine to 20 mg ephedrine (taken 3 times daily)—the results are synergistic.[122] In other words, the effects of each are greater than the sum of their individual effects. When aspirin—300 mg of it per each ephedrine/caffeine dose—is thrown into the equation, the results are further enhanced.[68]

Aside from burning fat, this stack has also been shown to have "nutrient-partitioning" effects: animals fed the mixture obtained the same growth on a 20% lower energy intake but gained 10% more muscle and 30% less fat than animals that were not fed caffeine and ephedrine.[13, 216]

Aside from turning calories into heat instead of storing them as fat, the combination may actually cripple the body's ability to form fat. Caffeine, by itself,

TRIED AND TRUE: BODYBUILDING'S TOP TEN SUPPLEMENTS

SUPPLEMENTS•TRIED AND TRUE: BODYBUILDING'S TOP TEN SUPPLEMENTS•TRIED AND TRUE: BODYBUILDING'S TOP TEN SUPPLEMENTS•TRIED AND TRUE: BODYBUILDING'S TOP TEN SUPPLEMENTS•TRIED AND TRUE: BODYBUILDING'S TOP TEN SUPPLEMENTS•TRIED AND TRUE: BODYBUILDING'S TOP TEN SUPPLEMENTS•TRIED AND TRUE:

CHAPTER 4

increases blood adrenaline levels, thereby increasing lipolysis (the breakdown of fat). The use of caffeine and/or ephedrine may also increase strength and "focus" during workouts—a lot of bodybuilders take these compounds for this reason.

Some studies have suggested that one of the most potent aspects of the caffeine/ephedrine/aspirin stack is simply appetite suppression; in fact, up to 75% of the "fat-burning" effects of this powerful stack may have to do with appetite suppression, which is something supplements with the potential to burn fat, such as HMB, CLA, and pyruvate, *may not* help with. In fact, I think that's probably why this stack is so popular—it helps you stick to your diet and gives you a perceived "energy boost."

This stack can help you get cut *if* you use it along with a proper *and disciplined* exercise and nutrition program, but I would definitely not use it all the time; in fact, when I'm cutting up, I try not to take it more than every other day, and I try not to use it for any more than a few weeks—I save it for when I really need it. I recommend you take the same approach if you want to experiment with these compounds. Studies indicate an effective dose is 200 mg of caffeine, 20 mg of ephedrine, and 300 mg of aspirin, 3 times a day. If aspirin irritates your stomach, use the herbal equivalent, willow bark, or leave it out of the stack altogether. Just ephedrine and caffeine is a potent stack, too.

Remember, if you have any medical conditions, especially heart trouble, do <u>not</u> use caffeine and/or ephedrine without consulting your doctor first!! Also, do not exceed the recommended dosage of any drugs or herbal products that contain caffeine or ephedrine!

"The use of caffeine and/or ephedrine may also increase strength and 'focus' during workouts..."

POST-WORKOUT CARB/PROTEIN SUPPLEMENTS WORK WONDERS!

Here's a total no brainer—a surefire way to improve recovery, boost energy levels, and probably even accelerate muscle growth: all you've got to do to score big here is slam down a high-carb, protein-rich supplement right after you train. Simple, huh?

Make no mistake, there are a lot of things that are complicated, vehemently debated, pondered, and hypothesized about bodybuilding supplementation, but this is one thing virtually all experts agree on—it's even backed by solid university studies. There's really no question about it—if you're training hard, trying to pack on new muscle mass, you need to feed your body protein and carbs within an hour after your workout!

Scientific data show that right after you get done training, your body needs nutrients, and it's *ready* for them, too. It stands to reason the most important time to feed the body is right after you've expended a significant amount of fuel—when you work out, your body burns up amino acids, glycogen, glucose, and enhances the breakdown of a whole cornucopia of substrates. And that super-anabolic hormone insulin that I've already mentioned several times in this book, is ready to go to work as soon as you get done training—and your muscles are very "receptive" to insulin activity at this time as well—it's a match made in heaven (perhaps literally).

A great post-workout supplement should contain around 50-100 grams of carbohydrates (a mixture of high- and low-glycemic index carbs) and an ample dose of protein—30-50 grams. Simply combining a few scoops of protein powder with a big glass of juice would fulfill this requirement, and believe me, if you consume this after every workout, you will definitely notice a difference! You'll have more rapid recovery; your muscles will be fuller, tighter, and firmer; and I'd bet good money that you'll have less muscle soreness and be stronger the next time you train.

So, this "top ten" supplement can be almost any ole thing—milk protein and a glass of Tang or a Carnation Instant Breakfast drink mixed with milk and egg whites; a lot of supplements fit the bill here, but if you want to take *full* advantage of this post-workout "window of opportunity," you might want to consider taking your post-workout supplement to a more "high-tech" level. For example, I think adding five grams of creatine monohydrate to this protein and carb drink would be a *grand* idea and would produce even better results in all of the areas I mentioned (recovery, muscle fullness, enhanced strength in your next workout, etc.). And, if you want to step it up yet another notch, throw in some important amino acids like glutamine and taurine, some sodium phosphate, chromium, along with a slew of vitamins, minerals, and antioxidants—heck... I can think of at least two dozen nutrients that could be an important part of this post-workout drink.

Here's what a lot of bodybuilders do: take one of the popular meal-replacement products on the market, such as Myoplex Plus, and mix it with a serving (or two!) of Phosphagen HP. (Vanilla Myoplex Plus and a serving of fruit-punch Phosphagen HP in 16 oz of cold water is great!) This supplement stack delivers 42 grams of quality protein, 60 grams of carbohydrates, as well as gram quantities of glutamine, taurine, AKG, and over 2 dozen vitamins, minerals, and antioxidants. It's a fantastic way to feed your body after a workout!

So what do the studies say about post-workout supplementation? Well, scientific research, going back over a decade, shows consuming a carbohydrate-rich drink, within 60 minutes following exercise, substantially increases the rate of muscle glycogen synthesis and replacement.[130, 232] Obviously, by more quickly and fully replacing glycogen stores, you could help your body recuperate faster from your last bout of exercise and refuel for the next bout.

TRIED AND TRUE: BODYBUILDING'S TOP TEN SUPPLEMENTS

SUPPLEMENTS-TRIED AND TRUE: BODYBUILDING'S TOP TEN SUPPLEMENTS-TRIED AND TRUE: BODYBUILDING'S TOP TEN SUPPLEMENTS-TRIED AND TRUE: BODYBUILDING'S TOP TEN SUPPLEMENTS-TRIED AND TRUE: BODYBUILDING'S TOP TEN SUPPLEMENTS-TRIED AND TRUE: BODYBUILDING'S TOP TEN SUPPLEMENTS-TRIED AND TRUE:

More recently, scientists have carefully examined the effects of a post-workout carbohydrate/protein supplement. What they discovered is that carbohydrates mixed with protein may cause a greater insulin release than carbohydrates alone.[304] More insulin released, along with these nutrients, means more key substrates, like glycogen, amino acids, creatine, etc., get escorted into muscle cells, *which is a damn good thing!* In a study at the University of Texas, researchers specifically looked at combining carbohydrates with protein (specifically a mixture of dextrose, maltodextrin, and milk- and whey-protein isolates). What they discovered is this simple supplement blend increased the rate of glycogen synthesis following exercise by 40%, versus carbohydrates alone. Not only that, the total muscle glycogen saturation, four hours after exercise, increased as well. Basically, this study offers strong evidence that carbs *plus* protein is the way to go!

Other studies offer evidence that consuming a post-workout carbohydrate- and protein-containing supplement can help reduce post-workout cortisol levels,[50] producing a potent, anti-catabolic effect.

Here's another bit of information that supports the use of a carbohydrate- and protein-containing post-workout drink: studies have documented that amino acids and dipeptides (found in whey protein) help increase the absorption of water from the intestines.[65, 108] This increase in water absorption is significant; therefore, putting protein in your post-workout supplement may not only help replace glycogen stores, it may also help rehydrate and volumize your muscles!

There's just no getting around it—within an hour after you work out, you'd better slam a high-carbohydrate, protein-rich supplement. You can make it simple, or you can go the high-tech route.

What about consuming a high-protein and carbohydrate whole-food meal as an alternative to a supplement? Well, I don't think that's such a good idea. Let's say you were to eat a couple chicken breasts, some rice, and vegetables (a balanced "bodybuilder meal") after you work out—what type of effect would that have? Because whole foods are digested much more slowly and even whole-food sources of protein, like chicken, contain some fat, digestion would be slower, the insulin response would be lower, and the "punch" of this post-workout carb/protein consumption would not be the same. Even a relatively small amount of fat and/or fiber can decrease the rate of gastric emptying, slowing the absorption of food into the system and compromising glycogen synthesis rates. Not only that, but whole foods, like those I just mentioned, require quite a bit of water for digestion. Rather than rehydrating the system, such as with a protein and carbohydrate supplement, a whole-food meal may draw water out of the system. A supplement is much more quickly assimilated than whole foods.

As I mentioned, there are a variety of strategies you might try—one is consuming a creatine and carbohydrate drink right after a workout and then, within the hour, consuming a meal-replacement powder or another multinutrient supplement, like Phosphagain 2 mixed with fruit juice, which is rich in vitamins, minerals, creatine, protein, and carbs.

Some experts, including Torbjorn Akerfeldt, who pioneered the Anabolic Burst Cycling System, recommend consuming as much as 30% of your calories within 2 hours after your workout, as they believe this is when your body's protein machinery—your body's anabolic drive—can be substantially enhanced by feeding it carbohydrates, protein, and other important nutrients.

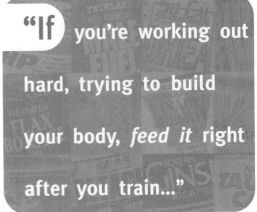
"If you're working out hard, trying to build your body, *feed it* right after you train..."

If you're working out hard, trying to build your body, *feed it* right after you train—I virtually guarantee you'll notice a difference!

GLUTAMINE—THE MOST IMPORTANT AMINO ACID FOR BODYBUILDERS

For decades, scientists have been fascinated with the many important functions and numerous possible applications of amino acid supplements. Since the early '80's, bodybuilders have also been "toying" with these building blocks of protein in an effort to gain more muscle. Many amino acid supplement fads have come and gone over the years, but the supplementation of the amino acid glutamine, in recent years, has become extremely popular, and rightfully so. Glutamine is, in essence, the mother of all aminos.

Technically speaking, glutamine is generally not considered an "essential amino acid" by nutritionists. It can be synthesized from a number of amino acids, notably glutamic acid, valine, and isoleucine. But in times of disease and stress (weight training is stress), certain parts of the body demand so much glutamine that the body can't manufacture enough. In these instances, glutamine supplementation could make a world of difference. In fact, in European hospitals, this amino acid is treated like a drug—it's routinely administered to patients suffering from stress or trauma (surgery, burns, disease, etc.). Studies have shown this type of glutamine supplementation can prevent muscle wasting—it produces a potent anti-catabolic effect.[156, 237]

Make no mistake, our bodies use a lot of glutamine every single day! For example, glutamine is required in mega-quantities to maintain the proper function of your immune system, kidneys, pancreas, gallbladder, and liver (basically, the whole gut). Glutamine is also an essential "nitrogen transporter"—it allows ammonia to be removed from some areas of the body (your brain and lungs in particular) and deposited into others (your intestines and kidneys). And, large amounts of glutamine are also used as the building blocks for what is most likely your body's

TRIED AND TRUE: BODYBUILDING'S TOP TEN SUPPLEMENTS

SUPPLEMENTS•TRIED AND TRUE: BODYBUILDING'S TOP TEN SUPPLEMENTS•TRIED AND TRUE: BODYBUILDING'S TOP TEN SUPPLEMENTS•TRIED AND TRUE: BODYBUILDING'S TOP TEN SUPPLEMENTS•TRIED AND TRUE: BODYBUILDING'S TOP TEN SUPPLEMENTS•TRIED AND TRUE: BODYBUILDING'S TOP TEN SUPPLEMENTS•TRIED AND TRUE:

CHAPTER 4

most powerful antioxidant, glutathione (which is made from glutamine, cysteine, and glycine). Glutamine also seems to be important for proper muscle glycogen deposition; although to be honest, I'm not sure why. I don't believe it's because glutamine increases insulin release, and I don't think it's being converted to a glucose-binding amino acid metabolite, like alanine.

As an added benefit, glutamine is also one of the few amino acids that causes extra growth hormone release; in fact, just a two-gram oral dose of glutamine was shown to cause a fourfold increase in growth hormone levels.[294] Whether or not that increase in growth hormone has any positive effects on body composition has yet to be determined, but it certainly couldn't hurt. I could go on and on, but suffice it to say, this amino acid is in high demand in your body—you need a bunch of it for a whole lot of things, *including* proper muscle metabolism.

Where Does All This Glutamine Come From?

Your body typically keeps a pretty hefty reserve of it in muscle tissue—muscle is actually a reservoir of stored glutamine; in fact, 60% of the free-floating amino acids in every one of your skeletal muscle cells is made up of glutamine.

When the gut, immune system, and other "glutamine hogs" can't get enough of this vital amino acid through the diet, nor by manufacturing it, they rob muscle tissue of glutamine, and when this happens, you basically go into "catabolism" or muscle breakdown. One reason this happens is because glutamine helps maintain proper cellular hydration or cell volume. When muscle glutamine levels fall, the cell volume decreases, which is catabolic.[162]

> "...glutamine is also one of the few amino acids that causes extra growth hormone release..."

Obviously, we want to do whatever we can to keep that from happening, so glutamine supplementation certainly seems important. But, simply slamming down mega-doses of glutamine, in hopes that it will find its way into skeletal muscle, may not be the best idea. Studies show that between 50% and 85% of a large dose of glutamine, ingested orally, does not reach the bloodstream—a lot of it is gobbled up before it can get to your muscles.

So what's the best way to supplement glutamine (which I think virtually all serious bodybuilders should be doing)? Well, my theory, which is shared by a number of experts, is that feeding the body two to three grams throughout the day (not huge mega-doses) is a sound approach. Many of you are already doing this unintentionally. Did you know that most of the popular meal replacements on the market, including Myoplex Plus, and multinutrient products, like Phosphagain 2, contain over two grams of glutamine per serving? A lot of quality protein supplements, like

Designer Protein, are also fortified with glutamine; thus, every time you take one of these supplements, you also get an extra dose of glutamine. This is good.

The Principle of Glutamine Preservation

Research scientist Anthony Almada believes that at certain times (such as right after an intense workout or right before you go to bed), you can help satisfy the gut and immune system's "hunger" for large amounts of glutamine through precision supplementation, thus, preserving glutamine levels in muscle. If you provide the gut and the immune system with the glutamine they need, these systems won't have to "call out" the glutamine reserves—your body won't have to dip into glutamine that's stored in muscle and supporting cell volume and proper protein metabolism. (Follow me? When you think about it, it really does make sense, and I think it's a very good approach.)

This is the theory behind a product Anthony Almada developed in 1993 called GKG® the Glutamine Preservation System® Actually, GKG was the first supplement promoted as a "cell volumizer" (a term that is widely used in sports nutrition today). The focus of glutamine preservation is just what it sounds like—preserving important levels of glutamine in muscle tissue. Almada's unique glutamine preservation formula not only included gram quantities of glutamine but also glutamine precursors (compounds that support the formation of glutamine in the body), such as alpha-ketoglutarate (AKG) and important glutamine synthesis cofactors. These include the mineral manganese and yeast RNA, which also help support the immune system, which is sometimes weakened by high-intensity training.

More recently, Almada developed the supplement CytoVol™ which expands the scope of GKG's glutamine-preservation/cell-volumizing formula, with the addition of other cell-hydrating compounds such as the amino acids alanine (which is also in high demand by working muscles), glycine, and inositol. Recent studies have shown that glycine, in combination with glutamine, induces cell-volumizing effects which are greater than those caused by glutamine alone.[286] During fasting (while you're sleeping) and after meals, glutamine appears to be released from muscle to maintain blood sugar concentrations. Alanine may help preserve muscle glutamine concentrations by being converted to blood glucose (it actually "lends" carbon atoms to make glucose) during periods of calorie restriction, such as dieting or prolonged times between meals.

How Much Glutamine?

Although scientific studies have not determined the exact amount of glutamine needed to support optimal muscle metabolism, there is no question, amongst the various bodybuilding and scientific experts, that glutamine supplementation is important. Precisely how much glutamine is required for a bodybuilder (not critically ill hospital patients, who have been the focus of most glutamine research) to support

TRIED AND TRUE: BODYBUILDING'S TOP TEN SUPPLEMENTS

SUPPLEMENTS•TRIED AND TRUE: BODYBUILDING'S TOP TEN SUPPLEMENTS•TRIED AND TRUE: BODYBUILDING'S TOP TEN SUPPLEMENTS•TRIED AND TRUE: BODYBUILDING'S TOP TEN SUPPLEMENTS•TRIED AND TRUE: BODYBUILDING'S TOP TEN SUPPLEMENTS•TRIED AND TRUE: BODYBUILDING'S TOP TEN SUPPLEMENTS•TRIED AND TRUE:

optimal muscle metabolism, enhance cell volume, and support the immune system has yet to be determined. However, my guess is that in addition to a diet rich in high-quality protein, bodybuilders could benefit from consuming at least an additional ten grams of glutamine a day. As I already mentioned, some of this can be obtained through meal-replacement products and protein powders. You can also go to the health-food store and buy a pure glutamine supplement and add an extra two or three grams to each of your protein drinks or just mix it with water and consume it with a regular-food meal. This may very well help out. I use CytoVol— I take a serving right after I work out and another right before I go to bed.

Here's one more tip—Duchaine, Almada, and I all believe there's a possibility that loading up on supplements like glutamine, in combination with a potent insulin-releasing carbohydrate for five to seven days, might help increase muscle-cell volume (by super-saturating glutamine stores in muscle cells). Thus, if you're just starting out on a glutamine supplement like CytoVol, I recommend you take four servings a day, in divided doses throughout the day. (Be sure to take one dose immediately after training and one right before going to bed.)

If you're not already using a glutamine supplement, consider giving it a try— the expert opinion, real-world evidence, and scientific data which support glutamine supplementation are quite compelling.

ANTIOXIDANTS—THEY REALLY ARE BODYBUILDING SUPPLEMENTS

Over the last 16 years, I've had the opportunity to closely observe the unique behavior of a species known as *the bodybuilder*. Although you might suspect that this particular breed would behave in a manner similar to other Homo sapiens, it has been my observation that the bodybuilder displays character traits that differ significantly from the "average Joe."

Here's an example: antioxidant supplements have become extremely popular amongst mainstream health and fitness enthusiasts. Literally millions and millions of Americans use antioxidant supplements every day. However, the bodybuilder, in general, has determined that since antioxidant supplements are good for "non-bodybuilders," they can't possibly be good for weight trainers, and they generally regard supplements with purported antioxidant properties right up there with *Aloe vera* and seaweed, in terms of muscle-enhancing potential.

But, nothing could be further from the truth—powerful antioxidants *really* are bodybuilding supplements. Here's why: intense weight-training exercise damages muscle tissue, which, in turn, sets in motion a sequence of metabolic events that often result in an increase in muscle size and strength. Now, think about it—do you really believe it's possible to specifically target only muscle fibers when we exercise, or do you think it's likely that an intense workout damages not just muscle tissue but, in reality, many other systems in your body? (Go ahead... think about it... I'll wait. Well, what do you think?)

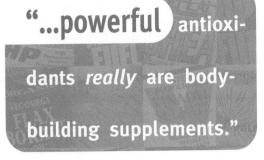

"...powerful antioxidants *really* are body-building supplements."

The truth is, a brutal workout takes its toll, not just on your muscles but on *your entire body!* Fortunately, the use of potent antioxidants can help mitigate this problem—they can help minimize the amount of free radicals that damage cells in your body following exercise, and I'm convinced the proper use of antioxidants can improve your recovery time, reduce muscle soreness, postpone fatigue, strengthen the immune system, and over the *long term*, can help you get better results faster from the time you spend exercising.

What Are Antioxidants?

Antioxidants are a class of chemical compounds (many are vitamins) that attack substances in your body known as "free radicals" and pro-oxidants. These aggressive molecules circulate in your body—they basically go around screwing up the function of cells and other molecules that move in the blood. Technically, free radicals are molecules that lack the appropriate electrons necessary to be stable—they indiscriminately kill cells, destroy enzymes, and produce toxic chemicals which disrupt cellular membranes. It is suspected that free radicals are involved in numerous diseases, including cancer, and they are associated with the aging process and even death itself. Other diseases that might be caused by free radicals include Alzheimer's disease, immune deficiency, arthritis, diabetes, and heart disease, to name only a few.

Here's a vivid example of free radicals at work: I'm sure you've taken a peach or an apple and cut it up and left it out in the open—before too long, it becomes discolored. Well, guess what's happening there? It's "oxidizing"—that means free radicals from the oxygen it's exposed to are disrupting the natural, healthy structure of the peach or apple. Now, visualize that happening to the cells in your body. It's not a pretty picture, is it?

Anyway, scientific research has demonstrated that strenuous exercise increases the number of free radicals roaming around in your body.[253] Thus, many experts are calling for increased antioxidant supplementation by bodybuilders, and I agree with that wholeheartedly—now more so than ever before, since over the past year, I have had a chance to examine this issue in great detail.

As you might suspect, the body has a natural antioxidant system of its own, and the more you exercise, the more your body increases the production of these natural antioxidants, but I'm convinced (as are numerous scientists and doctors) that you can improve your body's ability to squelch free radicals by consuming antioxidant supplements.

TRIED AND TRUE: BODYBUILDING'S TOP TEN SUPPLEMENTS

CHAPTER 4

SUPPLEMENTS•TRIED AND TRUE: BODYBUILDING'S TOP TEN SUPPLEMENTS•TRIED AND TRUE: BODYBUILDING'S TOP TEN SUPPLEMENTS•TRIED AND TRUE: BODYBUILDING'S TOP TEN SUPPLEMENTS•TRIED AND TRUE: BODYBUILDING'S TOP TEN SUPPLEMENTS•TRIED AND TRUE: BODYBUILDING'S TOP TEN SUPPLEMENTS•TRIED AND TRUE: BODYBUILDING'S TOP TEN SUPPLEMENTS•TRIED AND TRUE:

The Best Antioxidants

Some of the most effective antioxidants, which I think all bodybuilders should be using each and every day as a part of their supplement program, are Vitamins C, E, carotenes (like beta-carotene and lycopene—tomatoes are full of this red stuff), N-acetyl-cysteine (NAC), selenium, and perhaps lipoic acid. Other compounds, like conjugated linoleic acid (CLA) may also have potent antioxidant activity, as do proanthocyanidins (found in high concentrations in pine bark and grape seed extracts), curcumin and other curcuminoids (found in the spice turmeric), the amino acids methionine and cysteine, and green tea catechins.

Most antioxidants function primarily the same way. They have the ability to "share" electrons with free-radical molecules in the body. By lending one of their electrons to the free radical, they stabilize and "disarm" it. Even though each antioxidant pretty much functions in the same manner, typically what makes them unique is where the antioxidant is found in the body and how it supports antioxidant functions.

Vitamin C, for instance, is found mainly in the aqueous (water) environments in the body due to its water-soluble nature. Vitamin C not only acts as a direct antioxidant, but it's also responsible for regenerating the oxidized form of Vitamin E in the body. Thus, it helps to support Vitamin E's antioxidant activity.

Vitamin E, on the other hand, being a fat-soluble vitamin, along with the carotenes, works its "magic" mainly in the lipid environments of the body, including: bodyfat stores, cell membranes, and specific areas of organs and hormonal glands.

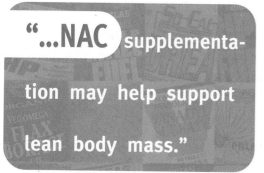

"...NAC supplementation may help support lean body mass."

Now, lipoic acid is somewhat unique, in that it is both water *and* fat soluble. For this reason, lipoic acid can act virtually anywhere in the body. Therefore, it is becoming well known as the "universal antioxidant." Besides having powerful antioxidant properties itself, lipoic acid can help regenerate Vitamin C *and* Vitamin E from their oxidized forms.

The mineral selenium plays a crucial role in helping to maintain adequate activity of the antioxidant enzyme glutathione peroxidase (the most powerful endogenously produced antioxidant) in the bloodstream. The amino acids glycine and cysteine, with help from glutamine (another role for glutamine!), work together to produce and maintain glutathione—the most abundant water-soluble antioxidant inside of cells. All of these nutrients are vital to the activity and efficiency of this natural antioxidant system. Studies have shown that age-related decreases of glutathione can actually be halted by diets rich in methionine (a precursor to cysteine) and cysteine.[58] Studies in animals and humans have shown that intense exercise can deplete glutathione in the blood and tissues, which may "allow" free-radical attacks to rev up after training and may prolong recuperation. Consistently low levels of selenium in the bloodstream have also been connected to forms of cancer.

The naturally occurring plant extract antioxidants (proanthocyanidins from grape seed and pine bark extract, curcumin, and green tea catechins) are similar in action. My guess is that these compounds are used by the plant sources from which they originate as their own natural antioxidant protection. Plants produce free radicals, as do humans, and if they weren't controlled, the plants would whither and die sooner, rather than later. Proanthocyanidins appear to have the unique ability to increase intracellular Vitamin C levels, as well as scavenge free radicals and delay the destruction of connective tissues.[169, 245]

Last, but definitely not least (as a matter of fact, probably on the *top* of the list in terms of effectiveness), is NAC, which has been shown to help increase glutathione levels by up to 500%.[133] Research shows NAC supplementation (200 mg, 4 times a day, with 800 mg on the morning of the test) virtually eliminates the exercise-related changes in glutathione status by preventing the increase of oxidized glutathione in the blood.[49]

Yet another very recent study has also suggested NAC supplementation may help support lean body mass.[140] In this recent study, published in the *Journal of Molecular Medicine*, researchers looked at the effects of repeated bouts of anaerobic exercise on both the ratio of lean body mass to bodyfat and immune function. Interestingly, it was discovered that repeated bouts of intense anaerobic exercise were actually associated with a decrease in lean body mass; it also, as expected, caused a suppression of immune-cell function. But, when researchers supplemented some of the exercising test subjects with NAC, they revealed the decreases in lean body mass and immune-altering effects of these tough workouts were almost completely prevented. Scientists involved in this study speculated that the positive results were not just because of NAC's ability to scavenge free radicals but also its ability to support higher levels of glutamine in the bloodstream, which aids in repairing damaged tissue. Because the method they used to measure body mass reflects the quantity of contents found in all body cells, this study also suggests that cysteine (as NAC) may indirectly exert a cell-volumizing effect. Other studies showing NAC to be capable of reducing inflammatory/catabolic molecules lend support to NAC's potential to preserve body mass. In this study, relatively low levels of NAC supplementation were used. Subjects took only 400 mg/day 3 days per week. This dosage is too low if you ask me, but you don't want to take too much NAC either—there is evidence an excess intake of NAC, in the area of 2,000 mg/day, may actually act as a pro-oxidant (a compound that makes free radicals)![143]

If you read my *1996 Supplement Review*, you might remember I highly recommended NAC supplementation; I still stand behind that advice. Try using 200-400 mg of NAC 2 or 3 times a day, with or between meals.

TRIED AND TRUE: BODYBUILDING'S TOP TEN SUPPLEMENTS

SUPPLEMENTS•TRIED AND TRUE: BODYBUILDING'S TOP TEN SUPPLEMENTS•TRIED AND TRUE: BODYBUILDING'S TOP TEN SUPPLEMENTS•TRIED AND TRUE: BODYBUILDING'S TOP TEN SUPPLEMENTS•TRIED AND TRUE: BODYBUILDING'S TOP TEN SUPPLEMENTS•TRIED AND TRUE:

There are several "pre-stacked" antioxidant formulas available on the market which contain a number of these important ingredients in quantities that I'm convinced produce a powerful antioxidant effect. Among them is a product called Recoup, which is made by Protech Nutrition as well as Antioxidant by Nature's Way, Super Antioxidant Companion by Solaray, Ultra Mega by GNC, and C+ Antioxidant Botanicals by Jarrow Formulas. Although I think many of the formulas on the market are good, I have yet to find the "perfect" antioxidant formula especially designed for bodybuilders. Gram quantities of Vitamin C are essential (3-6 grams/day), as are substantial quantities of lipoic acid (200-600 mg/day), selenium (100-200 mcg/day), beta-carotene (100-200 mg/day), NAC (400-1,200 mg/day), Vitamin E (500-1,000 IU/day), and proanthocyanidins (200-300 mg/day, pine bark or grape seed extract).

Antioxidants, Good—Free Radicals, Bad (Simple, Huh?)

Consuming a high-potency antioxidant supplement will <u>not</u> increase your bench press by 20 lbs in 20 days, and it most likely won't even produce a noticeable increase in muscle mass or fat loss in a month, but I cannot emphasize enough how important the *long-term* use of antioxidant supplements is for your success in bodybuilding. Make no mistake, antioxidants are *bodybuilding* supplements—they help protect not only your muscles but your entire system against the damage caused by intense exercise. Indeed, recent studies confirm that the use of antioxidant supplements by athletes is warranted.[32, 99, 253] We don't have all the answers yet as to which antioxidants work best, nor how or why, but the evidence is mounting. So, listen up, *bodybuilders*—just because antioxidants are popular with mainstream health and fitness enthusiasts doesn't mean they're too "ordinary" for us—use 'em—you can't go wrong.

VITAMINS AND MINERALS—THEY'RE NOT EXCITING, BUT THEY'RE VITALLY IMPORTANT

You want to build muscle and burn fat, right? Well, then you'd better make sure your body is in *top working order*. Did you know that if your body is deficient in just one of the essential vitamins or minerals, over a thousand chemical and enzymatic processes in your body could be impaired? It's true! Having the proper amounts of all the important vitamins and minerals available when and where your body needs them is extremely important. Each and every vitamin and mineral is responsible for literally thousands of biochemical reactions, including: the formation of hormones, converting food energy to "chemical energy" (which is needed by your system to function), and building and reinforcing the immune system—in other words, virtually everything you can think of.[197] If you don't feed these important micronutrients to your body *every day*, in the right amounts, you'll never reach your fullest potential.

I'll give you the lowdown on virtually every vitamin and mineral you need to know about in Chapter 6, "The Wide, Wide World of Vitamins and Minerals: What They Are and What They Do." Please read that chapter! This is important stuff, friend!

For now, suffice it to say that these nutrients are incredibly important—there are literally hundreds and hundreds of studies which have been done showing the vital role vitamins and minerals play in proper biological function.

I would definitely say that vitamins and minerals are tried and true—they're hardly a supplement fad; in fact, they're supplements everyone, especially bodybuilders, should use every day! I stand behind this recommendation with my fullest conviction!

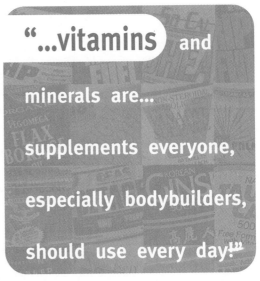

"...vitamins and minerals are... supplements everyone, especially bodybuilders, should use every day!"

MEAL-REPLACEMENT POWDERS (MRP'S)—THE BODYBUILDER'S "FAST FOOD"

Any bodybuilder who knows anything at all about building a lean, muscular, healthy body knows that optimal nutrition is incredibly important. Let's face it—trying to force your body to do things it doesn't want to do requires extraordinary measures. (You can't eat "normal" if you don't want to look "normal"!) When you think about it, what we are doing as bodybuilders is really trying to force our bodies to get bigger, *yet smaller* at the same time. That is, we are trying to make our muscles bigger while making the "fat compartments" of our bodies smaller—it's not something our systems were designed for. More muscle and less fat was not something that was conducive to the survival of our ancestors, and we're living in bodies that were forged from tens of thousands of years of evolution, so it's an issue we have to deal with. The era in which humans have not had to endure regular periods of famine is a mere speck on the timeline of human existence.

I don't mean to confuse you or go off on a tangent, but what I am trying to make clear is that your body was not designed to build muscle and lose fat at the rate at which you and I want it to; in fact, our bodies were actually designed to store fat and prevent the excessive accumulation of muscle tissue. You see, muscle burns more calories, and those of us who have a higher metabolic rate (although considered lucky today) were the first to die when a famine hit, way back when.

In more recent years, human beings have found themselves in a world where there's more than enough of the *wrong kinds* of foods readily available for their consumption. This has led to a variety of problems, including: high rates of obesity, diabetes, heart disease, and cancer.

TRIED AND TRUE: BODYBUILDING'S TOP TEN SUPPLEMENTS

SUPPLEMENTS•TRIED AND TRUE: BODYBUILDING'S TOP TEN SUPPLEMENTS•TRIED AND TRUE: BODYBUILDING'S TOP TEN SUPPLEMENTS•TRIED AND TRUE: BODYBUILDING'S TOP TEN SUPPLEMENTS•TRIED AND TRUE: BODYBUILDING'S TOP TEN SUPPLEMENTS•TRIED AND TRUE: BODYBUILDING'S TOP TEN SUPPLEMENTS•TRIED AND TRUE:

CHAPTER 4

As bodybuilders, our concerns go beyond trying to avoid health problems. We are faced with the extremely complicated task of feeding our bodies in a manner that allows us to maximize our potential to build muscle, while at the same time, avoiding the excess accumulation of bodyfat.

Of course, one of the strategies we employ, in an effort to change our bodies, is resistance exercise—there's no question that it works, but weight training alone will not produce the results you're looking for. You *have to* combine an intense training program with optimal nutrition; in fact, I think food—the way you feed your body—may have more to do with how you look and feel than you even realize.

Food *literally* has "drug-like" effects. When you eat, a whole cascade of hormonal reactions occurs, which you can control by consuming different foods at certain times. Food, like drugs, has "side effects." If you eat improperly, one obvious side effect is the accumulation of bodyfat. Another side effect of "food abuse" is unstable energy levels. Everyone has experienced this—if you don't eat the right things at the right times, your energy levels go up and down throughout the day.

Of course, you don't need a prescription for food, but maybe you should! Literally tens of thousands of people die each year, prematurely, because they misuse or abuse food. (Think about it—it's true!)

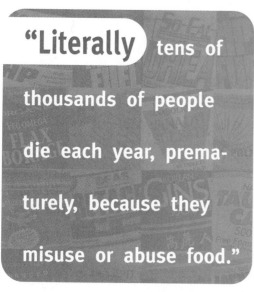

"Literally tens of thousands of people die each year, prematurely, because they misuse or abuse food."

Understanding the Problem

Many experts contend this whole problem could be solved if we all just learned how to "eat right." These experts offer recommendations like consuming this or that amount of leafy, green vegetables each day; eating a certain amount of grains and dairy products; and so on. Now, I consider myself to be a relatively smart person, but to be honest, I've never been able to figure out exactly what the hell these nutrition "experts" are talking about. The fact that Americans, as a population, are getting fatter and more out of shape each year tells me that no one else understands what the heck these experts are talking about either.

I'm convinced most people will never learn how to "eat right." In today's busy world, few of us have time to shop for and prepare multiple nutritionally balanced, complete whole-food meals each and every day. And even if we did, I still don't think that would be optimal. Think about this—the amount of Vitamin C found in two identical-looking oranges at your local grocery store can vary enormously. How long ago was the fruit picked? What type of soil was it grown in? What part of the country did it come from? It's almost impossible to predict the nutrient value of various whole foods.

Not only is it virtually impossible to reliably predict the amount of vitamins and minerals in various whole foods, it's also very difficult to keep track of the calorie content. Remember, as bodybuilders, the number of calories we consume is one of the most important (yet poorly controlled) aspects of making our bodies look the way we want them to. If you consume just a couple hundred calories less than you need each day to maintain proper muscle metabolism or anabolic drive, you'll never get bigger and stronger. On the other hand, if you consume just a few hundred calories too many a day, in no time at all, your body will become smooth, and over a period of months, you'll get downright fat.

Not even supplements like creatine and HMB will help you reach your full muscle-building potential if you're not getting the energy (calories) you need. And not even the most powerful fat-burning supplements (not even the caffeine/ephedrine/aspirin stack) will help you get "ripped" if you're taking in more calories than your body burns.

Keeping track of the calories you consume from whole-food sources is more difficult than you might think—a chicken sandwich with lettuce and tomato from one restaurant may contain 700 calories, yet at another, it may contain only 300 (because of the difference in portion sizes). A plain baked potato can contain as few as 100 calories or as many as 300—unless you carry around a food scale and weigh just about everything before you eat it, you never really know how many calories you're consuming.

This is probably old news to most of you—especially if you've been bodybuilding for quite a while, like I have. The bottom line is that it's very difficult to maintain "optimal nutrition" day in and day out. From my personal experience, and the observations I've made based on feedback from literally hundreds and hundreds of bodybuilders, I've learned that most of us have enormous flaws in our "big-picture" nutrition programs. Many bodybuilders consume too many calories (others don't eat enough), and not enough bodybuilders take advantage of such things as proper meal patterning, portion control, and multiple feedings.

Virtually every credible bodybuilding expert these days agrees that the best way to approach bodybuilding nutrition is to consume numerous (five, six, or even seven) nutritious "meals" each day. This strategy differs significantly from the typical American diet—most "regular people" eat two or three big meals a day, which is not the best way to maximize the anabolic effects of insulin, maintain proper muscle metabolism, or even keep your energy levels up. The bad news is, eating six regular food meals a day can be a real pain.

High-Tech Superfoods Offer a Solution

Meal-replacement powders or "engineered foods" or "total-nutrition" products—whatever you want to call them—offer a simple solution to this somewhat complex problem. That's why they have become such popular sports supplements.

REVIEW•SPORTS SUPPLEMENT REVIEW, 3RD ISSUE•SPORTS SUPPLEMENT REVIEW, 3RD ISSUE•SPORTS SUPPLEMENT REVIEW, 3RD ISSUE•SPORTS SUPPLEMENT

•SPORTS SUPPLEMENT REVIEW, 3RD ISSUE•SPORTS SUPPLEMENT REVIEW, 3RD ISSUE•SPORTS SUPPLEMENT REVIEW, 3RD ISSUE•SPORTS SUPPLEMENT REVIEW, 3RD ISSUE•SPORTS SUPPLEMENT REVIEW, 3RD ISSUE•SPORTS SUPPLEMENT REVIEW, 3RD ISSUE•SPORTS SUPPLEMENT REVIEW, 3RD ISSUE•SPORTS SUPPLEMENT

TRIED AND TRUE: BODYBUILDING'S TOP TEN SUPPLEMENTS

SUPPLEMENTS•TRIED AND TRUE: BODYBUILDING'S TOP TEN SUPPLEMENTS•TRIED AND TRUE: BODYBUILDING'S TOP TEN SUPPLEMENTS•TRIED AND TRUE: BODYBUILDING'S TOP TEN SUPPLEMENTS•TRIED AND TRUE: BODYBUILDING'S TOP TEN SUPPLEMENTS•TRIED AND TRUE:

But do these "superfoods" really do anything that food itself doesn't do? Ya know... the answer to that question is, "Probably not." Meal replacements probably don't do anything that food itself doesn't do, but think about what that means. Food literally has miraculous, *even drug-like*, effects on your body. Without food, you would obviously perish, and without precision nutrition, you'll never be able to build the perfect body.

Don't underestimate the incredible difference improving your core nutrition program can make. This *is* something meal-replacement powders can help you do. Think of it this way: let's say you took an entire grocery cart full of whole foods (like fruits and vegetables, milk, meat, etc.) and you put them in some type of "magic" food processor that extracted all of the valuable nutrients—the good things your body needs—and put them in one place and took all of the "junk"—the excess calories, the *saturated* fat, and other garbage—and got rid of it. Then, if you took all of the "good stuff" and combined it in precise ratios, what you would have is a high-tech, custom-designed food—a precision nutrition formula that offered you the positive biochemical effects of food, without the negative. Well, that's what this whole meal-replacement powder concept is all about—designing new, better ways to feed your body!

For this new nutrition concept to be practical, these new superfoods have to meet certain criteria. For example, they have to be convenient (it's well established that people eat what is convenient for them); these "superfoods" have to taste good (people eat what tastes good—that's a fact); and they have to be economical. (Think about this—why do up to 50 million people a day eat fast-food hamburgers? They're convenient, inexpensive, and to many people, they taste good. Most things that are high in saturated fat and loaded with salt "turn on" the palate.)

Basically, the ideal "high-tech" meal-replacement powder should not only be extremely high in the nutrients bodybuilders need and not contain excess calories, it should also taste good, be priced right, and it should offer convenience.

Fortunately, there are a number of quality sports supplements on the market that fit this criteria. Unlike a few years ago when a lot of the multinutrient products on the market were filled with inferior ingredients, didn't taste very good at all, and upset most people's stomachs, today's products are a completely new breed. And, no one company has a "world exclusive" on the technology to build a quality total-nutrition product. However, some of these products are more complete than others, and some taste better than others. (Of course, taste is an individual thing—what is delicious to me might not be so "scrumptious" to you.) And, these products are usually a pretty good value—the best ones cost around $2-$3 per serving, which when you consider all the nutrition they provide, is pretty reasonable. Two or three bucks is not much for a "complete meal"; in fact, that's probably less than most regular people spend on fast-food lunches that are loaded with saturated fat and empty calories.

Are They Right for You?

Could you benefit from using a meal-replacement powder that was specifically designed for bodybuilders? Well, to answer that question, you just have to think about your eating habits. Do you eat "perfectly" day in and day out? Do you usually consume protein and carbohydrates at the same time (which is a good idea—especially within an hour after your workout)? Do you know how many calories you're consuming each day? (Tip: a lot of people are experimenting with a new diet called the Anabolic Burst Cycling System, which calls for a high consumption of calories for two weeks, then switching over to a low-calorie diet for two weeks. Guess what? The system doesn't work *unless* you keep track of your F-in' calories! And one of the best ways to do that is by consuming meal-replacement powders for some of your meals!)

On a typical day, I have two or three meal-replacement powder "shakes," and then I try to consume a few balanced, whole-food meals. The great thing about eating like this is my "supplement" meals are so high in nutrients and low in calories that my other meals can be a little "less disciplined." I can eat some "fun foods" and still stay lean and muscular.

Using meal-replacement powders is really great for me because I don't have any time to waste—I usually don't even want to take a 20- or 30-minute break for lunch. I'd rather just take three minutes to mix a packet of a total-nutrition powder with water (occasionally I use skim milk) in a blender, mix it up, and drink it. Then, my body's fed, my stomach doesn't feel all bloated and "bogged down," and I'm right back to work.

Meal-replacement powders can also offer huge advantages to people who travel a lot—have you ever been stuck at a hotel and had to order from room service and all they had were crappy club sandwiches, cheeseburgers, and French fries? It sucks. I can't tell you the number of times I've blown my diet when I've been on the road.

Another one of the great things about meal-replacement powders is that they offer a level of "completeness" a lot of bodybuilders are looking for. For example, with just 3 servings a day of EAS' new supplement, Myoplex Plus Deluxe™, I get almost 130 grams of quality protein (including ion-exchanged whey) and 150% of the U.S. RDA for virtually every essential vitamin and mineral. I also get eight grams of glutamine, as well as a big dose of taurine. Myoplex Plus Deluxe even takes the concept of total nutrition a step further by providing an ample dose of conjugated

> "...my 'supplement' meals are so high in nutrients and low in calories that my other meals can be a little 'less disciplined.'"

93

TRIED AND TRUE: BODYBUILDING'S TOP TEN SUPPLEMENTS

SUPPLEMENTS•TRIED AND TRUE: BODYBUILDING'S TOP TEN SUPPLEMENTS•TRIED AND TRUE: BODYBUILDING'S TOP TEN SUPPLEMENTS•TRIED AND TRUE: BODYBUILDING'S TOP TEN SUPPLEMENTS•TRIED AND TRUE: BODYBUILDING'S TOP TEN SUPPLEMENTS•TRIED AND TRUE: BODYBUILDING'S TOP TEN SUPPLEMENTS•TRIED AND TRUE:

linoleic acid (CLA), vanadyl sulfate, and a number of other key micronutrients, which are contained in EAS' bodybuilding formulas V2G™ and GKG®. Basically, with Myoplex Plus Deluxe, you get a total-nutrition product/meal-replacement powder that's already combined with V2G, GKG, CLA, and whey protein. This is one of EAS' newest products, but it's already very popular—obviously, bodybuilders like you and me can appreciate the significance of the added convenience and value of this "pre-stacked" supplement. Myoplex Plus Deluxe is probably the most complete meal-replacement powder on the market—I don't know of any others that I'd recommend more highly, but as I've already explained, you should feel free to experiment and choose whichever works best for you.

Lean-Mass Stimulators

One subcategory of meal-replacement powders is a kind of multinutrient product called "lean-mass stimulators." These include products like Phosphagain® by EAS, Lean Gainer™ by Champion Nutrition, Creatine Fuel Plus™ by TwinLab, PhosphaMass™ by Pro Performance, and a product called PhosphaGold™ by Weider Nutrition. These supplements contain practically the same vitamin and mineral blend as the high-protein meal-replacement products, and they usually contain around five or six grams of creatine monohydrate per serving. Usually, they're lower in protein (Phosphagain 2 has 25 grams of protein, compared to Myoplex Plus Deluxe's 42 grams), and they're lower in calories. Lean-mass stimulators, being multinutrient products, are good to use as "mini-meals" or snacks between big meals, or if you mix them with milk, they actually make a pretty decent meal by themselves.

Which Is Right for You?

As far as how to decide which one of these products is right for you, I simply recommend trying a variety of them: a number of health-food stores sell single packets—try Myoplex Plus, Myoplex Plus Deluxe, Rx Fuel™, Metaform™, Pro Rx™, Perfect Rx™, and so on, and compare them. I recommend that you go with a quality brand (I'll tell you later in this book about which companies I think you can trust and which ones you need to watch out for), but other than that, just use the one you like best. (I've tried virtually every one of these total-nutrition products, and I believe that EAS' meal-replacement powders—Myoplex Plus and Myoplex Plus Deluxe, are very good. But I'm pretty biased.)

The bottom line is, meal-replacement powders are one of my top ten supplements not because they produce some amazing "steroid-like" effect but because they help improve your nutrition program by taking *a lot* of the guesswork out of it. Let's cut right to the chase—if you don't feed your body right, no matter how hard you work out, you're never gonna look your best. And, for a lot of bodybuilders, meal-replacement powders make "eating right" a lot less complicated.

Essential Fatty Acids—Fats That Make Muscle!

It wasn't that long ago that the word fat was considered a "four-letter word" by bodybuilders and serious fitness buffs. The ability to completely eliminate fat from your diet would have earned you a "bodybuilding badge of honor." *Cut the fat, and you'll lose fat—fat makes you fat*—were the mottos. But guess what? We cut the fat, and we felt like crap! In contrast to what experts everywhere were saying, when we slashed the fat out of our diets, it became more difficult to lose fat, our testosterone levels dropped, insulin function became impaired, muscle growth was slowed, and we lost energy!

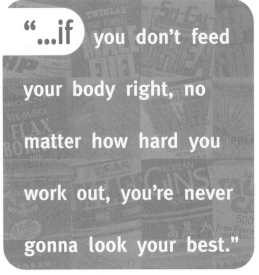

"...if you don't feed your body right, no matter how hard you work out, you're never gonna look your best."

Unfortunately, the bad rap fats get in the media caused us to "throw the baby out with the bath water," so to speak. To simply say that "fat is bad" is erroneous. In reality, there are good fats and bad fats; in fact, some fats are essential to life itself, not to mention optimal muscle and fat metabolism! But, trying to explain which fats you need, which ones you don't, and how they can benefit your health and exercise performance is not a simple thing to do. There are so many stigmas and half-truths attached to what fats are and what they do. Trying to sort it all out can be confusing and complex. However, in this section, I'm going to try to take this complicated subject and make it simple. I'll give you just the information you really need to know and leave it at that. Okay? Good.

Here's the deal: saturated fats are the bad ones. They really don't play any important role in the body except to be burned as energy. Quite simply, you don't need saturated fats at all, but the typical American diet is rich in saturated fat—it's what's in butter, cheese, beef, etc. Saturated fat is solid at room temperature (like Crisco), and it's the crud that can lead to a number of problems like heart disease, cancer, insulin resistance, and even a greater likelihood of gaining bodyfat (even if your total calories are the same as someone on a low-saturated-fat diet). Try to consume as little saturated fat as possible. Simple.

Unsaturated fats are usually liquid at room temperature—they are considered much healthier. Two particular types of unsaturated fats are considered *essential fatty acids* or "EFA's." These are ones that *cannot* be made by the body and are necessary for thousands of biochemical reactions to take place in the body. These fatty acids are called linoleic acid (sometimes called an omega-6 fatty acid) and linolenic acid (omega-3). In the ideal metabolism, linoleic and linolenic acid are the only dietary fats you need.

TRIED AND TRUE: BODYBUILDING'S TOP TEN SUPPLEMENTS

SUPPLEMENTS-TRIED AND TRUE: BODYBUILDING'S TOP TEN SUPPLEMENTS-TRIED AND TRUE: BODYBUILDING'S TOP TEN SUPPLEMENTS-TRIED AND TRUE: BODYBUILDING'S TOP TEN SUPPLEMENTS-TRIED AND TRUE: BODYBUILDING'S TOP TEN SUPPLEMENTS-TRIED AND TRUE: BODYBUILDING'S TOP TEN SUPPLEMENTS-TRIED AND TRUE: BODYBUILDING'S TOP TEN SUPPLEMENTS-TRIED AND TRUE: BODYBUILDING'S TOP TRUE:

CHAPTER 4

The body uses linolenic acid to make two other essential fatty acids, "docosahexaenoic acid" and "eicosapentaenoic acid." These last two fatty acids are commonly found in fish oil.

Cold-water fish (which have a higher bodyfat content than warm-water fish), such as salmon, mackerel, and trout, have "advanced" forms of linolenic acid (docosahexaenoic and eicosapentaenoic). Low-fat fish like haddock, sole, and flounder contain almost insignificant amounts of these important fatty acids. (Shellfish are generally not a good source, either.)

Now, you can either eat a lot of fish, or you can make sure you eat oils high in linolenic acid to allow your body to make its own eicosapentaenoic and docosahexaenoic acid. The best vegetable source of linolenic acid is flaxseed or linseed oil.

Good sources of linoleic acid include canola oil, safflower oil, sunflower oil, and soybean oil. Generally speaking, Americans get a lot of this type of oil in their diets from eating processed foods.

Primrose oil and borage oil, both used by some bodybuilders, contain decent amounts of both types of essential fatty acids.

What Do EFA's Do?

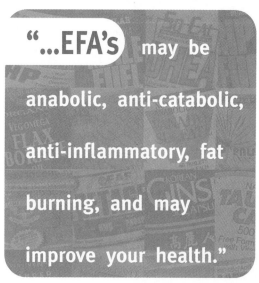

"...EFA's may be anabolic, anti-catabolic, anti-inflammatory, fat burning, and may improve your health."

One of EFA's main roles is as a structural component of all cell membranes. EFA's are also necessary for the formation of vital chemicals in the body called "prostaglandins," which are hormone-like substances that play a role in an enormous variety of functions, including: the proper regulation of blood pressure, heart function, allergic response, inflammation, nerve transmission, and even steroid hormone production. Yep... that's right—if your diet lacks the optimal amounts of these two fatty acids, your body won't even be able to maximize testosterone production! In fact, extremely low-fat diets (like many athletes follow) can cause a decrease in testosterone levels. In one study, researchers examined the effects of a very low-fat diet (which was unquestionably low in EFA's) against that of a moderate-fat diet—a 7% dietary fat intake versus a 36% fat intake. Researchers found that free testosterone levels were increased by 22% in the latter group (the ones consuming more reasonable amounts of fat) versus the fat-deprived subjects.[229] In another study, researchers showed a 19% reduction in free testosterone when test subjects' diets were reduced from a 40% fat intake to a diet that contained 18% of its calories from fat.[128] Even a small decrease in dietary fat, from 37% to 25%, was shown in yet another study to decrease free testosterone production by 13%.[112]

Now, I'm not saying that to boost your testosterone, all you have to do is eat more fat. The point I'm emphasizing is scientific studies offer strong evidence that dietary fat has a direct effect on your body's testosterone production. My guess is that the enhancement of testosterone production in these studies was due primarily to a greater intake of EFA's. I think a diet that is 20% fat, if it's high in EFA's, would optimize testosterone production.

So you're not "sold" on fats quite yet... well, let me see what else I can do to convince you...

How about if I told you supplementing the diet with EFA's may decrease catabolism and increase growth hormone secretion? Scientific evidence indicates that *is* the case.[75] And, just in case you're one of those bodybuilders who *cares* about maintaining a great-looking, *healthy* body, you might be interested to discover EFA's have been shown to cause a decrease in total serum cholesterol and an increase in HDL (good cholesterol).[93] EFA's may even help accelerate fat loss.

EFA's may also improve the action of insulin[33, 218] and enhance the oxygen use and energy transformation required for optimal performance.[40, 291] Basically, EFA's may be anabolic, anti-catabolic, anti-inflammatory, fat burning, and may improve your health. *That's* why I'm calling them one of a select few tried and true supplements—one of the top ten supplements you should use!

EFA Supplements

So just exactly how should you supplement your diet with EFA's? Well, the most popular method used by bodybuilders right now is to consume a supplement called flaxseed oil. This stuff is very high in linolenic acid, but is actually not a very good source of linoleic acid. Soybean oil and safflower oil, on the other hand, are relatively good sources of linoleic acid, but they are low in levels of linolenic acid. And fish oils are good sources of the active omega-3 metabolites of linolenic acid: namely, eicosapentaenoic acid and docosahexaenoic acid.

Another EFA supplement that's becoming very popular with bodybuilders is a "designer fat" called Udo's Choice (named after Dr. Udo Erasmus, who wrote a great book called *Fats That Heal, Fats That Kill*). Udo's Choice is available by calling 1-800-446-2110, and it can also be found at a lot of specialty health-food shops. If you use Udo's Choice, I recommend one tablespoon three times per day.

Alternatively, I would recommend creating your own EFA concoction by mixing one cup of flaxseed oil with one cup of safflower, borage, or primrose oil. Then take one tablespoon of this mixture with a protein drink, meal-replacement powder, or regular meal, two or three times a day—this is an excellent way to get a quality source of essential fatty acids in your diet.

There's no question in my mind that EFA supplementation is very important to bodybuilders, and I think over the next few years, we'll see some exciting, new

TRIED AND TRUE: BODYBUILDING'S TOP TEN SUPPLEMENTS

SUPPLEMENTS•TRIED AND TRUE: BODYBUILDING'S TOP TEN SUPPLEMENTS•TRIED AND TRUE: BODYBUILDING'S TOP TEN SUPPLEMENTS•TRIED AND TRUE: BODYBUILDING'S TOP TEN SUPPLEMENTS•TRIED AND TRUE: BODYBUILDING'S TOP TEN SUPPLEMENTS•TRIED AND TRUE: BODYBUILDING'S TOP TEN SUPPLEMENTS•TRIED AND TRUE: BODYBUILDING'S TOP TEN SUPPLEMENTS•TRIED AND TRUE:

CHAPTER 4

discoveries in this area. For example, one relatively newly discovered fatty acid, called CLA (conjugated linoleic acid), has been shown to support a significant increase in fat loss and an increase in lean body mass.[212] I use CLA and EFA's every day. (I'll tell you more about the fascinating effects of CLA in Chapter 9.)

So, the next time you hear the word "fat," keep in mind that not all fats are bad. Avoid saturated fat, and consume whole-foods rich in EFA's. For example, two or three times a week, have a six-ounce serving of salmon or trout, and use flaxseed oil or safflower oil in salad dressings, sauces, etc. And, try not to let your dietary fat intake drop below 15%. If you supplement your diet with EFA's, I think you'll really notice a difference. If you're skeptical, give this recommendation a try for a month, and see what happens. If your muscles start feeling fuller, your strength goes up, and you just feel better, you'll know you stumbled onto something good!

SUMMARY

Okay—in this chapter I told you about the supplements I think are tried and true—the best of the best—the ones I would highly recommend to any and all serious bodybuilders. A supplement stack consisting of a quality whey-protein powder and/or meal replacement, creatine monohydrate *plus carbs*, HMB, glutamine, antioxidants, vitamins, minerals, and EFA's, can't fail—it is the *crème de la crème*—the foundation of the most effective bodybuilding supplement programs in existence. And, despite my reputation as "Mr. Controversy," you can rest assured that eight out of ten bodybuilding experts, who know *anything* about supplementation, would agree the supplements reviewed in this chapter are as close to a "sure thing" as you're going to get. Give these supplements a try—use one of them, all of them, or cycle them. These top supplements are tried and true. They worked for me, and they'll work for you. (Oh shit, does that rhyme? How dorky. I didn't mean to do that... let me try again...) These supplements are good. Try 'em. (Is that better?)

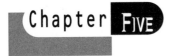

Chapter FIVE

Supplements
That Suck

Unfortunately, not all supplements work—in fact, the truth is *a lot* of the crap that proliferates on the bodybuilding market doesn't do diddly. And, since it's my job to call a spade a spade, in this chapter, I'll reveal what I believe are some of the worst bodybuilding supplements on the market—the ones which are, in my opinion, "bad news."

Some of the supplements that found their way into this chapter did so primarily because of *the way they are marketed*—not merely because of their effects or lack thereof. That is, the advertising claims for some of these products or the claims made for them in "articles" in certain magazines are distortions of the truth (lies).

"...last year we tested six different HMB supplements that didn't contain any beta-hydroxy beta-methylbutyrate..."

SUPPLEMENTS THAT DON'T CONTAIN WHAT THEIR LABELS CLAIM

I can't think of anything that sucks more than a supplement that doesn't even contain what it claims on the label; unfortunately, this is a widespread problem in the bodybuilding supplement business. Because the market is so fragmented and there are so many small supplement companies popping up left and right and because most of the muscle magazines accept advertising from virtually anyone (*Muscle Media* is the **ONLY** one that tests companies' products to make sure they contain what their labels claim before we run their ads), this problem is getting worse and worse as far as I can tell.

Here are a few brutal examples: last year we tested six different HMB supplements that didn't contain any beta-hydroxy beta-methylbutyrate (the real HMB). Not a speck! This included a product called HMB/K+ manufactured by Dews Research and distributed by an outfit called Twenty First Century Nutrition; a product called GMB; a bogus product put out by the Conan Corporation; another put out by

SUPPLEMENTS THAT SUCK

EMENTS THAT SUCK•SUPPLEMENTS THAT SUCK•SUPPLEMENTS THAT SUCK•SUPPLEMENTS THAT SUCK•SUPPLEMENTS THAT SUCK•SUPPLEMENTS THAT SUCK•SUPPLEMENTS THAT SUCK•SUPPLEMENTS THAT SUCK•SUPPLEMENTS THAT SUCK•SUPPLEMENTS THAT SUCK•SUPPLEMENTS THAT SUCK•SUPPLE

Molecular Nutrition; another by Castlewood Nutritional Systems; and yet another by Dexter Sports Supplements, which put out a bogus HMB product under the name Power Star. This same company produced a phony supplement called "CCLA" which we had analyzed—the supplement contained 0% CLA! It was simply ordinary vegetable oil. (Unbelievable, huh?!)

And, check this out—we recently tested several batches (lot numbers 84505 and 85450) of a creatine supplement put out by a company called USA Sports Labs. Their creatine product, called Creatine Plus, contained virtually no creatine at all! And one of their protein supplements called "X-Plode Powder" contained only 5 grams of protein per serving, when the label claim was 50 grams per serving! (The lot number on the batch we tested was 6440.) We were also unable to find any active yohimbine in the product, when it claimed it contained 750 mg of yohimbe per serving.

This is a problem a lot of the information providers and "experts" in this industry ignore, probably because it's such a difficult issue to deal with. It's almost impossible to "police," and many supplement industry insiders believe that even bringing up the issue will fuel consumers' skepticism that sports supplements, or *any* supplements, are for real. Basically, they're afraid they'll lose money by exposing this problem. The muscle magazine publishers are in the same boat—if they blow the whistle on these dirtbags, they'll lose tens of thousands of dollars in ad revenue! (You wouldn't believe the amount of ad money I have turned down from companies which wanted to advertise in *Muscle Media*, but their products just weren't good enough. You see, I'm determined to be *part of the solution* to our industry's weaknesses, rather than part of the problem!)

> "...I have tested and exposed literally dozens and dozens of fraudulent, mislabeled supplements..."

Over the past seven years, I have tested and exposed literally dozens and dozens of fraudulent, mislabeled supplements through my publications. There is no question that these "bad apples" give a black eye to the entire supplement industry, but I think the best way to deal with this is to just get it out in the open, expose and make an example out of those companies which think they're going to get away with ripping you off. We've got to make them accountable for their deceptive practices. And, hopefully, these disreputable companies will learn this is <u>not</u> the right way to do business.

I wish I could give you a listing of every supplement on the market that doesn't contain what its label claims, but unfortunately, that would probably be impossible. The best advice I can give—the advice I give my friends who are shopping for supplements—is to go with a reputable brand name, such as my company (EAS), Weider, Schiff, TwinLab, Next Nutrition, Ultimate Nutrition, Beverly International, or American Bodybuilding. I have tested numerous products from each of these companies, and I believe the consistency and quality are there.

One of the points I cannot emphasize enough is that these discount, bargain-basement supplement distributors who sell products at extremely low prices or offer deals that are "too good to be true" are often up to no good. In an effort to make a quick buck, they'll substitute expensive, important ingredients with very cheap, worthless "fillers."

Believe me, folks, there's a lot of this going on and, like I said, the best advice I can give is to stick with a reputable brand. Sure, not every single product is going to meet label claims *exactly*—sometimes a supplement that is supposed to contain 30 grams of protein per serving will have 28 or maybe 32 or maybe some of the other vitamins and minerals are off by a little bit here and there, but it's easy to tell when a diligent effort is being made to maintain quality.

CREATINE "BOOSTERS"

Now, how could a product that contains creatine or one that's supposed to enhance the effects of creatine be a supplement that sucks? Well, this category of supplements gets a "sucks" rating primarily because there is simply no evidence that these products do what their marketing materials claim. For example, one company distributes a product that's actually called "Creatine Booster." They claim "Creatine Booster uses tried-and-true principles of enzyme physiology to stop the endogenous creatine shutdown that is thought to be a major cause of creatine's short-lived benefits." This product supplies arginine, glycine, and methionine—the base amino acid elements of natural creatine production. The company claims these substrates help maintain a greater natural production of creatine. They even go on to say this will help extend the effects of creatine above and beyond what normal supplementation can do. This, my friends, is what you call unsubstantiated hype.

Our bodies normally produce only about one or two grams of creatine per day on their own.[19] If we take supplemental amounts of creatine, between five and ten grams per day, the natural feedback mechanism may shut down creatine production regardless of what substrates you ingest.[241] But, if you stop supplementing with creatine, your body starts making creatine again. It's as simple as that.

Several companies contend, "Krebs cycle intermediates are the answer." Survey says, "Not." The "Krebs cycle intermediates" used in one creatine product are nothing more than a variety of B vitamins. True, some B vitamins play a role in energy production through the Krebs cycle; however, there is absolutely no evidence to suggest these same vitamins could improve the uptake or effectiveness of creatine monohydrate. Dr. Paul Greenhaff (the creatine guru at the University of

SUPPLEMENTS THAT SUCK

CHAPTER 5

EMENTS THAT SUCK•SUPPLEMENTS THAT SUCK•SUPPLEMENTS THAT SUCK•SUPPLEMENTS THAT SUCK•SUPPLEMENTS THAT SUCK•SUPPLEMENTS THAT SUCK•SUPPLEMENTS THAT SUCK•SUPPLEMENTS THAT SUCK•SUPPLEMENTS THAT SUCK•SUPPLEMENTS THAT SUCK•SUPPLEMENTS THAT SUCK•SUPPLE

102

Nottingham) tells me that simply loading more B vitamins into the system would have no effect on creatine efficiency. There's simply no research to support this theory.

Claiming better results by using creatine citrate is another slight-of-hand marketing approach. Marketers claim creatine citrate is more effective because it is "more soluble" and supposedly "more easily absorbed." It is more soluble in water than creatine monohydrate; however, one molecule of creatine citrate contains roughly half the amount of actual creatine than a molecule of creatine monohydrate. Dr. Paul Greenhaff tested creatine citrate head to head with creatine monohydrate. He found, through muscle biopsy studies, that creatine citrate and creatine monohydrate were absorbed into the system at similar rates. Now, keep in mind that creatine citrate contains a lot less actual creatine. Dr. Greenhaff found it was necessary to supply subjects with much more creatine citrate versus creatine monohydrate to obtain the same muscular saturation. Thus, it would be more expensive to use creatine citrate due to the extra amount needed. Creatine citrate also tastes awful—like battery acid.

Since EAS researchers first introduced creatine monohydrate to bodybuilders, they have been aggressively exploring theories and methods for making creatine monohydrate supplementation even more effective. Although other supplement companies claim to have discovered "magic formulas" that supposedly make creatine monohydrate work better (like those discussed above), none have offered any evidence (like a university study) to demonstrate any degree of efficacy above and beyond plain creatine monohydrate.

Certainly, there is nothing wrong with trying to develop a theory. I don't fault any researcher (and I use that term loosely in this context) for trying to come up with an idea—a hypothesis of how creatine might be combined with other nutrients to make it more effective. However, I do think it *sucks* to claim your product is effective, that it enhances the effects of creatine, when you have virtually *no scientific proof* whatsoever to support that claim. I mean, make no mistake, these companies flat out tell you their products are the best thing going. It's downright deceptive, and although it's standard practice in this arena to market supplements in this manner, it certainly wouldn't fly with the FTC (Federal Trade Commission) which stipulates you must be able to *substantiate* claims made in marketing materials.

Such blatant disregard for the facts and substantiation is far too common in the bodybuilding supplement market. Unfortunately, the FTC only goes after the big cats. They've got only so much time, and their resources are relatively limited, so most of these small companies can get away with making deceptive claims of greater creatine efficacy without getting busted.

Despite the inability of other "enhanced" creatine product pushers to validate their claims, there really does appear to be a way to make creatine work even better. And, several new studies (which I reviewed in Chapter 4 under the creatine section) offer strong evidence that the effects of creatine can be enhanced, but the only way that's been university tested is combining creatine with a high-glycemic carbohydrate (a carb that causes a rapid and significant release of the anabolic hormone insulin). This is the basis for EAS' Phosphagen HP formula—the first scientifically validated product that has been tested head to head against regular creatine and been shown to produce better results.[104, 265]

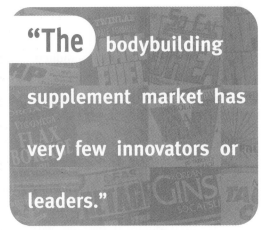

"The bodybuilding supplement market has very few innovators or leaders."

So, even though some of these enhanced creatine products contain creatine, which is a great supplement, I say they suck because they are deceptively marketed.

KNOCK-OFF SUPPLEMENTS SUCK

Okay... I'll admit I'm getting really biased on this one. But, hear me out. (You didn't think you were going to pick up one of my books and not get bombarded with my opinions and beliefs, did you?)

The bodybuilding supplement market has very few innovators or leaders. Make no mistake, the majority of the companies in this market are just trying to make a buck any way they can. Usually, when one company comes out with a product that is "hot," dozens of other companies try to jump on the bandwagon. I call these "me, too" products or "knock offs."

Now, there's a reason I'm very biased and "down" on knock-off products, and most of it has to do with the fact that my products have been the most "copied" sports supplements in history! My company, EAS, follows the philosophy, "innovate, don't imitate." For example, Phosphagen was the first creatine monohydrate product on the market (now there are at least 100 others), and EAS' Phosphagen HP was the first university-tested supplement to combine creatine with an insulin-releasing carbohydrate and other key nutrients to enhance the effects of creatine. EAS was also the first to bring the scientifically designed, university-tested product HMB to the market, and we pioneered the "lean-mass-stimulator" category with the development of Phosphagain, *the* low-calorie mass gainer, a product that has been shown in scientific studies to help bodybuilders gain size and strength without putting on fat. We were also first to the market with CLA, and our scientists started the "cell-volumizing" supplement craze.

A company called Next Nutrition that is owned by a guy named David Jenkins (by the way, despite what some people have heard, I have absolutely <u>no</u> financial/ownership interest in Next Nutrition) was the first to come out with a high-quality, ion-exchanged/whey-peptide protein supplement. I believe Dan Duchaine discovered

SUPPLEMENTS THAT SUCK

EMENTS THAT SUCK•SUPPLEMENTS THAT SUCK•SUPPLEMENTS THAT SUCK•SUPPLEMENTS THAT SUCK•SUPPLEMENTS THAT SUCK•SUPPLEMENTS THAT SUCK•SUPPLEMENTS THAT SUCK•SUPPLEMENTS THAT SUCK•SUPPLEMENTS THAT SUCK•SUPPLEMENTS THAT SUCK•SUPPLEMENTS THAT SUCK•SUPPLE

that compound during the course of his research and worked with Jenkins on the development of this unique protein. Since Designer Protein has come out, at least 30 knock-off products have hit the market. Of course, all the imitators claim their "knock offs" are as good or better than the original, but how convenient... they never have any proof to support their "hype."

The only product EAS has come out with that was "inspired" by another product, and I admit it, is Myoplex Plus. As you may or may not know, I introduced the "meal-replacement" or "engineered-food" concept, along with a doctor in California, to bodybuilders in July of 1991. Before long, the meal-replacement product we introduced (I can't say the name of the product nor the name of the doctor I worked with, even though most of you know what I'm talking about, because of some silly legal issues) became a top seller. But, when I had the opportunity to get involved with EAS, I agreed to turn my rights to this popular engineered food over to another group and let them run with it.

Anyway, in this case, I feel that since I helped create the category and since I knew the product so well, it would not be inappropriate to come out with our own version of that supplement—our own meal-replacement powder that I believe is extremely high in quality and is now a very popular supplement.

My big problem with the companies that knock off EAS' products in particular is that these companies don't contribute to furthering the science of sports nutrition. On the other hand, when you buy a product from EAS, a portion of every dollar you spend goes directly to fund university research programs. For example, last year we signed a deal to provide a $772,000 research grant to the University of Nottingham in England, under the direction of Dr. Paul Greenhaff, quite likely the world's leading creatine expert. This research effort will undoubtedly uncover new ideas about how to use the incredibly powerful supplement creatine to get even better results. And, during the course of this research, many issues which pertain to drug-free enhancement of the muscle-building process will be explored.

At any given time, as many as ten separate university studies are being conducted at prestigious institutions around the world, such as Wichita State University, Kent State University, Creighton University, University of Memphis, University of Nebraska, State University of New York at Stony Brook, Iowa State University, Western Illinois University, and University of Wisconsin at La Crosse, etc., which have been funded by EAS. We even allocate funds to

> **"...the imitators claim their 'knock offs' are as good or better than the original, but... they never have any proof to support their 'hype.'"**

study products we don't sell, such as pyruvate (EAS is the only company I know of that has funded studies on pyruvate to examine the effects of <u>reasonable</u> dosages of the compound and its efficacy in athletes). We're also studying other supplements which we don't have any financial interest in, such as Endurox (Siberian ginseng) as well as funding research to evaluate what type of weight-training programs work best.

Think about this: in order for EAS to continue to invest in this kind of scientific research (research which is benefiting all of us!), we obviously must sell products. And, every one of these knock-off supplements that hits the market and tries to steal business from EAS—the ones that pirate our product ideas and come out with their knock-off versions—are actually taking money away from scientific research!

If this were the way the pharmaceutical industry were run, make no mistake, there would be virtually no advancements in medicine—no new treatments for cancer or AIDS—no new antibiotics, etc. But, fortunately, the pharmaceutical industry is run quite differently from the supplement business. When a drug company invests a large amount of money in the development of a product, the laws say they have <u>exclusive</u> rights for up to 20 years to recoup their investment and make a profit, which they can then invest back into research in an effort to find even more products that work. In the pharmaceutical industry, and many others, investing in technology and inventing is encouraged. But, that's not the case in the bodybuilding supplement business, which I think is a mistake.

From what I know, knock-off products are rarely as good as the original, and to me, they're based on sleazy business—it's actually a lazy way to make a living. There's no thinking or innovating involved. And, the more these knock-off products proliferate (the more people buy them), the worse off the industry actually is.

When you invest in EAS supplements, remember that a portion of every dollar you spend on these products goes to fund university research studies. It's our goal to answer questions about bodybuilding supplements that have gone unanswered for far too long. And, it's time to do the right thing—to spend the money required to develop new, truly powerful products. Obviously, your support and loyalty to the EAS brand would be greatly appreciated.

SUPPLEMENTS THAT DON'T COME WITH A MONEY-BACK GUARANTEE

Once again, this is a category that you may not have expected to see in this chapter, but think about it—even the best supplements don't work for every single person—even steroids, the most powerful muscle builders in the world, don't work for some people for some unknown reason. When you really get down to it, even though a lot of scientific studies show creatine works, and even if it helps your training partner gain 10 lbs of solid weight in 14 days and boost his bench press by 25 lbs... doesn't that supplement suck if it doesn't work for you? Honestly, what works or doesn't work for **YOU** is the ultimate determinant of what sucks and what doesn't, right? Come on... admit it... it's true!

Wouldn't it be nice if every bodybuilding supplement you purchased came with an unconditional, lifetime money-back guarantee? If that were the case, and if companies actually honored the guarantees they make (which some companies don't!), then in actuality, you could never get ripped off. Every time you tried a new supplement, you would have nothing to lose because if it didn't work for you, you could just get your money back. Isn't this the way it should really be? If it were this way, the whole industry would be better off because people like you, and me, who like to try new supplements all the time, would not have as many reservations about experimenting with different compounds to try to find the ones that work best for *us*. As it stands now, when you make a decision to try a supplement, you're saying to yourself, "I'm going to take a gamble... I'm going to take some of this hard-earned money of mine and take a chance that spending it on this or that supplement is a wise investment." The truth is, that's what you're doing when you buy supplements from most companies—you're just rolling the dice and hoping you'll be a winner.

If what I'm saying here doesn't make sense, then ignore or even criticize me for making the following plug; in fact, if what I'm saying here doesn't make perfect sense to you, write me a letter and explain why it wouldn't be right for every company in the supplement industry to offer a lifetime money-back guarantee. And you know what I'll do? I'll sit down, cover a copy of this F-in' book with flaxseed oil, and eat it!

Okay... here's my plug... my company, Experimental and Applied Sciences (EAS), is the **ONLY** company in the bodybuilding supplement industry that offers an <u>authentic</u>, unconditional, lifetime money-back guarantee. In fact, I offer the same guarantee for every product I sell. It's the way I've always done business and the way I always will. You see, it's my belief that the goal of any business should *not* be just to get customers but to *keep* them. This is true in all types of businesses but is especially important to a company selling supplements, where you really don't make that much money on each sale. Success in this industry requires *repeat business* from loyal customers.

That's why all my companies offer a rock-solid, no B.S., money-back guarantee on anything and everything we sell. If you subscribe to *Muscle Media* or purchase one of our supplements and you're not completely satisfied—if you don't think you've received good value in exchange for the hard-earned money you've invested in one of our products, you're entitled to a refund. That's all there is to it. My guarantee is a *promise* from me to you and a reflection of how confident I am our products are top quality.

At EAS and *Muscle Media*, when a customer is dissatisfied or has a complaint about our service or one of our products, we look at that as a chance to go above and beyond what is expected and gain that customer's loyalty for years to come, instead of seeing it as an opportunity to give someone the shaft. We have literally thousands and thousands of loyal customers—fellow bodybuilders who trust us to do the right thing, and that, probably more than anything else, is the secret to our success.

Unfortunately, not all companies feel this way— many companies believe offering a guarantee will cost them money—it will cut into their profit margin. Perhaps they are not as confident about their products as I am. As you may or may not know, EAS has a relatively small product line that is very focused and very specialized.

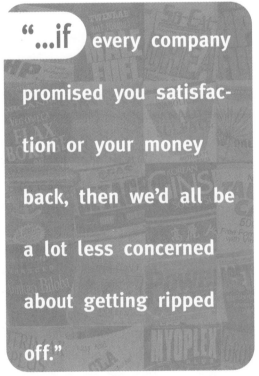

"...if every company promised you satisfaction or your money back, then we'd all be a lot less concerned about getting ripped off."

We only sell products which science shows could offer an advantage to weight trainers and other serious athletes—products that could help us all get better results faster from the time we spend working out. Some companies have as many as a thousand different products in their line—at this time, EAS offers only about a dozen.

To make things even more complicated, I've heard from a number of *Muscle Media* readers who have warned me about one new bodybuilding supplement company from Canada that claims to offer an unconditional money-back guarantee but just gives you the run-around when you try to take them up on their offer. Man... how low can these guys go?!

Anyway, I could go on and on, but I think you'll agree that if every company stood behind its products with as much confidence, pride, and integrity as EAS does—if every company promised you satisfaction or your money back, then we'd all be a lot less concerned about getting ripped off. The bottom line is I would like to encourage more companies to stand behind their products and take care of their customers. They need to realize that offering an unconditional money-back guarantee might force them to cough up some bucks now, but it's a better *long-term* strategy for business success.

HIGH-CALORIE WEIGHT GAINERS

In the late 1980's and early '90's, the bodybuilding supplement industry went through what I call "mega-calorie mania." This was when the hottest bodybuilding

107

•SPORTS SUPPLEMENT REVIEW, 3RD ISSUE•SPORTS SUPPLEMENT REVIEW, 3RD ISSUE•SPORTS SUPPLEMENT REVIEW, 3RD ISSUE•SPORTS SUPPLEMENT REVIEW, 3RD ISSUE•SPORTS SUPPLEMENT REVIEW, 3RD ISSUE•SPORTS SUPPLEMENT REVIEW, 3RD ISSUE•SPORTS SUPPLEMENT REVIEW, 3RD ISSUE•SPORTS SUPPLEMENT

SUPPLEMENTS THAT SUCK

CHAPTER 5

ements that suck-supplements that suck-supplements that suck-supplements that suck-supplements that suck-supplements that suck-supplements that suck-supplements that suck-supplements that suck-supplements that suck-supplements that suck-supple

108

supplements were super-high-calorie weight-gain formulas. First, there was a product that contained 900 calories per serving; then one came out that contained 1,200 calories; the next step in this evolution was a product that contained 2,000 calories per serving. Believe it or not, there was one company that came out with a product that contained 10,000 calories per serving (even though a "serving" was equal to almost an entire bucketful of this crap/powder)!

Back then, all you had to do to top your competition was come out with a product that allegedly contained more calories than the competing brand. It was really a ridiculous trend.

Today, high-calorie weight-gain supplements are not nearly as popular as they once were—as a matter of fact, the majority of these weight-gain supplements have been taken off the market because they stopped selling. But, there is still some confusion—I get quite a few letters from bodybuilders who still think one of these high-calorie weight-gain formulas is the answer to putting on quality muscle mass fast. The truth is, these formulas helped more bodybuilders gain <u>more fat</u> than anything else.

Typically, these formulas contain a relatively small amount of low-quality protein and are loaded with sugar and trace amounts of various ingredients that are purported to have bodybuilding effects. They're not even "good nutrition."

> **"...weight-gain formulas... *suck* compared to the quality total-nutrition supplements which are widely available."**

A few years ago, I would have said that high-calorie weight-gain formulas were so-so, but today *they suck* compared to the quality total-nutrition supplements which are widely available.

If you need to add extra calories to your diet, just take a quality meal-replacement product, like Myoplex Plus, mix it with whole milk, and you'll have a 500+ calorie shake with around 60 grams of *quality* protein, an ample dose of simple and complex carbs, and a broad array of other important nutrients. Consuming a few of these drinks each day and eating a healthy, whole-food diet, which is balanced in quality proteins and carbohydrates, is the best way to increase your calorie intake.

HOMEOPATHIC SUPPLEMENTS

Homeopathic products are derived from plant, mineral, and animal sources. To anyone unfamiliar with homeopathic science, it sounds like the whole thing's based on Chinese herbal medicine or something similar, but that's not the case.

In a nutshell, followers of homeopathy believe if you take something in large amounts and it causes a negative reaction—a disease—then taking small amounts of the same substance will cure you! One comparison which comes to mind is the hung-over "partier" who takes a shot of alcohol in the morning to feel better. That's not exactly homeopathy, but in a basic sense, it is similar.

Likewise, homeopaths believe if you take a really, really small amount of a particular hormone, it will somehow stimulate your body to produce more of that particular hormone. Many homeopathic bodybuilding supplements allegedly contain growth hormone, luteinizing hormone, follicle-stimulating hormone, thyroid-stimulating hormone, etc. Maybe they do, maybe they don't. Here's the problem: according to most homeopaths, the smaller the amount of a compound you put in a homeopathic supplement, the more effect it has. Sound crazy? (It does to me.) Likewise, the amounts of these hormones, if they're even in the "supplement," are so small they're difficult to test for using conventional laboratory methods.

"Homeopathic" is actually defined in Stedman's Medical Dictionary as "Denoting an extremely small dose of a pharmacological agent, such as might be used in homeopathy; more generally, a dose believed to be too small to produce the effect usually expected from that agent." For instance, some homeopathic "remedies" list a number or "strength" on the label. This number may be, for instance, 10X or 24X. This means the product has been diluted 10 times or 24 times. They actually take a certain amount of an active ingredient, mix it with water and alcohol, shake it (a process called *succussing*). Then, they take some of the diluted mixture, mix it with some more alcohol or water, and "succuss" it again. They then repeat this process 10 times (10X), 24 times (24X), or even a hundred times (100X)! Each successive dilution has less active ingredient in it. In fact, according to homeopathic medicine, the most potent solution is the one that contains *no molecules of the original substance*. Duh, so what does that tell you?

So if the supplements really did contain those hormones, because the amounts of these compounds would be so small, the FDA or the DEA wouldn't pay much attention to them. Hence, I don't think you would be breaking any laws by selling or using the stuff.

For instance, a company called American Nutriceuticals makes a product called "Probestan" which allegedly contains chrysin, which I reviewed in Chapter 3. Chrysin may prevent some of your body's natural testosterone from aromatizing into estrogen, thus elevating your body's natural testosterone levels. Well, we had Probestan tested by an independent laboratory, and they couldn't find *any* chrysin in the sample.

If you're a practicing homeopath, that's just what you'd expect to find. However, if you're like me and believe in more "conventional science," you would want to see a hefty amount of chrysin in the sample.

Another example of a homepathic supplement, with alleged bodybuilding applications, is called Andropro from Nuremberg Labs in France. It is supposed to

SUPPLEMENTS THAT SUCK

EMENTS THAT SUCK•SUPPLEMENTS THAT SUCK•SUPPLEMENTS THAT SUCK•SUPPLEMENTS THAT SUCK•SUPPLEMENTS THAT SUCK•SUPPLEMENTS THAT SUCK•SUPPLEMENTS THAT SUCK•SUPPLEMENTS THAT SUCK•SUPPLEMENTS THAT SUCK•SUPPLEMENTS THAT SUCK•SUPPLE

CHAPTER 5

SUPPLEMENTS THAT SUCK•SUPPLEMENTS THAT SUCK•SUPPLEMENTS THAT SUCK•SUPPLEMENTS THAT SUCK•SUPPLEMENTS THAT SUCK•SUPPLEMENTS THAT SUCK•

contain luteinizing hormone which, as some of you probably know, is a substrate to testosterone production in the body. We had Andropro tested; no luteinizing hormone was detected. But, I guess that's homeopathy.

According to Trevor Cook, President of the United Kingdom Homeopathic Medical Association, homeopathic remedies work because their potions and mixtures have a "specific electromagnetic frequency" and these frequencies somehow activate the body's "vital forces" and allow it to heal itself.

This doesn't make much sense to me, and it doesn't make sense to the American Medical Association (AMA), which publicly denounced homeopathy. (Not that I agree with everything the AMA says.) They believe any perceived benefits of homeopathic medicines are caused by the "placebo effect." (You *believe* it works; therefore, you "feel it.")

Hey, maybe I'm wrong, but I just don't think homeopathic supplements will help with your bodybuilding endeavors.

BROAD-SPECTRUM AMINO ACID TABLETS

Amino acids are the building blocks of protein. They are essential material for the body to manufacture muscle tissue, so how could a supplement which contains these important nutrients suck? Well, what it comes down to is that I think amino acid pills (which were incredibly popular a few years ago) don't do jack squat. In fact, a lot of these tablets must be put together with a super-hydraulic, high-compression press. The end result is a rock-hard tablet that won't even dissolve in your stomach—they go straight through you. And, even if they do dissolve, consuming handfuls of amino acid tablets that contain a broad spectrum of amino acids just doesn't do anything to help your bodybuilding efforts. I don't know any bodybuilders who are so deficient in protein intake that consuming 5, 10, or even 20 of these tablets a day is going to make any difference. It's an insignificant "dose."

What's even worse is that broad-spectrum, <u>free-form</u> amino acids are not only cumbersome, they are also poorly absorbed through the intestine compared to actual whole-protein sources, such as whey protein, chicken, milk, etc. Scientists have discovered that small protein peptides (which are two or three amino acids connected together) are probably more readily absorbed into the bloodstream than actual free-form aminos. For that reason, if you're looking to increase your overall quality-protein intake, a natural protein source, such as whey protein, chicken, fish, or even isolated soy protein, would be the way to go. Only if you're trying to supplement individual amino acids, like glutamine and taurine, would you ever want to use a free-form amino acid supplement.

Taking one scoop of a quality ion-exchanged whey protein powder or whey peptides is far superior to consuming amino acid tablets. I challenge anyone to offer evidence that this is not the case.

PRODUCTS THAT CONTAIN TOKEN AMOUNTS OF EVERYTHING AND EFFECTIVE DOSES OF NOTHING

One of the classic nutritional product scams is to list every imaginable ingredient on your label, touting the product as the be-all, end-all—the only product you'll ever need for performance enhancement. These products claim to contain effective doses of supplements like creatine monohydrate, DHEA, L-glutamine, taurine, lipoic acid, vanadyl sulfate, chromium, OKG, etc. After performing a thorough chemical analysis on a few of these "all-in-one" products, I discovered some interesting things, such as a typical dose of creatine monohydrate was a pitiful, inconsequential 186 mg/serving. Other ingredients which I mentioned were likewise in "token" amounts. These types of products suck because they are deceptive and ineffective. I take pleasure in not recommending them.

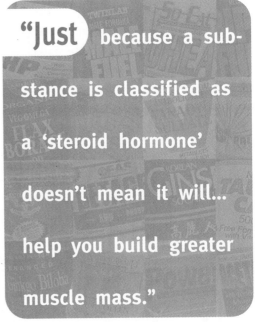

"Just because a substance is classified as a 'steroid hormone' doesn't mean it will... help you build greater muscle mass."

SUPPLEMENTS THAT JUST DON'T WORK

Obviously, any supplement that doesn't work sucks! In this group of compounds, you could include once popular bodybuilding supplements like boron, which is still marketed by some morons as a testosterone enhancer, even though it was shown to cause an increase in testosterone only in post-menopausal women. (It does not have this effect in young, healthy men.) Here's a quick rundown on some other relatively popular supplements that are marketed as having "bodybuilding benefits":

Pregnenolone—This is one of the new class of hormonal compounds which can now be sold as dietary supplements due to the Dietary Supplement Health and Education Act of 1994. A contention made by supplement companies selling pregnenolone (especially those marketed to athletes) is that pregnenolone is a precursor to testosterone and, therefore, will enhance serum testosterone levels. I'm not at all convinced this is true. As a matter of fact, I'm pretty sure it's not.

Although pregnenolone is considered a steroid hormone, so is cortisol (which is responsible for breaking down muscle), as well as estrogen (the "female hormone"). Just because a substance is classified as a "steroid hormone" doesn't mean it will act like testosterone and help you build greater muscle mass.

As far as it leading to greater testosterone production in the body, I strongly doubt this happens. Although pregnenolone is indeed a precursor to DHEA, which in turn can be converted to testosterone, it is also a precursor to a female hormone called progesterone, which can be converted to cortisol or aldosterone

•SPORTS SUPPLEMENT REVIEW, 3RD ISSUE•SPORTS SUPPLEMENT REVIEW, 3RD ISSUE•SPORTS SUPPLEMENT REVIEW, 3RD ISSUE•SPORTS SUPPLEMENT REVIEW, 3RD ISSUE•SPORTS SUPPLEMENT REVIEW, 3RD ISSUE•SPORTS SUPPLEMENT REVIEW, 3RD ISSUE•SPORTS SUPPLEMENT REVIEW, 3RD ISSUE•SPORTS SUPPLEMENT

REVIEW•SPORTS SUPPLEMENT REVIEW, 3RD ISSUE•SPORTS SUPPLEMENT REVIEW, 3RD ISSUE•SPORTS SUPPLEMENT REVIEW, 3RD ISSUE•SPORTS SUPPLEMENT REVIEW, 3RD ISSUE•SPORTS SUPPLEMENT

SUPPLEMENTS THAT SUCK

CHAPTER 5

EMENTS THAT SUCK•SUPPLEMENTS THAT SUCK•SUPPLEMENTS THAT SUCK•SUPPLEMENTS THAT SUCK•SUPPLEMENTS THAT SUCK•SUPPLEMENTS THAT SUCK•SUPPLEMENTS THAT SUCK•SUPPLEMENTS THAT SUCK•SUPPLEMENTS THAT SUCK•SUPPLEMENTS THAT SUCK•SUPPLEMENTS THAT SUCK•SUPPLE

(a hormone that causes water retention). Whether pregnenolone ends up as cortisol, estrogen, or testosterone is, basically, governed by the pituitary gland, which coordinates the many hormones in our bodies.

You see, the pituitary gland works through very sensitive feedback loops. If it senses that the level of testosterone in the body is too high, it will slow down production until it once again reaches equilibrium. By the same token, if it realizes that the body is deficient in cortisol, it will upgrade production of cortisol to once again reach normal levels. Suffice it to say, just because you're taking a precursor to a hormone like testosterone does not mean your body will simply convert it to testosterone just because that's what you want it to do.

I'm not convinced pregnenolone will do anything to help bodybuilders gain more muscle size and strength. I think it is probably more likely that using pregnenolone will have precisely the opposite effect.

Mexican Yam—This supplement is supposed to contain DHEA, but it doesn't. It has never been shown to do anything except go very well with roasted pig.

Colostrum—This is one of those supplements that actually makes me grin. If most people knew what this was, they wouldn't go anywhere near it. Colostrum is a thin, milky substance which is secreted in mother's milk the first few days of breast-feeding a newborn. It's rich in IGF-1 (insulin-like growth factor 1), as well as nutrients that are used by newborns to help kick start their immune systems and develop the proper gut enzymes to assure proper digestion. If you're not a newborn, your gut will destroy the active goodies in colostrum, delivering nothing but a few vitamins and minerals to your system.

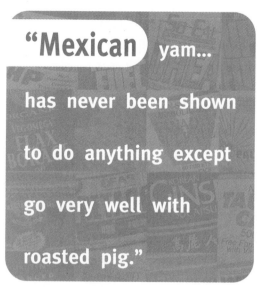

"**Mexican** yam... has never been shown to do anything except go very well with roasted pig."

GHB—GHB, or gamma hydroxybutyrate, despite its somewhat similar sounding name, has **ABSOLUTELY NOTHING** to do with HMB (beta-hydroxy beta-methylbutyrate). These are two completely different supplements that have virtually nothing in common!

In early 1990, GHB was a very popular supplement with bodybuilders—it was purported to increase growth hormone secretion and possibly lower cortisol levels—claims that were not completely without substantiation.[96] But, what bodybuilders quickly discovered is that GHB has an interesting little "side effect"—*it makes you stoned!* Yes, indeed—shortly after taking a substantial dose, many people experience a "pleasantly buzzed," almost euphoric state. But, if you take too much, you get sick as a dog, experience uncontrollable projectile vomiting, and eventually, you F-in' pass out (literally go into a short-term coma), especially if you take GHB while consuming alcohol. Because of these nasty side effects, on November 8, 1990, the FDA made it illegal to manufacture and distribute this compound. In more recent years, some states have classified it as a controlled drug, but today, its popularity in nightclubs is at an all-time high. Apparently, some people like the effect it causes—getting them significantly goofed up for the night, with reportedly no hangover the next day. (On the streets it's now called "G" or "Liquid X.")

Some people believe GHB does not have addictive potential, like other "party drugs," but I don't think that's true. I've known a number of people who've destroyed their lives because they got hooked on GHB. And, there is some research which indicates it is addictive.[91] In my opinion, this stuff is extremely addictive, and you should stay away from it.

Also, now that GHB has been "banned," manufacturers have gone "underground"—home-brewed batches of GHB may vary significantly in potency—that "one capful" you took last week at your friend's party might only be one-tenth as potent as "one capful" that somebody hands you tomorrow night at the techno-club. Thus, the "dosage" which felt cool last time could make you puke your guts out next time.

All in all, I can't see how GHB would be a valuable supplement to any bodybuilder—if you use this stuff to get stoned, watch out—you might get hooked on it, you might pass out and drown in your own vomit (I'm not kidding!), or, who knows, you may feel great and have a really fun night—it's a roll of the dice.

Beta-Sitosterol—This is a plant sterol supplement. It's derived from insoluble wheat germ oil extracts and is supposed to assist the body in production of various hormones, such as growth hormone. It's also purported to help prevent the absorption of dietary fat. Unfortunately, there's no evidence to support this claim.

Diosterol—This is just another plant sterol derivative, with the unique marketing approach that it is brought all the way from the jungles of Africa. No documentation. Not even any good theory. In my opinion, worthless.

Glandulars—Use of glandular preparations in all areas of nutrition supplementation, including bodybuilding, has been popular for many years. These substances have shown incredible lasting power considering that every nutrition "expert" I know thinks glandulars are a bunch of hogwash. I mean, the idea of eating the freeze-dried extract from a bull's balls in order to increase your testosterone levels would appear to be wishful thinking at best.

The main argument against glandulars is that most proteins are completely destroyed in the gut. They are broken down into base amino acids before they are absorbed. If this is the case, then obviously any active-hormone content a glandular

REVIEW•SPORTS SUPPLEMENT REVIEW, 3RD ISSUE•SPORTS SUPPLEMENT REVIEW, 3RD ISSUE•SPORTS SUPPLEMENT REVIEW, 3RD ISSUE•SPORTS SUPPLEMENT REVIEW, 3RD ISSUE•SPORTS SUPPLEMENT

•SPORTS SUPPLEMENT REVIEW, 3RD ISSUE•SPORTS SUPPLEMENT REVIEW, 3RD ISSUE•SPORTS SUPPLEMENT REVIEW, 3RD ISSUE•SPORTS SUPPLEMENT REVIEW, 3RD ISSUE•SPORTS SUPPLEMENT REVIEW, 3RD ISSUE•SPORTS SUPPLEMENT REVIEW, 3RD ISSUE•SPORTS SUPPLEMENT REVIEW, 3RD ISSUE•SPORTS SUPPLEMENT

SUPPLEMENTS THAT SUCK

EMENTS THAT SUCK•SUPPLEMENTS THAT SUCK•SUPPLEMENTS THAT SUCK•SUPPLEMENTS THAT SUCK•SUPPLEMENTS THAT SUCK•SUPPLEMENTS THAT SUCK•SUPPLEMENTS THAT SUCK•SUPPLEMENTS THAT SUCK•SUPPLEMENTS THAT SUCK•SUPPLEMENTS THAT SUCK•SUPPLEMENTS THAT SUCK•SUPPLE

CHAPTER 5

preparation may have is lost during oral ingestion and subsequent digestion. The problem with this blanket supposition is that it may not necessarily be true.

Now I'm not saying I believe in the efficacy of glandulars; I'm just saying that there are studies out there which show that whole proteins can be absorbed in active form when taken orally.[6, 92] Take thyroid extract for example. Original thyroid medications were developed by extracting thyroxine from the glands of cattle and sheep. Now the synthetic form is used, but it's still an active protein hormone which is taken orally.

The real problem with glandulars on the market currently is that they just don't contain enough of the true hormone or enzyme you are looking for. The methods of extraction and purification used just aren't reliable, and the amount of raw glandular material it would take to create a truly potent product is cost prohibitive. Because gastrointestinal absorption is so limited, you'd need mega-doses of the pure active hormone to make an impact.

As far as I know, there are no studies done on humans using glandular extracts which show ANY beneficial effects for any kind of athlete, let alone hardcore bodybuilders.

Neonatal Glandular Extracts—This is a nice new twist on the glandular preparation scam. The contention is that by extracting glandular preparations from embryonic tissues, the activity of the hormones found in the tissue is much higher and has a greater effect. This is just plain hogwash. First, to actually extract enough embryonic glandular tissue to make a product which contains "viable" amounts of hormones would be cost prohibitive; therefore, my guess is these products don't contain much of what they say they contain. Secondly, the process of stabilizing active hormonal extracts and having them survive the gut system on their way into the bloodstream is, at best, highly unlikely. I don't use them.

Orchic Testosterone Extract—This is one of those products that makes you think of going out for a plate of Rocky Mountain Oysters. This is an extract made from powdered bull testes—obviously, another glandular supplement. The extract is supposed to contain active testosterone and be taken sublingually. Once again, you run into the problems of keeping testosterone viable during manufacturing. This stuff's never been tested. I don't believe it's effective at all.

Digestive Enzymes—These beauties have been around forever (or so it seems). You walk into a health-food store and there is a whole friggin' section dedicated to enzyme preparations. Now before I get carried away and go off on a rant, let me say that digestive enzyme products do have their place. I mean, there are people out there who have enzymatic deficiencies—whether it's a genetic metabolic error or a problem secondary to surgery. These people can benefit from the use of oral enzyme supplementation. For instance, the use of oral pancreatic enzyme replacement (the enzymes responsible for breaking down fat into its absorbable form) is well documented[37, 110] and accepted in the medical community. If you must have your pancreas removed, a little oral pancreatic enzyme preparation will go a long way.

One other subgroup which is much larger and may also benefit from enzymatic supplementation is made up of lactose-intolerant individuals. Taking a lactase supplement with any dairy product can help you digest the milk sugar and avoid unwanted gas.

But for healthy individuals, with properly functioning guts, forget it. There is just no documentation out there to warrant all of the claims being made about how taking enzymes will help you "more effectively utilize the nutrients you eat" or "help keep your digestive tract clean by avoiding the buildup of undigested food." I'm sorry, but this is reality! Our bodies have been doing a pretty good job of digesting the foods we eat a long, long time. I don't see why they would all of a sudden stop doing their jobs.

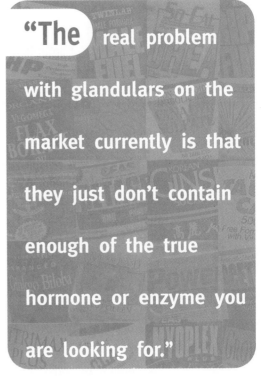

"The real problem with glandulars on the market currently is that they just don't contain enough of the true hormone or enzyme you are looking for."

And regarding performance enhancement, they may help you improve your two-capsule curls and your tilt and swallow, but that's about it. If you need pancreatic enzymes, your doctor will guide you. If you are lactose intolerant, use Lactaid as directed with milk. Other than that—who cares?

Sublingual Amino Acids—The contention here is that sublingual amino acids will be absorbed more quickly, thus, increasing blood concentrations more effectively. Once again, this has never been shown to be true. To my knowledge, there are no studies looking at sublingual amino acid delivery. If you look at it from a strictly biological point of view, amino acids are rather large molecules with very poor lipid solubility and are probably not absorbed very well at all sublingually. Not only that, but typically effective dosages of even important free-form amino acids, such as glutamine and taurine, are in gram quantities.

Desiccated Liver—Taking desiccated liver tablets is equivalent to taking badly contaminated amino acid tablets. You see, desiccated liver tablets are formed by vacuum drying at low temperatures. This process is effective for preserving all nutrients in a given substance; however, as far as the liver goes, I don't think that concentration mechanism is such a good idea. The liver is basically the

115

•SPORTS SUPPLEMENT REVIEW, 3RD ISSUE•SPORTS SUPPLEMENT REVIEW, 3RD ISSUE•SPORTS SUPPLEMENT REVIEW, 3RD ISSUE•SPORTS SUPPLEMENT REVIEW, 3RD ISSUE•SPORTS SUPPLEMENT REVIEW, 3RD ISSUE•SPORTS SUPPLEMENT REVIEW, 3RD ISSUE•SPORTS SUPPLEMENT REVIEW, 3RD ISSUE•SPORTS SUPPLEMENT

SUPPLEMENTS THAT SUCK

CHAPTER 5

EMENTS THAT SUCK•SUPPLEMENTS THAT SUCK•SUPPLEMENTS THAT SUCK•SUPPLEMENTS THAT SUCK•SUPPLEMENTS THAT SUCK•SUPPLEMENTS THAT SUCK•SUPPLEMENTS THAT SUCK•SUPPLEMENTS THAT SUCK•SUPPLEMENTS THAT SUCK•SUPPLEMENTS THAT SUCK•SUPPLEMENTS THAT SUCK•SUPPLE

garbage can of the body, filtering all of the toxins and heavy metals from the bloodstream throughout your lifetime. Although the liver does contain high levels of iron and fat-soluble vitamins, any benefit you might get from those substances found in these tablets would be far outweighed by the other toxic materials you would be ingesting along with them. These rate even below broad-spectrum amino acid tablets.

Medium-Chain Triglycerides (MCT)—This particular supplement *almost* had its "15 minutes of fame" back in the late '80's and early '90's when it was promoted as a fat burner and muscle builder. Today, "whatever" pretty much sums up my take on MCT—it's just not something I'm interested in, simply because I don't believe it's important for bodybuilders.

In terms of exactly what MCT is, in case you're interested (which I'm not), MCT is like normal fat in a way but it differs in its configuration; thus, it is absorbed and processed in the body slightly differently than regular fat, which must be broken down, combined with a protein, shuttled through something called the "lymph system" to the liver, and broken down into free fatty acids, which are either stored as bodyfat or converted to glucose and used as fuel. MCT, on the other hand, can enter the bloodstream directly, be converted immediately to glucose and used as fuel—much like dietary carbohydrates.

Back in the days of mega-calorie mania, bodybuilders who were convinced they needed to consume 8,000-10,000 calories a day to grow sometimes used MCT as a source of calories. Anyway, I don't want to go on and on about this—the bottom line is that although MCT is slightly different than regular fats, it's my opinion that it is not going to help you build muscle nor accelerate fat loss.

> **"Ecdysterone...** is a valuable hormone, *if you're an insect."*

Gamma Oryzanol/Ferulic Acid (FRAC)—They're advertised as being anabolic agents. It's claimed that the Japanese have used gamma oryzanol on their athletes for years. Supposed "research studies" have been done comparing gamma oryzanol head to head with very high doses of anabolic steroids "over 100 times the therapeutic dose." The results allegedly showed an average weight gain of 6.5 lbs for steroid users and 5 lbs for gamma oryzanol users. I'm sorry folks, but I just can't buy this. I mean, there's no way a test would ever be performed on humans using 100 times the therapeutic dose of steroids. And as for the effects of gamma oryzanol and its intermediate ferulic acid, they may be exactly the opposite of the ones claimed by distributors. The substance has been linked to actual decreases in secretion of luteinizing hormone, which can lead to decreases in testosterone production.

Pantocrine—This is one of a long line of weird "Russian supplements." It's an extract from the antlers of the male spotted deer found in Russia. It's supposed to increase muscular performance, but there really isn't any evidence to support that belief. There have been all kinds of rumors concerning pantocrine use during the Barcelona Olympics in '92, but none of it's been proven. What's more, there's reason to believe that taking pantocrine, either orally or via injection, could cause anaphylactic shock (a severe allergic reaction that may possibly lead to death). This is true anytime you introduce a foreign animal protein into your system. I can't think of any reason why I'd recommend pantocrine.

Ecdysterone—This is a valuable hormone, *if you're an insect*. It has been marketed as a bodybuilding supplement for years, but I just can't buy into the theory that this stuff is anabolic.

Dong Chong (Jing Zhi Dongchongxiacao)—With the possible restrictions on the herb ephedra on the horizon, supplement marketers are digging deep to find new stimulants and thermogenic aids that might act as alternatives. One of these is known in the market as "Dong Chong." Apparently, the active compound in this nutrient is called "*Cordyceps sinesis*." Studies using this compound, on laboratory animals, show it may enhance energy production—possibly in a manner like other compounds that mimic the effects of your body's fight-or-flight hormone, adrenaline (a "neuro-hormone").

Apparently, after you take a few grams of this stuff, you get a powerful "speed-like" effect that is reportedly similar to ephedrine.

It was rumored that this stuff was an herb, but in actuality, it's a fungus that grows on a certain caterpillar found in Sichuan, China, after the friggin' thing dies.

This stuff does have some speed-like effects, but if that's what you're looking for, stick with ephedra or just drink some strong coffee. I wouldn't mess with this stuff.

Smilax Officianalis—This is a plant sterol which has been on the marketplace for many years. As I've mentioned previously, certain plant constituents: namely, flavanoids, can have some bio-activity; however, the sterols in smilax have not been shown to cause any type of testosterone or performance enhancement. Smilax does absolutely nothing.

Shark Cartilage—Shark cartilage first became popular in 1992 when a slick marketer began pushing the substance as a possible cure for cancer. The reasoning was that sharks are the "only animals that don't get cancer." Well, sharks do get cancer, and there haven't been any legitimate studies to support the use of shark cartilage as a cancer fighter.

SUPPLEMENTS THAT SUCK

ments that suck•supplements that suck•supplements that suck•supplements that suck•supplements that suck•supplements that suck•supplements that suck•supplements that suck•supplements that suck•supplements that suck•supplements that suck•supple

Bodybuilders began to show an interest in shark cartilage because of its alleged effect on promoting the healing of damaged cartilage. Although some studies have been performed which show some effectiveness in this area,[155] it is only a small component of shark cartilage which appears to be the active agent in connective tissue health. The agent is glucosamine, which is becoming very popular in its purified form. Taking shark cartilage for joint health would be like eating four pounds of cheese to get your daily dose of CLA.

Inosine—This is a nucleic acid and it, along with other nucleic acids, forms the substance of DNA. Every living cell contains inosine, and people who use supplemental forms do so in hopes of increasing energy and exercise endurance. But a very recent study found no beneficial effects of inosine supplementation on aerobic or anaerobic performance.[260] In fact, it appeared that inosine actually lessened endurance due to increases in uric acid production.

The trouble is, inosine, <u>taken</u> <u>orally</u>, has never been shown to be effective at increasing endurance. One study was done looking at effects of <u>intravenous</u> inosine on the oxygen-carrying capacity of the blood—and it showed a nice increase. However, the results were never duplicated with oral inosine supplementation.[51]

There's no real evidence to suggest that inosine would help bodybuilders (or anyone else, for that matter).

Dibencozide—Dibencozide is a coenzyme of Vitamin B_{12}. When B_{12} is ingested, the body converts it into dibencozide. Dibencozide then assists the body in protein synthesis and the formation of red blood cells.

Because of these properties, Soviet scientists suspected it might help malnourished children gain weight and height. A 1969 study confirmed those beliefs.[262] However, American supplement manufacturers made an intuitive leap: they assumed that since it helped malnourished kids grow, it would help healthy athletes put on muscle.

Anyhow, dibencozide sales flourished briefly in the late '80's but quickly fizzled out soon after. Athletes thought they could achieve greater protein synthesis, increased appetite, and have a greater sense of well-being. I don't think dibencozide is all that great even though I used to use it. Besides, even if it were useful, it'd be damn hard to find any; real dibencozide is extremely oxygen, light, and temperature sensitive. Once it's exposed, it rapidly converts to ordinary B_{12}.

Exsativa—I don't know where this one came from... Exsativa is a blend of oats, nettle root, and Vitamin C. It's supposed to increase testosterone levels, and some poor jokers even use it as an aphrodisiac. Again, there's no evidence to support the claims of Exsativa distributors.

Coenzyme Q10 — There is no disputing the crucial role coenzyme Q10 (CoQ10) plays in energy production throughout the body. It has also been documented to have potent antioxidant characteristics.[257, 292] All of that is fine and dandy, but will taking oral doses actually help athletes perform better?

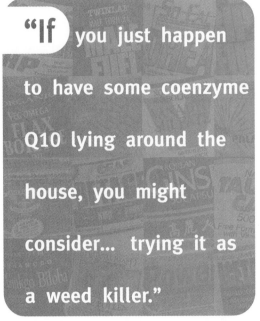

"If you just happen to have some coenzyme Q10 lying around the house, you might consider... trying it as a weed killer."

The answer appears to be NO! And for that reason, my stance on this supplement has not changed since I put it on the "F" list in the *1996 Supplement Review*. As a matter of fact, I have come across even more evidence to suggest coenzyme Q10 has no effect on exercise performance in healthy individuals and may even hinder it.

One very solid study using a double-blind, cross-over design looked at the effects of 300 mg/day of coenzyme Q10, plus a few other nutrients, on the performance of 11 elite triathletes. No significant differences were noted in ANY performance parameters between the coenzyme Q10 group and the placebo group.[256] One other study performed on untrained men using 150 mg/day reported similar results.[222]

Not only does this stuff not help, it may actually hurt your muscle-building efforts! A new study involving coenzyme Q10 and 15 healthy males showed that the stuff, under conditions of intense exercise, may actually cause cell damage secondary to possible <u>pro</u>-oxidant activity when taken in supplemental amounts.[165]

Don't waste your time or money on this one! If you just happen to have some coenzyme Q10 lying around the house, you might consider mixing it with a little water and trying it as a weed killer.

SUMMARY

I could go on and on about this subject—I could talk forever about supplements that suck because it's a topic I'm very passionate about and one that really drives me crazy. There are so many products on the market that I think are rip-offs—that I think *suck*. Those include ones that don't contain what their labels claim; knock-off products that are often inferior imitations of the original; supplements that don't come with a money-back guarantee; products that contain ingredients that just don't work; supplements that are based on a false premise (like high-calorie weight-gain products, which is a totally outdated bodybuilding-nutrition theory); and supplements that are based on science that I just don't believe is valid, such as homeopathy.

SUPPLEMENTS THAT SUCK

EMENTS THAT SUCK•SUPPLEMENTS THAT SUCK•SUPPLEMENTS THAT SUCK•SUPPLEMENTS THAT SUCK•SUPPLEMENTS THAT SUCK•SUPPLEMENTS THAT SUCK•SUPPLEMENTS THAT SUCK•SUPPLEMENTS THAT SUCK•SUPPLEMENTS THAT SUCK•SUPPLEMENTS THAT SUCK•SUPPLEMENTS THAT SUCK•SUPPLE

CHAPTER 5

The best advice I can offer at this point is to educate yourself about what is and isn't real in the bodybuilding supplement industry. Arm yourself with knowledge. Be skeptical and watch out for these fly-by-night operations that are only out to make a quick buck.

In updates to this book, and in future issues of my magazine *Muscle Media*, you can rest assured you'll get a great deal of up-to-date input on supplements that I think are a waste of money—ones that don't warrant your attention—ones that, in my opinion, *suck*.

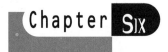

The Wide, Wide World of Vitamins and Minerals: What They Are and What They Do

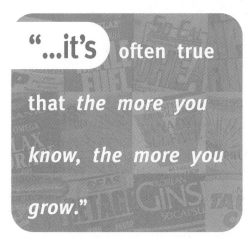

"...it's often true that *the more you know, the more you grow.*"

Accumcording to the U.S. Department of Agriculture, roughly 39% of all Americans use vitamin and mineral supplements daily. According to *my* estimates, over 80% of all bodybuilders regularly use vitamin and mineral supplements of one kind or another. (Folks like us tend to be extremely compulsive and adamant about taking care of our bodies and doing anything possible to maximize our muscle-building and fat-loss efforts.) But, I've discovered most bodybuilders don't really understand what the individual vitamins and minerals are nor what they do. Even though it's not absolutely essential that you have an understanding of this issue, I believe those of you who are into the "nuts and bolts" of bodybuilding nutrition and supplementation will find this to be very valuable information. Truthfully, if you read and perhaps reread this chapter, you'll know more about the aspects of nutrition than most bodybuilders on the planet. And, when it comes to bodybuilding, it's often true that *the more you know, the more you grow*.

WHAT ARE VITAMINS AND MINERALS?

In a broad sense, vitamins and minerals are considered "essential" dietary nutrients—meaning our bodies don't make them; therefore, they must be obtained from the diet or supplementation. Another term typically used by scientists and clinical texts to categorize vitamins and minerals is "micronutrients" because they're needed by the body in only very minute quantities compared with requirements for carbohydrates and protein. ("Micro" means small.) Although only small amounts of these nutrients are used by the body, they play a vital role in maintaining the proper biological functioning of everything from muscles to memory. Vitamins and minerals contribute to good health, muscle growth, and proper fat burning by regulating the metabolism and assisting the

121

•SPORTS SUPPLEMENT REVIEW, 3RD ISSUE•SPORTS SUPPLEMENT REVIEW, 3RD ISSUE•SPORTS SUPPLEMENT REVIEW, 3RD ISSUE•SPORTS SUPPLEMENT REVIEW, 3RD ISSUE•SPORTS SUPPLEMENT REVIEW, 3RD ISSUE•SPORTS SUPPLEMENT REVIEW, 3RD ISSUE•SPORTS SUPPLEMENT REVIEW, 3RD ISSUE•SPORTS SUPPLEMENT

THE WIDE, WIDE WORLD OF VITAMINS AND MINERALS: WHAT THEY ARE AND WHAT THEY DO

MINERALS: WHAT THEY ARE AND WHAT THEY DO•THE WIDE, WIDE WORLD OF VITAMINS AND MINERALS: WHAT THEY ARE AND WHAT THEY DO•THE WIDE, WIDE WORLD OF VITAMINS AND MINERALS: WHAT THEY ARE AND WHAT THEY DO•THE WIDE, WIDE WORLD OF VITAMINS AND MINERALS: WHAT THEY ARE AND WHAT THEY DO•THE

biochemical processes that release energy from digested food. If you don't take in enough of these vital micronutrients to maintain proper biological levels, deficiency symptoms, which include muscle weakness, connective-tissue deterioration, and suppression of the immune system, just to name a few, will appear.

Vitamins are "organic" compounds, which means they are produced naturally in both vegetables and animals and are therefore found in abundant quantities in both of these food sources. The main function of vitamins in the system is to act as "coenzymes" (i.e., substances that enhance the action of proteins which induce chemical reactions). Enzymes are catalysts in all chemical reactions that take place in the body. These reactions include energy metabolism and muscle building, to name only two of thousands. As coenzymes, vitamins are an essential component of enzymatic activity—without vitamins, enzymes simply wouldn't work; you wouldn't build muscle, and your body wouldn't be able to convert the food you eat into all the magnificent chemicals that make up the human body. (Bottom line—these little dudes are very important!)

Vitamins are either fat soluble or water soluble, depending on whether fat- or water-based molecules transport the vitamin through the bloodstream. Fat-soluble vitamins include A, D, E, and K. Because these vitamins have an affinity for fat, they can be stored in both adipose (fat) tissue and in the liver, extending their functional life span in the body and strongly decreasing the chance of developing deficiencies. The water-soluble vitamins include all of the B vitamins and Vitamin C; they aren't stored in the body for more than a few hours, so daily intake is a must.

Way back in 1911, there were only two known vitamins: a fat-soluble vitamin called "A" and a water-soluble vitamin called "B." Within a decade, another vitamin was isolated and called "C." In the early 1920's, another fat-soluble element was discovered in Vitamin A. This was then designated as "Vitamin D." By 1948, all of the currently known vitamins had been defined.

Minerals are *in*organic in nature, meaning they are *not produced* by plants nor animals. They can, however, be found in food sources (e.g., iron in red meat, calcium in milk, and potassium in bananas.) Minerals are extremely important for your body to work right. They are essential for neural conduction (dats your brain, mon), muscular contraction, fluid balance, and energy production. Many minerals also serve as building blocks for body tissues, such as calcium and phosphorus for bones.

Minerals are subcategorized as either "bulk" or "trace" depending on the amount needed by the body. Bulk minerals include calcium, magnesium, phosphorus, potassium, and sodium and are typically needed in close to gram quantities. Trace minerals, on the other hand, may be required in quantities as little as a few micrograms (that's one one-thousandth of a milligram). These include chromium, cobalt, copper, iron, selenium, silicon, and zinc.

Before 1941, there was no such thing as an established Recommended Daily Allowance (RDA). There were no guidelines whatsoever regarding necessary intakes of vitamins and minerals to maintain health. Because of this, many of the rations prepared for foot soldiers in World War II were incomplete and did not provide sufficient vitamins and minerals. Foot soldiers became sick and even died due to nutrient deficiencies in the field. This prompted a government group called the Food and Nutrition Board to establish human vitamin and mineral needs to avoid deficiency, hence, the RDA.

The RDA is defined as "the levels of intake of the essential nutrients that, on the basis of scientific knowledge, are judged by the Food and Nutrition Board to be adequate to meet the known nutrient needs of practically all healthy persons." Basically, the RDA's were established *to avoid deficiency syndromes*. The Food and Nutrition Board has never taken a close look at what *optimal* intake levels should be. By optimal, I mean not just avoidance of disease but optimizing all parameters of health and performance. For that reason, I consider the RDA's a starting point and a safety net, but they're not to be taken as scripture for optimal intake levels.

All right, enough scientific mumbo jumbo—here's a list of every vitamin and mineral I could think of, along with a brief description of what each of these nutrients does:

> "...the RDA's were established *to avoid deficiency syndromes.* ...they're not to be taken as scripture for optimal intake levels."

The VITAMINS

CAROTENES

Almost everyone has heard of beta-carotene, but it's only one of a group of 300 vitamin-like nutrients called carotenes. These unique nutrients have a variety of functions in the body, including pro-Vitamin A activity and powerful antioxidant potential.

Of all the carotenes, beta-carotene is most readily converted to Vitamin A in the body. Despite a bit of bad press which beta-carotene has received over the past year or so, I believe it is the safest and most effective way to meet your Vitamin A requirements. It's nontoxic, is only converted to Vitamin A in the body as needed, and has much greater antioxidant activity than pure Vitamin A.[154] In order to avoid any of the possible, although unlikely, side effects caused by beta-carotene supplementation,

THE WIDE, WIDE WORLD OF VITAMINS AND MINERALS: WHAT THEY ARE AND WHAT THEY DO

CHAPTER 6

MINERALS: WHAT THEY ARE AND WHAT THEY DO·THE WIDE, WIDE WORLD OF VITAMINS AND MINERALS: WHAT THEY ARE AND WHAT THEY DO·THE WIDE, WIDE WORLD OF VITAMINS AND MINERALS: WHAT THEY ARE AND WHAT THEY DO·THE WIDE, WIDE WORLD OF VITAMINS AND MINERALS: WHAT THEY ARE AND WHAT THEY DO·THE

THE WIDE, WIDE WORLD OF VITAMINS AND MINERALS: WHAT THEY ARE AND WHAT THEY DO·THE WIDE, WIDE WORLD OF VITAMINS AND MINERALS, WHAT THEY ARE AND WHAT THEY DO·THE WIDE, WIDE WORLD OF VITAMINS AND MINERALS, WHAT THEY ARE AND WHAT THEY DO·THE WIDE, WIDE WORLD OF VITAMINS AND

I recommend combining it with extra doses of Vitamins C (1 gram), E (400 IU), and selenium (100 mcg).

As for the antioxidant effects of carotenes, lycopene (a rather obscure carotene found in tomatoes and palm oil) has been shown to have the highest activity level.[70]

I think your best overall source of mixed carotenes—including beta and lycopene—is palm oil extract. Don't worry about the saturated fat content; the fat's almost completely removed during the extraction process.

Supplementation with carotenes is important to avoid a deficiency, to help you meet your Vitamin A needs, and to supply antioxidant protection.

Although it's virtually impossible to overdose on beta-carotene, you may experience one quirky side effect if you take too much. Consuming gram doses can actually make your skin turn orange—making you look a little like the "great pumpkin." This happens because fat-soluble carotenes—which are naturally endowed with a bright-orange hue—become concentrated in the fatty layer right below the skin. This is not harmful; it just makes it hard to find shirts that don't clash with your face.

Dosage: Around 120 mg/day of beta-carotene is plenty. Alternatively, a gram of carotenes extracted from palm oil per day should get the job done.

VITAMIN A

Vitamin A has never been on the top of my supplement list. And now with the upsurge in beta-carotene popularity, Vitamin A is perceived as almost obsolete. However, because beta-carotene is unable to synthesize enough Vitamin A in the body to create supraphysiological levels, Vitamin A may have a place for use in special situations. Nonetheless, pure Vitamin A supplementation above the RDA levels will probably do nothing to enhance muscular performance or development.

One situation where Vitamin A seems to be helpful is with acne. Short-term supplementation with mega-doses of pure Vitamin A (300,000-500,000 IU) has been widely used for many years in the treatment of various acne conditions.[146] It appears to help eradicate acne by blocking the buildup of certain proteins which can clog the pores of your skin. The problem with this treatment is that mega-doses of Vitamin A can become very toxic and damage the liver.

"...Vitamin C has a multitude of beneficial biological effects, many of which are substantiated by high-quality clinical research."

Vitamin A is also used as the base of various skin creams, the most popular being "Retin-A."

Some experts suggest combining a much lower dose of Vitamin A (30,000 IU) with Vitamin E and zinc citrate. This may be just as effective and is definitely safer because Vitamin E and zinc citrate potentiate the effects of Vitamin A, and since a lower amount of Vitamin A is needed, the toxicity is decreased.

One more point of interest is that Vitamin A has been shown to have some rather impressive antiviral activity.[201] In fact, it may actually help stave off the dreaded common cold.

Dosage: For daily maintenance, I suggest sticking with beta-carotene, around 120 mg/day. If you feel a cold coming on, try 50,000-75,000 IU/day of pure Vitamin A for 3-4 days. For help controlling acne, try 30,000 IU of Vitamin A plus 800 IU of Vitamin E and 40 mg of zinc citrate.

VITAMIN C

As I mentioned in the *1996 Supplement Review*, Vitamin C has a multitude of beneficial biological effects, many of which are substantiated by high-quality clinical research. These benefits range from Vitamin C's powerful antioxidant and immunosupportive effects to its role in ligament and tendon synthesis.[219, 234] And it has been documented to actually suppress the body's natural production of cortisol, thus supporting a stronger testosterone to cortisol ratio. All of this is obviously important stuff to those of us who are training and working hard and demanding that our bodies keep up.

I suggest that all hard-training athletes supplement their diets with at least three grams of Vitamin C a day, and I think there are specific times when you should consider doubling or even *tripling* that amount. One such time is when you are in any kind of moderate to severe calorie-restricted state. You see, what I have discovered while researching Torbjorn Akerfeldt's new Anabolic Burst Cycling System (see Chapters 15 and 16) is that when you suppress your calorie intake *and* continue to train hard, you create a catabolic biochemical environment. Not only does the body tend to crank up its free-radical production and decrease its natural antioxidant protection,[231] it increases the excretion rate of Vitamin C as well.[98]

This combination of reactions may account for much of the muscle wasting and propensity towards sickness that bodybuilders experience when cutting up. In order to combat this catabolic and immunosuppressive response, I suggest taking between six and eight grams of Vitamin C per day during your dieting phase. Take these in one- or two-gram doses throughout the day, with meals for greater absorption.

When looking for a C supplement, don't get caught up in the marketing hoopla over such expensive forms as "ester C." Studies indicate that plain old ascorbic acid

THE WIDE, WIDE WORLD OF VITAMINS AND MINERALS: WHAT THEY ARE AND WHAT THEY DO

MINERALS: WHAT THEY ARE AND WHAT THEY DO·THE WIDE, WIDE WORLD OF VITAMINS AND MINERALS: WHAT THEY ARE AND WHAT THEY DO·THE WIDE, WIDE WORLD OF VITAMINS AND MINERALS: WHAT THEY ARE AND WHAT THEY DO·THE WIDE, WIDE WORLD OF VITAMINS AND MINERALS: WHAT THEY ARE AND WHAT THEY DO·THE

(the chemical name for Vitamin C) is absorbed and utilized by the body every bit as well.[137]

Dosage: Take three grams daily during times of good health and low stress. Take up to eight grams a day when dieting down or when you feel a cold coming on.

VITAMIN D

With exposure to direct sunlight, the body can produce its own Vitamin D. For this reason, it's considered both a vitamin and a hormone. (Seems kind of weird, huh?) For those who have little exposure to sunlight, Vitamin D becomes an essential vitamin.

The main function of Vitamin D is regulation of calcium absorption. In other words, it's responsible for getting calcium into the bloodstream and delivering it to the bones for building purposes. Vitamin D deficiency has been strongly connected to decreases in bone strength and density.

One very recent study has documented the effects of Vitamin D on osteoarthritis in previously injured joints. Researchers found that individuals with long-standing joint injuries who used 400 IU/day (or slightly more) of Vitamin D reduced the progression of arthritis in their joints by 50% compared to individuals with an intake below 350 IU/day.[171]

So, although Vitamin D supplementation will probably not make any noticeable differences in day to day performance in the gym, it may help delay the progression of any trauma-related arthritis (which is unfortunately common to many long-time bodybuilders).

Dosage: In cold or cloudy climates, shoot for 600-700 IU/day. In sunny climates, 400-500 IU should be sufficient.

VITAMIN E

Best known for its antioxidant effects, this fat-soluble vitamin also had 15 minutes of fame when it was touted as the "anti-sterility" or "virility" vitamin back in the '80's. Unfortunately, this "virility" effect was not due to something as interesting as increased testosterone production; the effect was due to Vitamin E's ability to protect the cellular membrane of sperm.

Vitamin E's main function is indeed to protect all cellular membranes in the body from oxidative stress. One study showed 1,200 mg/day of E, taken for 14 days prior to an exhaustive exercise bout, virtually eliminated the white-blood-cell DNA damage typically seen following intense muscular activity.[114] This may help hard-training athletes maintain a stronger immune system, thus avoiding some of the typical consequences of overtraining: namely, infection and sickness.

Another interesting study showed that Vitamin E may play a role in insulin sensitivity. Ten healthy subjects who took 1,350 IU/day of E for 4 months showed significantly improved insulin sensitivity and glucose clearance.[211] Although no studies have been done to document benefits for the average person, proper insulin sensitivity—as you are most likely aware—is important for muscle building.

Dosage: For very active athletes, I suggest 1,200-1,500 IU/day. Stick with the natural *d*-alpha-tocopherol form, as it is the most biologically active.

VITAMIN K

This fat-soluble vitamin plays a crucial role in the process of blood *coagulation*. Without it, your blood would simply not clot, and even a minor scratch could continue to bleed indefinitely.

Vitamin K does have one other recently discovered function. It has been found to act much like Vitamin D, in that it helps modify a certain bone protein which causes this protein to bind with calcium, thereby strengthening the bone matrix.[269]

Due to the fact that Vitamin K requirements are only about 100-150 mcg/day (which you can get by eating a mere 3 oz of any number of green vegetables), deficiencies are very rare.

There's no documentation to suggest that excess Vitamin K supplementation will benefit bodybuilders in any way.

Dosage: 100-150 mcg/day. You can get this from three ounces of broccoli, spinach, or a small cup of green tea.

VITAMIN B₁ (THIAMIN)

This is a vitamin that is really rather one dimensional. Its sole known purpose is to act as a coenzyme that promotes proper energy production and nerve cell function. Both of these actions are obviously important in assuring proper muscle function. However, mega-doses of thiamin in healthy individuals do not appear to improve energy production nor neural function beyond what is considered normal.

A couple of interesting studies have shown that 3-8 *grams*/day of thiamin (the RDA is only 1.5 *mg*) may help improve mental function and memory in aging,

> " ...**mega-doses** of thiamin in healthy individuals do not appear to improve energy production nor neural function..."

"senile" individuals.[25, 177] It appears to do this by potentiating and mimicking the effects of acetylcholine (a neurotransmitter involved in memory).[176]

You can cover your RDA for thiamin by consuming a six-ounce bowl of oatmeal and a slice of toast with peanut butter. You should be well covered if you consume a high-quality meal-replacement powder or a high-potency multivitamin daily.

One final note for you hardcore "java-heads"—coffee may destroy thiamin. So make sure you take your multivitamin with something other than coffee.

Dosage: I suggest about 50 mg/day of thiamin. There is no known toxicity level, so don't worry about high-potency multivitamins that include mega-doses of this vitamin. Your body excretes excess water-soluble vitamins in the urine.

VITAMIN B$_2$ (RIBOFLAVIN)

Since Vitamin B$_2$ is found in meats, fish, poultry, and milk products, only strict vegetarians are typically at risk for riboflavin deficiency. Those of us who drink skim milk like it's water, eat poultry like we've got a chicken coop in the backyard, and/or eat tuna like we own stock in Star-Kist don't need to worry about our riboflavin levels.

After scouring the research, I found no documentation to suggest that mega-dosing this micronutrient will offer any substantial benefits to athletes. However, research has shown that increased energy expenditure and hard work increase riboflavin requirements.[280] Therefore, if you're a hard-training, strict vegetarian, you may want to supplement with 10-20 mg/day. The human intestine may be <u>un</u>able to assimilate more than 20 mg in a single oral dose.[193] Anything over that in a supplement will probably end up in your toilet. (The upside is you'll have pretty, bright-orange pee which looks really cool in the snow [hey, when you're out skiing, and you gotta go...].)

Dosage: 10-20 mg/day should be sufficient for hard-training athletes.

VITAMIN B$_3$ (NIACIN)

I'm not even sure niacin should be considered an essential vitamin because our bodies can actually synthesize it from the amino acid tryptophan. Even though strenuous training will increase your niacin requirement,[125] an intake of over 150 grams/day of quality protein (which every bodybuilder should be shooting for) supplies your body with more than enough niacin precursor to meet your physiological needs.

> **"Because** of Vitamin B$_6$'s close connection with amino-acid metabolism, your intake should vary with your level of protein consumption."

There isn't any evidence to suggest that mega-dosing niacin will increase your anabolic potential, but there are a couple of interesting therapeutic uses. It has been used for years to treat high cholesterol levels, but mega-doses can be hard on the liver and—because of its vasodilating effects—niacin can cause a dramatic "flushed" sensation and appearance, especially in the face.

(Back in the mid '80's, we used to pop a handful of niacin tablets while we were pumping up before bodybuilding contests. It helps bring out vascularity, but using too much made my face as red as a tomato and gave me a headache. Plus, it comes out in your sweat, and you smell like a huge vitamin pill [Pee-uuw!].)

The other therapeutic application may interest those of you who experience cramping problems—especially in the calf muscles. A very specialized form of niacin called "inositol hexanicotinate" has been used for many years in Europe to help treat chronic calf cramping and Raynaud's disease (which is caused by an abnormal degree of spasms of the blood vessels in a person's extremities). This supplement exerts its effects by increasing blood flow to peripheral tissues,[267] and this form of niacin is much easier on the liver and doesn't cause "flushing."

Dosage: For general health, consume at least 150 grams of quality protein and/or 25-30 mg of niacinamide a day. For treatment of cramping, start with about 500 mg of inositol hexanicotinate 3 times a day and work up to 1 gram 3 times a day after about 2 weeks.

VITAMIN B₅ (PANTOTHENIC ACID)

Pantothenic acid is sort of a "pseudo-vitamin." It's found so widely in the foods we eat on a daily basis that the scientists who named it used the Greek word *pantos*, which means "everywhere," as the root. There has never been a documented case of accidental pantothenic acid deficiency, except in connection with serious calorie deprivation.

This pseudo-vitamin plays a role as a typical coenzyme in energy production, but there are no studies which even vaguely address the issue of pantothenic acid's effects on exercise performance in regular or mega-doses.

Dosage: There's no RDA, but four to seven milligrams per day is considered sufficient.

VITAMIN B₆ (PYRIDOXINE)

This is one of the most thoroughly studied vitamins. Scientists have examined therapeutic applications of pyridoxine for everything from asthma to epilepsy. Although deficiencies are pretty uncommon, they are on the upswing due to the highly processed nature of most of the foods in our diets. Because of the important role of B₆ in so many vital bodily functions, a deficiency can be devastating.

THE WIDE, WIDE WORLD OF VITAMINS AND MINERALS: WHAT THEY ARE AND WHAT THEY DO

MINERALS: WHAT THEY ARE AND WHAT THEY DO•THE WIDE, WIDE WORLD OF VITAMINS AND MINERALS: WHAT THEY ARE AND WHAT THEY DO•THE WIDE, WIDE WORLD OF VITAMINS AND MINERALS: WHAT THEY ARE AND WHAT THEY DO•THE WIDE, WIDE WORLD OF VITAMINS AND MINERALS: WHAT THEY ARE AND WHAT THEY DO•THE WIDE, WIDE WORLD OF VITAMINS AND MINERALS: WHAT THEY ARE AND WHAT THEY DO•THE

CHAPTER 6

One result of a B_6 deficiency is a decrease in the uptake of amino acids by muscle cells. (This especially applies to hard-training athletes trying to maximize muscle gains.) Scientists believe this response may be due to significant reductions in growth hormone and insulin secretion.[9]

It's obviously important to avoid a deficiency, but current scientific information doesn't warrant mega-dosing. Because of Vitamin B_6's close connection with amino-acid metabolism, your intake should vary with your level of protein consumption.

Dosage: I recommend 0.10 mg/gram of protein intake. For example, if you're consuming 150 grams of protein, you should take 15 mg of Vitamin B_6 per day.

VITAMIN B_{12}

The active form of this water-soluble vitamin is not found in vegetable sources. (Researchers have found the form in sea vegetables and tofu to be virtually unusable by the body.) Only animal-derived foods contain viable amounts of B_{12}. For this reason, many nutritionists advise strict vegetarians to take a B_{12} supplement. Although this is probably sound advice, I have never heard of any vegetarian—bodybuilder or otherwise—who has ever experienced a B_{12} deficiency.

Even if you didn't consume a single speck of B_{12} for three years (the RDA is two micrograms per day), you probably wouldn't notice any of the typical signs of deficiency, which include anemia and neural dysfunction. It simply takes too long for your body to become depleted (five to six years).

There also isn't much support for the marketing claims of energy enhancements. In one study, researchers injected one milligram of B_{12} into subjects three times per week for six weeks and noticed no change in performance in pull-ups or leg lifts.[274]

Nonetheless, B_{12} supplementation (injections especially) is quite popular with bodybuilders who believe it helps boost energy levels, protect the liver, and increase appetite. I used to take huge doses of B_{12}, sometimes the injectable form, but I can't honestly say it did anything for me.

If you've been raised as a strict vegetarian from childhood and decide you need a B_{12} supplement, don't go for the injections. They cost more, hurt more, and have been shown to be no more effective than using the oral cyanocobalamin form at 500 mcg/day.[157]

Dosage: Eat a two-egg omelet and a tuna sandwich and you'll be covered for the day.

BIOTIN

Are you one of those rare individuals who still adheres to the Rocky Balboa school of protein supplementation? If so, you may be at risk for biotin deficiency.

You see, raw egg whites contain a protein called "avidin," which strongly binds to biotin in the gut, blocking all absorption.

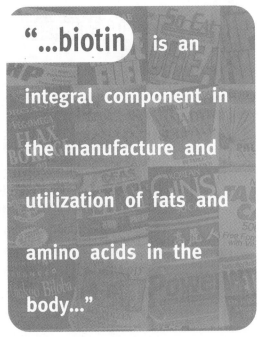

"...biotin is an integral component in the manufacture and utilization of fats and amino acids in the body..."

Because biotin is an integral component in the manufacture and utilization of fats and amino acids in the body, a deficiency is a bad thing. So I suggest avoiding raw egg whites and instead focusing on consuming your oatmeal, peanuts, and soy products—all of which are good sources of biotin.

As far as an application for bodybuilding, there has been some interesting work examining the effects of biotin on insulin sensitivity. One such study showed a significant lowering of fasting blood sugar levels and better blood glucose control overall in type II diabetics taking nine milligrams of biotin per day.[163] Only further research can tell us whether or not this would translate to improved blood sugar regulation and insulin function in healthy athletes.

Dosage: 500 mcg/day for general health. If you're diabetic or think you're hypoglycemic, try about ten milligrams per day and monitor your energy and blood sugar levels.

FOLATE

Folate (also known as folic acid) deficiency is the most common vitamin deficiency in the world. This is probably because the only really good sources of folate are beans and green, leafy veggies, and folate is very easily destroyed by light and heat. People just don't eat their beans and veggies like they should (me included), and when they do eat them, they typically cook the hell out of them, destroying any folate present.

Even moderate deficiencies can put you at risk for anemia, causing lethargy and muscular weakness. On the other hand, mega-doses of five to ten milligrams have been shown to exhibit mild antidepressant effects.[66] Nonetheless, as long as there's no deficiency, there's no evidence that folate supplementation can improve performance.

When looking for a multivitamin that includes folate, try to find one that contains the crystalline "folinic acid" form. Although the "folic acid" form will indeed do the job, folinic acid is the most easily absorbed, and research indicates it's the most effective in raising body stores of folate.[193]

Dosage: For general health, shoot for one milligram per day. If you have trouble with depression, seven milligrams per day may help improve your mood.

THE WIDE, WIDE WORLD OF VITAMINS AND MINERALS: WHAT THEY ARE AND WHAT THEY DO

MINERALS: WHAT THEY ARE AND WHAT THEY DO•THE WIDE, WIDE WORLD OF VITAMINS AND MINERALS: WHAT THEY ARE AND WHAT THEY DO•THE WIDE, WIDE WORLD OF VITAMINS AND MINERALS: WHAT THEY ARE AND WHAT THEY DO•THE WIDE, WIDE WORLD OF VITAMINS AND MINERALS: WHAT THEY ARE AND WHAT THEY DO•THE

The MINERALS

BORON

Scientists aren't absolutely sure what boron does in the human body. There's some evidence to suggest it might be useful in preventing or helping to treat osteoporosis and arthritis. One thing seems sure, though; despite the claims of some seedy supplement companies, boron supplementation has absolutely no effect on testosterone levels in men. As I've mentioned before, this alleged benefit of boron supplementation came about from the results of a single study that found increased testosterone production in post-menopausal women who began taking boron.[199] This study has no relevance to normal males.

There's relatively new evidence that boron may play a role in how calcium, magnesium, and phosphorus are metabolized; the exact role isn't clear yet, but exercise appears to exert a mediating effect.[174, 175]

Boron is contained in fruits and vegetables.

Dosage: There's no RDA for boron, but it seems a daily intake of between 1.5 mg and 3 mg/day is plenty.

> "...hard-training athletes... may benefit from... calcium supplementation."

CALCIUM

Calcium is by far the most abundant mineral in the body. It forms the structural matrix which gives the strength to our bones, fingernails, and teeth. Calcium also plays a vital biochemical role by helping regulate muscle contraction, heartbeat, blood clotting, and the release of certain neurotransmitters.

Not only is calcium important in all of these biochemical functions but it's also been suggested that supplementing with it may help promote gains in lean mass in athletes. One recent study in *JAMA* (*The Journal of the American Medical Association*) looked at the effects of calcium supplementation on bone mineral content and muscle mass in male athletes. Researchers found that bone mineral content in athletes—especially endurance athletes—was lower than in sedentary controls. The athletes' diets were supplemented with between 500 and 2,000 mg of calcium daily; the study showed that subjects not only increased bone mineral density but lean body mass as well.[144] Therefore, it appears hard-training athletes who lose more calcium may benefit from some degree of calcium supplementation.

The most common deficiency pertains mainly to female athletes; that's the development of osteoporosis (literally translated "porous bone"), which can cause bones to become weak and brittle, especially later in life. Studies actually show that many female athletes consume less calcium than the RDA, and because their needs are probably higher than the RDA, this can easily lead to calcium deficiencies, weak bone structure, and ultimately, stress fractures.[56] Stress fractures are quite common for female athletes.

One other point of interest is calcium's effect on blood pressure. Population studies show that individuals with chronically lower intakes of calcium tend to have higher blood pressure.[45] Calcium supplementation has been found to be especially helpful for blacks and individuals who are salt sensitive and those who show signs of hypertension.[178] So, if your blood pressure tends to run high, calcium supplementation may be a good idea.

Dosage: The current RDA for calcium is 1,000 mg/day for adults. Typically, those of us who consume a lot of dairy products will hit this RDA level with no problem. However, if you avoid dairy products, are a female athlete, or suffer from even mild hypertension, a calcium supplement may be a good idea. One way to supplement your calcium intake is by taking HMB. The active HMB molecule is actually bound to elemental calcium in order to create a stabilized compound. One gram of HMB contains 128 mg of calcium. However, when taking a straight calcium supplement, I would recommend using a calcium citrate form over the more common calcium carbonate, as it is better absorbed in the system and less likely to cause kidney stones if taken in supplemental amounts.[5] If you have high blood pressure, you might try taking in 500 mg/day.

CHROMIUM

Chromium has probably been the hottest mineral in the media and on the marketplace during the past seven years. It has been touted by patent holders and distributors alike as a remedy for everything from hypoglycemia to obesity. So, is chromium the real deal? What's fact, and what's fiction?

As with any nutritional element subjected to extensive media hype, chromium's actual scientific applications have been a bit overblown and misconstrued. I'll try to outline for you what the studies really show and what this stuff does and doesn't do.

Chromium's key function in the body is to act as a coenzyme in insulin action—it helps insulin do its job. At this point, I think it's safe to say science has shown chromium deficiencies indeed play a role in the development of both insulin-resistant diabetes and hypoglycemia. This, in turn, can lead to less-than-optimal muscle and fat metabolism. Numerous studies have indicated that supplementing the diet of non-insulin dependent diabetics and/or hypoglycemic individuals with at least 200 mcg of chromium per day can significantly decrease fasting glucose levels, improve glucose tolerance, lower overall insulin levels, and alleviate symptoms of hypoglycemia.[1, 7, 8, 191] You see, it appears that most of the population with intakes below 100

THE WIDE, WIDE WORLD OF VITAMINS AND MINERALS: WHAT THEY ARE AND WHAT THEY DO

CHAPTER 6

MINERALS: WHAT THEY ARE AND WHAT THEY DO•THE WIDE, WIDE WORLD OF VITAMINS AND MINERALS: WHAT THEY ARE AND WHAT THEY DO•THE WIDE, WIDE WORLD OF VITAMINS AND MINERALS: WHAT THEY ARE AND WHAT THEY DO•THE WIDE, WIDE WORLD OF VITAMINS AND MINERALS: WHAT THEY ARE AND WHAT THEY DO•THE WIDE, WIDE WORLD OF VITAMINS AND MINERALS: WHAT THEY ARE AND WHAT THEY DO•THE

134

mcg/day is probably marginally chromium deficient. By supplementing the diet with chromium, that deficiency is eradicated; thus, the symptoms are as well.

As far as bodybuilders are concerned, I think it is important to avoid a chromium deficiency because insulin resistance can lead to increases in bodyfat and can impair proper muscle metabolism. There have been some studies which show chromium supplementation may, indeed, help people lose excess bodyfat and gain muscle.[138] Test subjects who consumed 200 mcg of chromium per day over a 10-week period lost 3.3 lbs of fat and gained 1.5 lbs of muscle, while the placebo group lost only .4 lbs of fat and did not gain any lean body mass. Keep in mind that these results used subjects who were not highly conditioned athletes and probably already had some type of insulin resistance and chromium deficiency to begin with.

There was a relatively recent study done with football players which showed that the subjects receiving chromium noticed no significant changes in body composition over and above the placebo group.[55] It was also noted that the urinary excretion of chromium in the chromium-treated group increased by 500%. Apparently, when the body reaches a saturation level of chromium, the rest is simply lost in the urine.

So, the science shows chromium supplementation does indeed produce an effect in some (but not all) athletes. I suspect it works best in those whose diets are deficient in this trace mineral and/or those who suffer from mild insulin resistance.

Dosage: There is no RDA for chromium; however, most experts agree you need at least 200 mcg/day. A recent study which showed positive results used 1,000 mcg/day. Hard-working athletes may want to make sure they get at least 300 mcg/day. There are several forms of chromium, including: chromium picolinate, chromium citrate, chromium chloride, and chromium polynicotinate. The picolinate form is the most widely used; however, there has been some controversy as to its safety. Because there is no solid proof one form is better than another, I use chromium citrate. I see no harm in using a chromium supplement each day. It's included in many multinutrient bodybuilding supplements.

COPPER

There really isn't much to say about copper as it relates to bodybuilders, except that one study did show athletes probably have a higher demand for copper than nonathletes.[31]

Copper is important, however, in that it is an integral part of the function of two very important enzymes. The first, "superoxide dismutase," is one of the most powerful free-radical combatants in the body. The second is called "lysyl oxidase." This enzyme is responsible for cross linking collagen and elastin, which are connective tissue elements in the body. It has been shown that a copper deficiency may contribute to the development of aortic aneurysms, due to impaired lysyl oxidase activity.[145] An aortic aneurysm is when the main artery coming directly out of your heart actually pops and begins to leak. (This is not a good thing by the way.) It is believed that the aorta is weakened by this copper deficiency because collagen and elastin synthesis, which helps maintain the integrity of that artery, is impaired.

Dosage: The RDA for copper is 1.5-3 mg/day. If you use meal-replacement powders or a multivitamin, you're probably covering this requirement.

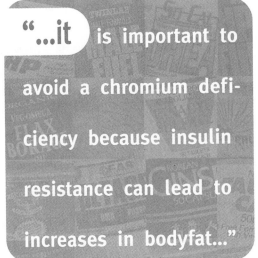

"...it is important to avoid a chromium deficiency because insulin resistance can lead to increases in bodyfat..."

IODINE

Iodine plays one major role in human metabolism: it helps in the production of thyroid hormones. Without adequate amounts of iodine in the system, the thyroid gland can't use the amino acid tyrosine to manufacture thyroid hormones. However, one recent study found that chronically excessive iodine intake can *block* the production of thyroid hormones.[85] Obviously, a correct balance is important.

Some symptoms of iodine deficiency (which is rare in the U.S.) are goiter, cretinism, growth retardation, and intellectual disability. The most common visible symptom is the enlargement of the thyroid gland, commonly known as goiter. When iodine levels are low, the cells in the thyroid gland become enlarged, so much so that the swelling is easily noticed.

Although goiter used to be quite common in the U.S., it has become almost nonexistent since the appearance of iodized salt back in the 1920's. (Manufacturers add iodine to salt solely in an attempt to prevent iodine deficiencies in the population.) However, there are still pockets of iodine-deficient people in the U.S. due to their ingestion of large amounts of "goitrogens"—foods like turnips, cabbage, mustard, soybeans, and peanuts that block iodine utilization and induce goiters.

Dietary sources of iodine include seaweeds and, of course, iodized salt.

Dosage: The RDA for iodine is about 150 mcg/day. I don't even think about taking extra amounts because salted foods are so common.

IRON

Iron is what I would consider a "big boy" in the realm of minerals. This mineral is so important that even a slight deficiency can cause impaired immune function,

THE WIDE, WIDE WORLD OF VITAMINS AND MINERALS: WHAT THEY ARE AND WHAT THEY DO

MINERALS: WHAT THEY ARE AND WHAT THEY DO-THE WIDE, WIDE WORLD OF VITAMINS AND MINERALS: WHAT THEY ARE AND WHAT THEY DO-THE WIDE, WIDE WORLD OF VITAMINS AND MINERALS: WHAT THEY ARE AND WHAT THEY DO-THE WIDE, WIDE WORLD OF VITAMINS AND MINERALS: WHAT THEY ARE AND WHAT THEY DO-THE

decreased energy levels, and decreased physical performance.[62, 81, 149] You see, without iron, your body couldn't transport oxygen from the lungs to body tissues. Iron is an integral component of a molecule called "hemoglobin," which is the portion of a red blood cell which actually binds to and carries oxygen to all of the body's cells. Hemoglobin is also responsible for picking up carbon dioxide (the metabolic byproduct from all cellular metabolism) and transporting it back to the lungs where it can be expelled.

An iron deficiency may lead to a condition called anemia. Anemia literally translated means "without blood," but, of course, anemia does not mean you are completely without blood; it just means that your level of red blood cells, or hemoglobin therein, is decreased. Thus, the capacity of your body to carry oxygen and produce energy is decreased.

Iron deficiency is actually the most common dietary deficiency in the United States—between 35% and 58% of young, otherwise healthy women suffer from an iron deficiency.[81, 149] I don't have any statistics on the exact level of iron deficiency among healthy males; however, there is scientific evidence which indicates that intensely training athletes have a much greater need for iron than sedentary individuals. This greater demand for iron is due in part to an increase in red blood cell turnover during exercise.[238, 255]

Although many Americans use iron supplements, it is important to recognize there are two types of iron available: "heme" and "non-heme." Heme iron is the type found in animal products and is more easily absorbed than non-heme iron, which is the type found in plants. If you'd rather not use an animal source of heme iron, one trick to increase the absorption of non-heme iron is to take it with at least 500 mg of Vitamin C. This can increase iron absorption fourfold.[61]

One final interesting note is that new methods are being developed to use blood levels of iron as a marker of both adaptation to training and acute inflammatory response to exercise. Measuring iron status appears to provide information as to the state of recovery, or lack thereof, experienced by athletes in both acute and chronic training programs. This use of iron as a biochemical marker may help athletes avoid overstress situations.[254]

> "...new methods are being developed to use blood levels of iron as a marker of both adaptation to training and acute inflammatory response to exercise."

Dosage: The RDA for iron is 10 mg/day for males and 15 mg/day for females. If you're a vegetarian or your diet does not contain much meat, you may want to consider supplementation, either through a meal-replacement product or a multivitamin with iron. I would suggest a daily intake of about 20-30 mg of heme-type iron, especially if you're feeling fatigued.

MANGANESE

Without adequate levels of the essential mineral manganese, animals in labs have suffered from impaired growth, skeletal abnormalities, and defects in fat and carbohydrate metabolism. It's not certain that human manganese deficiency will lead to the same metabolic problems, although I found one study which indicated a more optimal bone-matrix development with supplemental manganese (along with some other trace minerals).[242] The limited number of manganese deficiency studies on humans have shown loss of hair color, bone remodeling, reduced growth of hair and nails, skin rash, and reduced HDL (good) cholesterol.

Despite the lack of knowledge about manganese, it does seem to play an important role in various enzyme systems, including those which are involved in blood sugar control, energy metabolism, and thyroid hormone production. It also seems to increase the activity of the body's high-powered antioxidant, superoxide dismutase (SOD).[235]

Manganese has been used to treat certain conditions, although with mixed success. Some experts claim it helps heal strains and sprains. (Maybe through the actions of SOD, which may help remove superoxide radicals from the inflamed area, thus speeding the healing process. But, more likely, the sprain-healing theory can be attributed to the role manganese plays in the function of glutamine synthetase and the vital role of glutamine in the tissue-healing process.) Some experts also claim it helps combat epilepsy and lessens the severity of diabetes.

Whole-food sources of manganese include nuts; whole grains; dried fruits; and green, leafy vegetables.

Dosage: There's no RDA for manganese, but many experts recommend between two and five milligrams per day. However, for sprains, strains, or inflammation, you might want to experiment with between 50 and 200 mg/day, in divided doses for 2 weeks, followed by 15-30 mg/day until the injury heals.

MAGNESIUM

This mineral is typically overlooked as a necessary nutrient for muscular performance and function. You just don't see much in the scientific papers about magnesium or its effect on health and overall muscular performance. However, I believe magnesium ranks right up there with iron, as far as overall performance goes. You see, this mineral is involved in over 300 enzymatic reactions in the body, many having to

THE WIDE, WIDE WORLD OF VITAMINS AND MINERALS: WHAT THEY ARE AND WHAT THEY DO

MINERALS: WHAT THEY ARE AND WHAT THEY DO-THE WIDE, WIDE WORLD OF VITAMINS AND MINERALS: WHAT THEY ARE AND WHAT THEY DO-THE WIDE, WIDE WORLD OF VITAMINS AND MINERALS: WHAT THEY ARE AND WHAT THEY DO-THE WIDE, WIDE WORLD OF VITAMINS AND MINERALS: WHAT THEY ARE AND WHAT THEY DO-THE

do with ATP production for energy in the muscle cells. Not only that, but it actually functions at the ribosomal level to help promote protein synthesis in muscle cells.

Although magnesium is found in rather high levels in such common foods as seeds, nuts, whole grains, and leafy vegetables, deficiencies are not that uncommon in the United States. The RDA for magnesium is 350 mg/day, while the average intake is between 143 and 266 mg/day.

Signs of deficiency include fatigue, mental confusion, weakness, irritability, and problems with nerve conduction and muscle contraction, as well as muscle cramping.

As far as athletes go, there is scientific evidence showing strenuous physical activity (like weightlifting) may substantially increase the body's need for magnesium.[73] There is also scientific data which shows the effects of magnesium supplementation on muscular strength. In one study, subjects were supplemented at a level of 3.6 mg/lb of bodyweight/day for 7 weeks (this is 720 mg/day for a 200-lb male). At the end of the seven weeks, it was found that absolute strength as well as strength adjusted for bodyweight and lean body mass increased rather dramatically.[39] Researchers speculate that the mechanism of action was due to an increase in protein synthesis at the ribosomal level of the muscle cell. This is quite an interesting finding. However, I don't believe they ascertained whether or not subjects were deficient before the study began, and by supplementing, they simply reached non-deficient levels, or whether the 720 mg/day actually caused an effect over and above what the RDA would provide. Nevertheless, magnesium appears to be a *very* important mineral for weight trainers.

Dosage: *Muscle Media* "Strength Guru" Charles Poliquin, who suffered a heart attack around a year ago, was diagnosed as having a severe magnesium deficiency, which may have contributed to his heart problems. He now takes 1,000 mg/day of supplemental magnesium. I think a dosage of 500-1,000 mg/day would be good for most bodybuilders. I get most of my magnesium from the meal-replacement product I take—Myoplex Plus (3 servings contain 525 mg of magnesium). Almost all forms of magnesium are absorbed well, so if you decide to supplement, don't worry about which type you choose.

Molybdenum

Molybdenum is a mineral that plays a part in alcohol detoxification, uric acid formation, and sulfur metabolism. Sulfur, or more precisely, sulfites, are preservatives that were once commonly used in a lot of foods. Nowadays, their use is more restricted, but they do show up in wines and dried fruits. Although they don't normally present a problem, some people are allergic to them, and molybdenum may decrease this sulfite sensitivity.

There's also some evidence that molybdenum deficiency might play a role in causing some forms of cancer,[26] and high levels have shown an ability to fight tooth decay,[136] but there is no research showing this mineral has any unique bodybuilding applications.

Common whole-food sources of this trace mineral include legumes and whole grains.

Dosage: There's no official RDA for molybdenum, although the National Research Council estimates a safe and regular intake to be 75-200 mcg/day. Some experts recommend 200-500 mcg/day.

SODIUM

Sodium is the primary regulator of extracellular fluid volume. In other words, it has a lot to do with water balance in the body. It also helps regulate acid/base balance in the bloodstream and facilitates active cellular transport across all cellular membranes, including muscle cells. There's actually good evidence to suggest sodium is a necessary and vital component in helping to upgrade creatine transport across muscle membranes. (This is one of the reasons sodium phosphate is a component of the EAS Phosphagen HP formula.)

Our actual metabolic needs for sodium intake are around 500 mg of sodium chloride (common table salt) per day. However, a typical American daily intake ranges from 1,800-5,000 mg/day.[197] Intakes upwards of 3,000 mg/day may not be healthy. As most athletes and bodybuilders are aware, excess sodium intake can pull water from cells into extracellular space, resulting in edema, which is that smooth, puffy look we all try to avoid. Not only that, it can also aggravate hypertension (high blood pressure).

It's common practice in the bodybuilding world to restrict sodium intake when cutting up for a contest or photo shoot. Here's a tip—the body reacts very quickly to sodium restriction. When dietary intake is severely restricted, a hormone called "aldosterone" (which is responsible for sodium excretion regulation) increases, and the amount of sodium which is excreted from the system immediately decreases in an effort to maintain homeostatic (consistent) levels of sodium in the bloodstream. This feedback response takes place within a matter of 12-24 hours. Therefore, if you are going to restrict sodium to "dry out" and "tighten up" for a show or photo shoot, I suggest moderating your levels to approximately 1,000 mg/day for 1 week before the show and only severely restricting sodium within 12-20 hours before actual show time.

> **"There's** actually good evidence to suggest sodium is a necessary and vital component in helping to upgrade creatine transport..."

Dosage: For overall health purposes, I suggest restricting sodium intake to below 3,000 mg/day while following my above recommendations for contest or photo preparation.

POTASSIUM

This bulk mineral plays an important role in cellular transport and hydration—much like sodium. It actually works in concert with sodium to activate a mechanism in cells called the "sodium/potassium pump." This "pump" moves water and other nutrients back and forth between the interior and exterior of the cell, maintaining proper physiological balance, nerve function, and muscle performance.

Although potassium deficiencies are very rare in the United States, an important point to consider is the potassium to sodium intake ratio. Americans typically consume twice as much sodium as potassium. This imbalance may lead to major health problems, including cancer and cardiovascular disease.[134, 139] Some scientists recommend a dietary intake ratio of 5:1, potassium to sodium, in order to avoid promoting disorders and to maintain optimal cardiovascular health.

Foods high in potassium include asparagus, avocados, carrots, potatoes, bananas, and even chicken. For this reason, I doubt many bodybuilders suffer from a lack of potassium intake, especially since it has been shown that regular exercise can actually enhance the potassium-regulating mechanisms in the body.[172] However, if a bodybuilder is relying on the use of a diuretic, especially for contest or photo preparation, a potassium supplement may be needed as many diuretics tend to wash potassium from the system.

A word of caution: some bodybuilders use prescription potassium salts along with diuretics while cutting up for a contest or photo shoot. Used improperly and in excessive dosages, this can be very dangerous, due to the fact that highly concentrated potassium in the plasma can actually cause fatal cardiac irregularities.

One other interesting note is that potassium is typically excreted from cells into the bloodstream during intense muscular exercise. This decrease in intracellular potassium and increase in plasma potassium have been implicated in causing fatigue.[161] However, this increase in plasma potassium also acts to help increase vasodilation and perfusion of blood through muscular capillaries, which helps deliver nutrients to active muscles.[296] After exercise, potassium levels in the blood can drop far below baseline, as muscles reabsorb potassium. This sudden decrease in plasma potassium may restrict capillary blood flow and has been implicated in post-exercise cardiac arrest.

> "...it is important to meet potassium requirements and to attempt to maintain a healthy potassium to sodium ratio..."

I think the take-home message here is that it is important to meet potassium requirements and to attempt to maintain a healthy potassium to sodium ratio— I generally try to consume three to five times more potassium each day than sodium. However, messing with mega-supplementation, especially while using diuretics (particularly potassium-sparing diuretics like Dyazide, Aldactone, and Aldactazide), is not a good idea.

Dosage: Although there is no formal RDA for potassium, recommended intake for overall health is approximately 3.5 grams/day, but how much potassium you really need depends on your sodium intake. Due to the exercise response of potassium, my suggestion would be to take at least one gram of this daily dose directly following your workout to help maintain blood levels and increase peripheral blood flow to move lactic acid and other metabolic byproducts out of muscles, possibly helping accelerate the recuperation process. (This is another reason to use EAS' Phosphagen HP, which includes potassium phosphate, directly following a workout.)

SELENIUM

This trace mineral has become very popular over the past year for good reason. Its primary function in the body is to act as an antioxidant—it is an integral component of the very powerful antioxidant enzyme "glutathione peroxidase." Not only does it boost glutathione peroxidase functionality, it also seems to exert antioxidant activity on its own, as well as being involved in the production of thyroid hormones.[60] It appears most of the health benefits which have been assigned to selenium (including: decreased cancer rates,[123] decreased rates of fatal heart attacks,[147] enhancement of immune function,[141] as well as protection against the symptoms of rheumatoid arthritis[272]) have to do with selenium's potent antioxidant effects. This makes sense—lower levels of antioxidant activity in the body allow free radicals to run wild, wreaking havoc on the system, and causing an accelerated breakdown of cells.

It is interesting to note, however, that all these health risks are not necessarily due to depressed intakes of selenium and poor antioxidant function.

Supplemental selenium (in the form of sodium selen*ate*) has been shown in animal studies to act as an "insulin mimic." One animal study compared the action of sodium selenate to insulin in transporting glucose into muscle cells.[80] Although selenate did not match insulin action, there was a significant increase in glucose uptake with selenate supplementation. This action is the reason sodium selenate is part of EAS' V2G (vanadyl sulfate second generation) formula.

One study showed individuals with normal selenium concentrations in their blood who received 200 mcg of selenium per day as a supplement increased the ability of lymphocytes to kill tumor cells by 118%, as well as increasing the activity of white blood cells by 82.3%.[142] It would appear from this finding that the current RDA recommendation of 70 mcg/day is probably not optimal.

THE WIDE, WIDE WORLD OF VITAMINS AND MINERALS: WHAT THEY ARE AND WHAT THEY DO

MINERALS: WHAT THEY ARE AND WHAT THEY DO•THE WIDE, WIDE WORLD OF VITAMINS AND MINERALS: WHAT THEY ARE AND WHAT THEY DO•THE WIDE, WIDE WORLD OF VITAMINS AND MINERALS: WHAT THEY ARE AND WHAT THEY DO•THE WIDE, WIDE WORLD OF VITAMINS AND MINERALS: WHAT THEY ARE AND WHAT THEY DO•THE

As far as bodybuilding applications go, I think any time we can take a substance which decreases the oxidative damage in our bodies, secondary to exercise, the better off we are and the more quickly we can recover from exercise. Studies looking at selenium and its effects on athletic performance have been equivocal. However, its effects on oxidation activity following rigorous exercise have shown strong results.[208] One study concluded, "The administration of organic selenium partially compensates and decreases the intensity of oxidative stress following exercise."

Dosage: As I mentioned, the RDA for selenium is 70 mcg for men and 55 mcg for women. However, I think the literature confirms that an intake of closer to 200 mcg/day would be optimal for hard-training athletes.

SILICON

Next to oxygen, silicon is the most abundant element on earth. When I think of silicon, I think of computer chips and breast implants, not of a vital nutrient. But silicon is actually pretty important. It plays a role in bone and tendon formation. And studies have shown deficiencies can lead to poor connective-tissue integrity.[84, 198] It also seems to be necessary for healthy skin, ligaments, tendons, and bones, and a lot of people take silicon for those reasons.

Whole-food sources of this mineral include oatmeal and brown rice.

Dosage: Although no RDA has been established, estimated requirements for bone collagen synthesis are 5-20 mg/day.

VANADIUM

Vanadium, in the form of vanadyl sulfate—which is derived from the trace mineral—has been a popular bodybuilding supplement since it was introduced to the market in 1989. It has a reputation amongst bodybuilders for enhancing muscle fullness and for its ability to create good pumps and vascularity. But, what's the science behind this bright blue mineral?

Only recently has vanadium been included as an essential nutrient for human nutrition. There are still no known deficiency diseases; however, some researchers speculate that deficiencies may cause elevated cholesterol levels or faulty blood sugar control.

As far as bodybuilding and/or other sports applications go, the main effect which people are interested in is the ability of vanadium to mimic the actions of insulin. There have been a number of studies showing that oral supplementation of vanadyl sulfate can help sensitize muscle and liver tissues in non-insulin-dependent diabetics. This insulin sensitization has allowed the subjects of these studies to reach acceptable blood sugar levels without the use of insulin medications.[111]

Conclusive data as to whether or not vanadyl sulfate enhances muscle growth is not available, and studies measuring muscle fullness or an "improved pump" would be hard to design. Thus, the "scientific jury" is still out on vanadyl sulfate, despite its popularity with bodybuilders.

I suspect vanadyl sulfate is similar to chromium in that it "up-regulates" insulin action in some (but not all—why, I don't know) bodybuilders. Remember, insulin is responsible for carrying nutrients, like amino acids and glucose, into muscle cells (which increases cell volume, improves protein metabolism, and results in greater pumps). However, it's likely that vanadyl sulfate and chromium help dispose of glucose by different means: vanadyl at the receptor *inside* cells and chromium from the *outside* of cells.

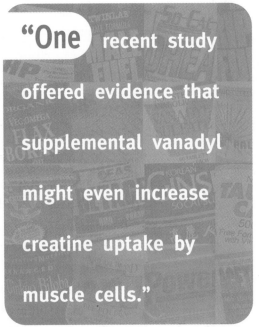

"One recent study offered evidence that supplemental vanadyl might even increase creatine uptake by muscle cells."

One recent study offered evidence that supplemental vanadyl might even increase creatine uptake by muscle cells.[226]

Dosage: I believe vanadyl sulfate is the best form of vanadium on the market now, in terms of safety and effectiveness. If you're interested in trying vanadyl sulfate to see if it works for you, I would suggest taking between 30 and 50 mg/day in divided doses with meals. As is the case with several trace minerals, consuming too much may be toxic, so be sure not to exceed the recommended dose.

ZINC

Zinc is a mineral involved in the action of several hormones, including: insulin, growth hormone, testosterone, and estrogen. It's also involved in more than 200 enzymatic reactions. Obviously, it is very important for the body to have adequate amounts of zinc, and recent research has indicated that people who exercise may need more zinc and, in fact, experience a higher risk of zinc deficiency.[63]

Severe zinc deficiencies are very uncommon in the United States. However, surveys indicate that average zinc intake is in the range of 47-67% of the RDA, especially in athletes. This may lead to a marginal zinc deficiency. Marginal zinc deficiencies can result in increased susceptibility to infection, poor wound healing, and certain skin disorders.[281]

Interestingly, a study showed that supplemental zinc, 25 mg/day, actually blocked the normal exercise-induced increase in free radicals in the bloodstream.[63] This antioxidant effect may be one of the things which accounts for zinc's apparent role in supporting immune function and preventing infection.

Good sources of zinc include oysters (which are loaded with 149 mg/3.5 oz), nuts, and oats.

Dosage: The RDA for zinc is 15 mg/day. I would recommend a dosage of 25-30 mg/day for hard-training athletes.

SUMMARY

As you can see, the wide, wide world of vitamins and minerals can indeed get a bit complex and confusing. Certainly, I've only begun to scratch the surface as to the thousands of biochemical functions that vitamins and minerals play in our bodies. But, like many other aspects of bodybuilding nutrition and supplementation, as long as you understand the basics (and the basics are that you should definitely be making sure you use a vitamin and mineral supplement of some kind each and every day!), you don't have to drive yourself crazy trying to understand every little detail.

To review, vitamins and minerals are micronutrients that are essential components of structures and functions in the body. No, taking a vitamin pill or capsule won't give you instant energy nor produce immediate results in terms of new size and strength, but if you feed your body with ample amounts of the broad spectrum of micronutrients that it needs, every day, week in and week out, my educated guess is that, over time, you will see and feel the difference. Who knows, your bodybuilding program may not be "firing on all cylinders" because of even the most minuscule deficiency in some vitamin or mineral.

Of course, many old-school nutritionists and dietitians will tell you that you can get all these important micronutrients from simply consuming a "balanced diet" (whatever the hell that is). The reality of it all is most of us, even those who are health conscious, do not consume, on a daily basis, adequate, much less "optimal," amounts of every vitamin and mineral our bodies need. Thus, supplementation is wise.

Typically, I rely on meal-replacement powders, such as Myoplex Plus, to deliver the majority of vitamins and minerals I need—two servings of Myoplex Plus (and many other meal-replacement products and multinutrient formulas on the market) contain a broad spectrum of quality vitamins and minerals.

The only vitamin I have regularly used in a "mega-dose manner" is Vitamin C, which I try to consume at least three grams of per day, with meals, and sometimes

> "Don't be a dingbat—make sure you are supplementing your diet daily with ample amounts of vitamins and minerals..."

I'll go up to as many as ten grams a day when I'm on a strict diet or if I feel like I'm getting run-down.

An alternate strategy would be to consume a daily vitamin and mineral capsule or tablet (even though I don't think all vitamin tablets contain what their labels claim, nor do they dissolve very well). A few of the vitamin and mineral supplements I would recommend include Soft-Gelatin Multiple by Nature's Life, Multivitamin with Iron by Nature's Way, Ultra Two by Nature's Plus, Country Life's Multi-100, and GNC's Multi-Gel.

Simply consuming a couple of these multivitamin and multimineral capsules in the morning with breakfast, and again in the evening with dinner, could take virtually all the brain work out of the numerous items we reviewed in this chapter.

The bottom line is, this stuff is very basic but not so basic you should overlook it. It doesn't have to be complicated; there are so many good vitamin and mineral formulas already available on the market, whether they are multinutrient formulas or capsules; it's really true that the work has already been done.

Don't be a *dingbat*—make sure you are supplementing your diet daily with ample amounts of vitamins and minerals; otherwise, I promise you will never reach your fullest potential, not only in bodybuilding but in terms of health, longevity, and well-being.

Okay... that's not so complicated after all, is it?

SPORTS SUPPLEMENT REVIEW, 3RD ISSUE•SPORTS SUPPLEMENT REVIEW, 3RD ISSUE•SPORTS SUPPLEMENT REVIEW, 3RD ISSUE•SPORTS SUPPLEMENT REVIEW, 3RD ISSUE•SPORTS SUPPLEMENT REVIEW, 3RD ISSUE•SPORTS

146

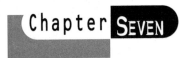

Chapter SEVEN

The Facts and Folklore of Herbal Supplements

Typically, I'm not the type of bodybuilder who pays much attention to "herbal medicine." Quite frankly, I find it to be a complicated and somewhat dubious field, but now that herbs are officially classified as "dietary supplements" according to the Dietary Supplement Health and Education Act of 1994, I figured I'd better include a crash course on herbs in this book.

If you have questions about how various dietary supplements that contain one or more herbs might help or hurt your bodybuilding efforts, then you'll probably find this information relevant and possibly even stimulating.

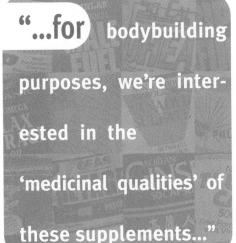

"...for bodybuilding purposes, we're interested in the 'medicinal qualities' of these supplements..."

WHAT ARE HERBS ANYWAY?

According to Webster's dictionary, an herb is, "A plant valued for its medicinal, savory, or aromatic qualities." Certainly, for bodybuilding purposes, we're interested in the "medicinal qualities" of these supplements—their potential to produce drug-like effects in some instances. In fact, a number of today's synthetic pharmaceutical preparations were originally discovered and prescribed as herbal extracts many, many years ago. For example, a drug called Digitalis, used to treat various types of heart disease, is prescribed by cardiologists worldwide, but it's actually an herb that was discovered about 100 years ago—it's derived from a plant called "Foxglove."[186]

Perhaps the herbs that are most frequently used by bodybuilders are guarana (which contains up to five percent caffeine by weight) and ephedra, also known as ma huang. (The *Ephedra sinica* form of this herb contains the thermogenic chemical ephedrine at a concentration of about two percent by weight of the whole herb. It's important to use the *sinica* species of this herb since the other types of ephedra may contain very little or no ephedrine.) These herbs are metabolized by the body into the same basic chemicals as the over-the-counter drugs caffeine and ephedrine, which have potent central-nervous-system-stimulating, appetite-suppressing,

THE FACTS AND FOLKLORE OF HERBAL SUPPLEMENTS

CHAPTER 7

FACTS AND FOLKLORE OF HERBAL SUPPLEMENTS•THE FACTS AND FOLKLORE OF HERBAL SUPPLEMENTS•THE FACTS AND FOLKLORE OF HERBAL SUPPLEMENTS•THE FACTS AND FOLKLORE OF HERBAL SUPPLEMENTS•THE FACTS AND FOLKLORE OF HERBAL SUPPLEMENTS•THE FACTS AND FOLKLORE OF HERBAL SUPPLEMENTS•THE FACTS AND FOLKLORE OF HERBAL SUPPLEMENTS•

and fat-burning properties—especially when they are used together, as they produce a profound synergistic effect."¹ These herbs are the "active ingredients" in many fat-loss supplements, such as SportPharma's Thermadrene™, TwinLab's Ripped Fuel™, and Metaform Heat™ by Weider Nutrition.

Make no mistake, there are definitely some herbs which have powerful effects, but as you'll discover in this chapter, most herbs aren't what I would call worthwhile bodybuilding supplements, as they don't have much potential to help us gain muscle, burn fat, or increase our strength, and since that's the focus of this book, I'll review these herbs from that standpoint.

BE SURE TO WATCH FOR "STANDARDIZED EXTRACTS"

One of the problems with herbal supplements is that you can't always be certain of the potency of the formulation. Depending on what part of the plant was used to make the herb, where it was grown, when it was harvested, and how it has been processed and packaged, it can be either very potent or virtually inert (chemically inactive).³⁰ One way the herbal industry has attempted to deal with this problem is to establish something known as a "standardized extract." What that means is the potency of an herbal extract is basically guaranteed. This potency will be expressed as a "standardized" level of the active compounds found in the herbal extract. This is usually expressed as a percentage of the total. For instance, a typical standardization level for ephedra is six percent. This means the ephedrine content of the herb has been increased by threefold from 2% in the whole herb to 6% in the extracted form, meaning 100 mg of the standardized herb would supply 6 mg of active ephedrine.

And, as if things weren't already complicated enough, unfortunately, as we've discussed in other chapters of this book, just because one of these products might say "standardized extract" on the label doesn't necessarily mean it is. Thus, I recommend that you go with a quality brand, such as Nature's Way, Herb Pharm, and Earth Friend Herb Co.—a small but very high-quality mail-order company in Mt. Shasta, CA (call 916-926-7978 to ask for their catalogue).

All right—let's get to the meat and potatoes of this chapter and explore the ancient science of herbs and how certain ones are being accepted as potent substances by the Western scientific community, and let's see if we can't figure out just which ones might help us get better results in our bodybuilding endeavors.

GINSENG

Ginseng falls into the category of herbal supplements known as "adaptogens." Simply put, adaptogens supposedly help the body adapt to higher levels of stress. This might mean increasing endurance or helping recovery rates. Of all the adaptogens, ginseng is the most famous and the most widely used. Since ginseng is very popular, particularly in the general-health market, a number of varieties have surfaced:

Indian Ginseng, also known as "*ashwagandha*," is a component of some supplements. It has been used in India for thousands of years as a "vitalizer" and can supposedly help treat symptoms of arthritis, asthma, bronchitis, cancer, etc. Animal studies have been promising, as have some human studies. Studies seem to indicate that children fed milk and Indian ginseng grew larger more quickly. Adults have shown improved serum cholesterol levels, as well as an increased number of red blood cells.

American Ginseng, or "*Panax quinquefolius*," has no proven beneficial effects, other than serving as a laxative. However, several hundred years ago, Indian tribes used this type of ginseng as an aphrodisiac and to treat colds and sore throats.

Korean Ginseng, also known as "*Panax ginseng*," is thought to have mild central-nervous-system effects. It's also thought to improve performance and stamina, as well as concentration and reaction times in the elderly.

Siberian Ginseng, or "*Eleutherococcus senticosus*," is the most popular type of ginseng—the one you typically see in little bottles on the checkout counter at health-food stores. It has been used in Russia for centuries because of its alleged immunostimulating effects. It's also thought to be a remedy for stress, fatigue, and complete nervous breakdown. Russian athletes and cosmonauts reportedly use it to enhance energy and alleviate stress. It has actually been suggested that ginseng may stimulate protein synthesis and cellular repair enzymes.[173]

As far as the scientific evidence regarding all types of ginseng, experts generally believe there's a lack of controlled research demonstrating its ability to improve or prolong endurance in humans.[16] I tend to agree—but some athletes swear by it.

Dosage: Varies according to the type of ginseng and the intended use. However, for many purposes, 100-200 mg of the powdered extract taken 3 times/day is recommended.

GERANIUM

Derived from a Bulgarian plant called *Geranium sanguineum*, this herbal extract has been shown to possibly have some potent antiviral effects. It can apparently suppress the growth of infectious viruses even after they have entered cells.[246]

> "It has actually been suggested that ginseng may stimulate protein synthesis and cellular repair enzymes."

149

THE FACTS AND FOLKLORE OF HERBAL SUPPLEMENTS

FACTS AND FOLKLORE OF HERBAL SUPPLEMENTS•THE FACTS AND FOLKLORE OF HERBAL SUPPLEMENTS•THE FACTS AND FOLKLORE OF HERBAL SUPPLEMENTS•THE FACTS AND FOLKLORE OF HERBAL SUPPLEMENTS•THE FACTS AND FOLKLORE OF HERBAL SUPPLEMENTS•THE FACTS AND FOLKLORE OF HERBAL SUPPLEMENTS•THE FACTS AND FOLKLORE OF HERBAL SUPPLEMENTS•

I could not find any indication in the medical literature nor any information from bodybuilders that would lead me to believe it has any performance-enhancing effects. But if you have a bad cold or the flu, it may well help speed your recovery.

Dosage: If you can find this one in the health-food store, you should probably take two or three times the recommended dosage to fight off an infection.

GRAPE SEED EXTRACT

This product is basically riding the coattails of the Pycnogenol (pine bark extract) boom. Grape seed extract is probably a better source of all the stuff that Pycnogenol claims to contain, including various potent flavone antioxidants. The gallic ester form of proanthocyanidins (the most potent free-radical scavengers) are found only in grape seed extract, not in pine bark extract.[245]

This product would probably be a valuable part of an overall antioxidant product or regimen which could help protect your hard-working muscles in the long run, but its use is not going to lead to immediate gains in mass or strength.

Dosage: 50-100 mg/day is probably sufficient for free-radical-scavenging effects in a hard-training athlete.

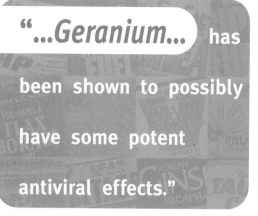

"...Geranium... has been shown to possibly have some potent antiviral effects."

CRANBERRY

Cranberry, either in pill form or in commercial juice, is often used to treat urinary-tract infections and may be useful in dissolving kidney stones and gallstones. Although cranberry juice has long been part of medicinal folklore, several studies have confirmed its effectiveness in fighting urinary-tract infections. For instance, researchers in one study found that after drinking cranberry juice for 21 days, 70% of the patients improved.[293]

Herbalists also claim cranberry not only kills the bacteria that cause urinary-tract infections but also actually prevents bacteria from adhering to cells, thereby allowing the bacteria to be flushed from the system.

Believe it or not, cranberry pills are "the rage" in hardcore bodybuilding circles, especially among steroid users, who believe it helps detoxify the kidneys.

Dosage: One to three grams of pure cranberry extract two to three times a day or several cups of pure cranberry juice, depending on the concentration. Avoid the sweetened cranberry juice as sugar can actually promote bacterial growth. If you'd rather go with pills, the recommended dosage is around one or two 500-mg capsules 2-3 times daily.

YOHIMBE

Okay, so far, we've reviewed a few herbs with antioxidant potential and even antibiotic characteristics but nothing thrilling. Now, yohimbe—or more specifically, yohimb*ine* hydrochloride (HCL)—may indeed be an herbal nutrient which will get your blood pumping—quite literally. Although this product has been on the market for quite some time, I think some of the new research information on this nutrient is going to help catapult it to a new level of popularity in the very near future.

The yohimbine hydrochloride chemical is found as a natural component of yohimbe bark. It is, apparently, this chemical extract which is the active component of yohimbe powder. Pure yohimbine hydrochloride has been used in the medical profession for a number of years to treat male impotence. Its action as an "alpha$_2$ adrenergic agonist" appears to increase the flow of blood into the penis, while at the same time preventing blood from flowing out. This would obviously have strong implications for male sexual function. It also appears to increase libido, and it's even been written in the *Physicians' Desk Reference* that it "may have activity as an aphrodisiac."

Not only does this stuff appear to improve sexual function and drive, it has also been shown to actually decrease fat synthesis in the body[192] as well as increase fatty acid mobilization from fat stores in women[27] (especially in the hips). The combination of these two effects may, indeed, position this herb/chemical as a viable aid to bodyfat loss.

As if these two rather attractive effects weren't enough, there appear to be other health benefits attached to the use of this product. Doses between 10 and 20 mg/day have been shown to decrease platelet aggregation in the bloodstream—which basically means it can help prevent arteries from becoming clogged and causing strokes or heart attacks. It has also been used in the treatment of congestive heart failure.[248]

Although further studies regarding its effectiveness as a sexual performance and libido enhancer are warranted, I think yohimbe/yohimbine holds some promise—expect to see it being used extensively in male potency products in the future. However, as I've reported before, yohimbe/yohimbine does <u>not</u> appear to increase testosterone production as some marketers contend.

There is, however, the ongoing concern that products containing yohimbe bark extract may or may not contain viable doses of the yohimbine HCL chemical. Always make sure to check the label of any products you purchase containing this ingredient to ascertain the actual amount of true yohimbine HCL. The safest way to assure that you have a quality product is to call the company and request a certificate of analysis, which they should be able to supply.

Dosage: The common dosage of yohimbine HCL used in the medical field is one 5.4-mg tablet 3 times/day. I suggest looking for products which mimic this

THE FACTS AND FOLKLORE OF HERBAL SUPPLEMENTS

FACTS AND FOLKLORE OF HERBAL SUPPLEMENTS•THE FACTS AND FOLKLORE OF HERBAL SUPPLEMENTS•THE FACTS AND FOLKLORE OF HERBAL SUPPLEMENTS•THE FACTS AND FOLKLORE OF HERBAL SUPPLEMENTS•THE FACTS AND FOLKLORE OF HERBAL SUPPLEMENTS•THE FACTS AND FOLKLORE OF HERBAL SUPPLEMENTS•

intake, but don't take the "more-is-better" attitude when using this product. Studies have shown that increased dosages may be less effective than the doses mentioned here.

TURMERIC

Turmeric is the major ingredient in curry powder, and it's also used in certain varieties of mustard. The herb is found in India, China, and Indonesia. Its active ingredient, curcumin, is prescribed as an anti-inflammatory agent in the treatment of numerous disorders, including: jaundice, bruises, chest pain, menstrual difficulties, etc.

I'm not at all convinced it cures any of those ailments, but it does appear to have uses as an antioxidant, anti-inflammatory, anti-carcinogenic, cardiovascular, hepatic, gastrointestinal, and anti-microbial agent.

The antioxidant effect of turmeric (or curcumin) is said to be comparable to that of Vitamins C and E (less effective than C and E but more effective than B or even superoxide dismutase). As far as its anti-inflammatory effects, it's said to be comparable to cortisone. However, this last property might be problematic for bodybuilders. Turmeric supposedly stimulates the release of glucocorticoids, increases the sensitivity of cortisol receptor sites, and increases the half-life of cortisol. Although these properties might help acute injuries heal, chronic use for a long-term injury could, theoretically, lead to protein catabolism.

On the other hand, turmeric seems to be an effective "liver protector," kind of like a supplement called silymarin. This liver-protecting characteristic is most likely due to turmeric's antioxidant properties.

Dosage: You'd have to eat a lot of turmeric to enjoy its healing powers, so curcumin supplements are generally used to treat illnesses. The general dosage for curcumin is 400-600 mg 3 times/day. To ingest an equivalent dosage using turmeric alone, you'd have to take roughly 8-60 grams 3 times/day.

DANDELION

Here is another herb which actually appears to have a viable bodybuilding application. Although it's known as dandelion in the U.S., this common plant is also known as "wet-a-bed" in other countries because of its diuretic action. Although the diuretic action is probably of greatest interest to bodybuilders, it is also generally regarded as a liver tonic and is used to treat fever, boils, heartburn, appendicitis, and various skin problems. Dandelion also contains the most Vitamin A of any known plant—14,000 IU/100 grams of raw greens.

Dandelion's beneficial effects on the liver have apparently been proven in laboratory studies.[268] It supposedly increases the flow of bile, which could alleviate such conditions as bile duct inflammation, hepatitis, gallstones, and jaundice. Dandelion's high choline content might be responsible for these liver-protectant properties.

Other studies demonstrate dandelion may be as effective a diuretic as furosemide (Lasix).[225] However, because dandelion replaces the potassium normally lost through diuresis, it doesn't seem to have the potential negative side effects of Lasix.

Other reported benefits of dandelion include anti-tumor and glucose-buffering properties, which might make it an effective herb for diabetics.

Because of its potassium-sparing diuretic action and its liver protection, I use this herbal supplement as an alternative to the prescription diuretics Aldactone and Lasix (which I used to use) to drop water before photos. A lot of bodybuilders I know use it for two days before contests or photo shoots. It actually works quite well.

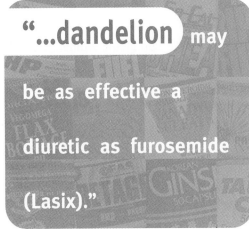

"...dandelion may be as effective a diuretic as furosemide (Lasix)."

Dosage: As powdered extract, 250-500 mg taken 3 times daily, with loads of water, works great! I wouldn't use it all the time though. Save it for when you need it.

GOLDENSEAL, BARBERRY, OREGON GRAPE, AND GOLDTHREAD

These four herbs appear to be interchangeable as far as their alleged healing powers go because they all contain high amounts of the active ingredient "berberine." Berberine is said to have a variety of beneficial effects, including: antibiotic activity, anti-infective activity (the ability to prevent bacteria from adhering to cells), immuno-enhancing effects, fever-lowering characteristics, and anticancer activity.

These herbs are also used clinically to treat infectious diarrhea, trachoma (an infection of the eye), and liver disorders (cirrhosis). Other possible uses include treating gonorrhea and syphilis, as well as being useful in treating symptoms of colds and flus.

Unfortunately, there haven't been any detailed studies done on berberine's effects. However, goldenseal, especially, is widely used as a potent "blood-cleansing" agent by people looking to clean their systems of drug residues to get ready for both urine and blood drug-screening tests.

Dosage: As powdered preparations vary widely in content, standardized preparations are recommended. Goldenseal appears to be the most widely available, so for treating ailments, 250-500 mg of powdered extract 3 times/day is what's generally

THE FACTS AND FOLKLORE OF HERBAL SUPPLEMENTS

CHAPTER 7

FACTS AND FOLKLORE OF HERBAL SUPPLEMENTS•THE FACTS AND FOLKLORE OF HERBAL SUPPLEMENTS•THE FACTS AND FOLKLORE OF HERBAL SUPPLEMENTS•THE FACTS AND FOLKLORE OF HERBAL SUPPLEMENTS•THE FACTS AND FOLKLORE OF HERBAL SUPPLEMENTS•THE FACTS AND FOLKLORE OF HERBAL SUPPLEMENTS•

recommended and up to a gram per day for emergency drug cleansing. Warning: higher doses than listed here might interfere with Vitamin B metabolism. Likewise, pregnant women are advised to avoid berberine-containing plants.

GUARANA

Guarana is basically just caffeine in herbal form. It contains between 2.5% and 5% of the popular stimulant—2½ times the amount found in the coffee bean. As far as I can tell, there's really no performance benefit (nor harm) in taking caffeine via guarana, rather than from coffee or caffeine tabs.

Some effects which appear to be specific to guarana are inhibition of platelet aggregation[42] (or thinning of the blood, much like aspirin), as well as possible alleviation of migraines (probably due to the caffeine) and diarrhea (probably due to its diuretic effects.)

All in all, guarana is just a "natural" source of caffeine. Caffeine increases endurance by increasing the breakdown of fat—it can allow you to train longer and burn more fat. And caffeine, as well as ephedra, can make muscle contraction more forceful by promoting greater neurotransmitter release from the nerve at the neuromuscular junction.

"...this type of herbal caffeine/ ephedrine/aspirin stack... is probably easier on the gastrointestinal system."

Dosage: 200-300 mg of caffeine is a typical dose. Check the "% standardization" of the guarana to assure proper caffeine ingestion. Guarana capsules at a dosage of 250 mg standardized to 5% caffeine contain only 12.5 mg of caffeine.

WHITE WILLOW BARK

The scientific name for this herb is *Salix alba*. This natural medicinal herb contains a substance called salicin. For centuries, it has been used as a natural cure to help break fevers, alleviate headaches, and reduce pain and swelling in joints. The discovery of the salicin nutrient in white willow bark actually led to the synthesis of today's modern aspirin compound, which contains acetylsalicylic acid. Fortunately, unlike aspirin, which when consumed in large quantities can cause stomach irritation and even ulceration, white willow bark contains certain bio-active nutrients which are actually good for the digestive system.

White willow bark is used in a number of preparations that also contain ephedra and guarana, which are natural forms of ephedrine and caffeine. Although this type of herbal caffeine/ephedrine/aspirin stack may not be as potent as the pure compounds, it is probably easier on the gastrointestinal system.

All in all, white willow bark is probably a safe and relatively effective aspirin substitute.

Dosage: I would recommend using a standardized extract that contains 200-300 mg of the salicin compound in the herbal thermogenic stack. To get a dosage equivalent to 200-300 mg of aspirin, you'd need to take 1,400-2,000 mg of white willow bark standardized to 15% salicin.

EPHEDRA

This extremely popular and versatile herb, due to its thermogenic (fat burning) and "stimulating" effects, has some viable bodybuilding applications. The Chinese first started using it over 5,000 years ago for respiratory ailments due to its bronchodilating effects. Nowadays, people throughout the world are using it for everything from the common cold to weight loss. For the purpose of this book, I'll focus on its effects on exercise performance, muscular biochemistry, and fat loss.

I'm sure almost everyone is familiar with ephed*rine* which is the main active chemical component of the herb ephedra. There are a number of different strains of the ephedra herb, and their ephedrine concentrations vary widely. They range from *Ephedra sinica* and country mallow (*Sida coritfolia*), which typically contain about 2% ephedrine by weight, to *Ephedra nevadensis* (Mormon tea), which contains virtually no ephedrine at all.

As I mentioned in the *1996 Supplement Review*, ephedrine is a beta-adrenergic agonist, which means it tends to increase the heart rate and overall thermic (or heat-producing) character of almost all tissues in the body, including muscle and fat tissue.[12] This means it can indeed help your body burn more fat.

Ephedra supplements work by releasing noradrenaline in the brain which exerts a stimulatory effect. The body dumps adrenaline from the adrenal glands into the blood, and the brain releases noradrenaline. This causes body temperature to increase and promotes the breakdown of fat cells, so fuel can be obtained and a person can fight, run, or perform a large amount of physical work.

Some studies show that 25 mg of ephedrine or the herbal equivalent can increase the metabolic rate by ten percent.

Although ephedra is definitely not as effective on its own as when it is combined with guarana and white willow bark, there is evidence to suggest it can still be helpful for fat loss and muscle maintenance. A study of obese women given 50 mg of ephedrine 3 times/day, combined with a low-calorie diet (1,000-1,400 calories per day) for 2 months, showed the ephedrine group lost more than 3 times as much

THE FACTS AND FOLKLORE OF HERBAL SUPPLEMENTS

FACTS AND FOLKLORE OF HERBAL SUPPLEMENTS·THE FACTS AND FOLKLORE OF HERBAL SUPPLEMENTS·THE FACTS AND FOLKLORE OF HERBAL SUPPLEMENTS·THE FACTS AND FOLKLORE OF HERBAL SUPPLEMENTS·THE FACTS AND FOLKLORE OF HERBAL SUPPLEMENTS·THE FACTS AND FOLKLORE OF HERBAL SUPPLEMENTS·

bodyfat as the control group on calorie restriction alone.[214] Its muscle-sparing effects during severe calorie restriction have also been well documented.[215]

There isn't a lot of evidence for performance-enhancing effects of ephedra/ ephedrine. Every clinical study I looked at found no direct effect of ephedrine supplementation on a wide variety of performance parameters, including: muscular strength, endurance and power, aerobic capacity, anaerobic capacity, and even perceived exertion.[69, 250] Even considering all the scientific information, some quality ephedra 30 minutes before workout time still helps motivate me to get my butt in the gym on those days when a nap sounds much more appealing.

One of the problems (besides the jitters it can give you) with chronic ephedra use is that your body becomes resistant to its effects rather quickly. The results of one study indicated that only one week of ephedrine use can significantly depress the beta-adrenergic-receptor response.[200] And this attenuation was still present 36 hours after the last dose of ephedrine. This means in order to maintain a good response, cycling is probably a good idea—maybe a one-day-on, one-day-off plan.

I mentioned in my last book that the FDA was cracking down on ephedrine sales. Well, they have continued to do so. It is illegal to sell ephedrine in several states now. I don't believe possession is illegal anywhere, but the sale is in certain areas. The FDA has been evaluating the safety of the herb ephedra and will likely soon mandate certain dosage limits.

Because ephedra/ephedrine tends to increase blood pressure and stimulate cardiac muscle, if you have trouble with your heart, are diabetic, have a thyroid dysfunction, or suffer from high blood pressure, I would NOT recommend using this product—it can aggravate and intensify preexisting health conditions. Highly stressed, easily excited, and/or chronically nervous individuals should also avoid ephedra. Even if you are perfectly healthy, do <u>not</u> exceed the recommended dosage! Insomnia, anxiety, or panic attacks may result from doses above recommended levels.

Dosage: 420 mg of ephedra standardized to 6% ephedrine alone or as part of the guarana/ephedra/willow bark stack 3 times/day, 30 minutes before meals.

Silymarin (Milk Thistle)

Milk thistle is an herb generally used as a liver protectant. Since oral anabolic steroids are metabolized in the liver, the drugs often cause a tremendous strain on the organ. I've known athletes who have been using anabolic steroids for years yet have normal liver enzyme levels—*perhaps* due in part to the regular use of silymarin. Studies also seem to support its use as a liver protectant in athletes who chronically overdose on acetaminophen (Tylenol).[202]

Although several research studies support its liver-protective properties, most experts believe it to be effective because it's a potent antioxidant.[120]

If I were taking steroids, I'd definitely take silymarin, either in its natural form or as LIV 52, a silymarin product that has other herbs thrown in for good measure.

Dosage: 500-1,000 mg/day of silymarin with meals, in 2 divided doses seems logical.

SMILAX OFFICIANALIS

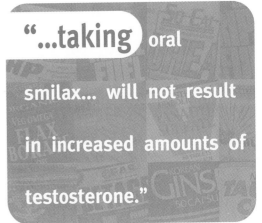

Smilax has been around the sport of bodybuilding about as long as the word "fraud." It's simply an herb that contains plant sterols. Note the spelling—s-t-e-r-o-l-s. Sterols are not the same thing as *steroids*. Although some sterols can mimic estrogen,[249] I don't believe sterols imitate testosterone. Certain sterols, when subjected to vigorous and complicated chemical procedures, can be turned into steroids, but the body can't do it. In other words, despite what some supplement companies say, taking oral smilax (or other sterols) will not result in increased amounts of testosterone. The body just doesn't have the enzymes to do the conversion.

I don't recommend smilax because I don't think it does anything.

Dosage: None is good.

FLAVONOIDS

Although flavonoids are derived from plant sources, much like the sterols previously mentioned, they are distinctly different compounds. Unlike most sterol products, there are a number of flavonoid compounds which appear to have some strong bio-activity.

There are over 4,000 different flavone compounds. Of all the different types of flavonoids out there, two are currently the most popular and best understood. These are "proanthocyanidins"—found in pine bark (Pycnogenol) and grape seed extract; and quercetins—found in citrus fruits and green tea.

Proanthocyanidins have very powerful antioxidant characteristics, and their free-radical-scavenging effects are better than most antioxidant vitamins.[119] They may also help protect connective tissue from disease and/or damage.[168]

Quercetins also have antioxidant characteristics, but their main uses in the marketplace have been as anti-inflammatory agents[83] or antiviral compounds.[22]

Although quercetins and proanthocyanidins are interesting, useful, and are selling like wildfire, I think they are small potatoes compared to the potential bodybuilding applications of certain flavones including various alkaloids found in *Tribulus terrestris* and something called chrysin (Duchaine's "Flavone X"—see

REVIEW•SPORTS SUPPLEMENT REVIEW, 3RD ISSUE•SPORTS SUPPLEMENT REVIEW, 3RD ISSUE•SPORTS SUPPLEMENT REVIEW, 3RD ISSUE•SPORTS SUPPLEMENT

•SPORTS SUPPLEMENT REVIEW, 3RD ISSUE•SPORTS SUPPLEMENT REVIEW, 3RD ISSUE•SPORTS SUPPLEMENT REVIEW, 3RD ISSUE•SPORTS SUPPLEMENT REVIEW, 3RD ISSUE•SPORTS SUPPLEMENT REVIEW, 3RD ISSUE•SPORTS SUPPLEMENT REVIEW, 3RD ISSUE•SPORTS SUPPLEMENT REVIEW, 3RD ISSUE•SPORTS SUPPLEMENT

Chapter 3). It's my guess there may be some interesting discoveries pertaining to performance enhancement and general health with these compounds over the next few years.

Dosage: A four-ounce cup of green tea two or three times a day with a meal will supply you with viable doses of many flavones. For a more progressive approach, look for a product containing *Tribulus terrestris*—make sure it is standardized to at least 20% alkaloid content.

BETA-SITOSTEROL

Beta-sitosterol is a plant sterol or phytoestrogen—a plant-derived estrogen. Some plant estrogens have estrogenic activity in animals but not by increasing estrogen production. Instead, they can influence estrogenic activity in a drug-like fashion. However, somewhere along the way, some people began to assume that the human body would take these plant sterols and use them to increase natural levels of hormones, most notably testosterone. This is garbage. Beta-sitosterol, or any of the other plant sterols or phytoestrogens, will not increase levels of testosterone. If anything, beta-sitosterol will affect estrogen levels. However, even this area is unclear. Certain phytoestrogens will influence the body to produce more estrogen. However, others will counteract the body's naturally occurring estrogen. How can it act in two different, seemingly opposite ways? No one is sure.

If science could somehow isolate beta-sitosterol's anti-estrogenic effects, it might make a useful bodybuilding supplement. As it stands now, it isn't. There is, however, some evidence to suggest phytoestrogens in general might help fight certain types of cancer, but that evidence isn't solid yet. Phytoestrogens also seem to play a role in inhibiting cholesterol absorption.[267]

> "The use of *Ginkgo biloba* does appear to be effective in increasing mental focus and concentration..."

Dosage: Bodybuilders shouldn't use it at all.

GINKGO BILOBA

Now here's an herb which I find quite intriguing and yet somewhat frustrating. Intriguing because I have read rave reviews from Charles Poliquin, *Muscle Media*'s "Strength Guru," about the effects this herb has on his mental focus and perceived exertion during workouts. Charles swears this really helps him focus during his workouts, which we all know is one of the keys to intensity and, ultimately, muscular adaptation and growth. Research supports this idea of increased mental focus and concentration. Study findings include improved blood flow to the cerebral cortex,[15] augmented alpha-brain-wave patterns that are linked to alertness,[4] as well as enhanced ATP synthesis in the brain[121] and improved glucose uptake.[95]

Unfortunately, I can't give you much firsthand feedback regarding the use of this herb because it gives me a terrible headache. Apparently, a lot of bodybuilders get headaches from using this stuff.

The use of *Ginkgo biloba* does appear to be effective in increasing mental focus and concentration, and in reality, some people probably don't have an adverse reaction to its use. If you feel you're really lacking concentration and focus in the gym, I would recommend giving this a shot, just keep the Advil handy.

Dosage: It is important to find a form of *Ginkgo biloba* which is standardized for 24% glycosides and 6% terpenes. This is commonly referred to as a 24/6 form of *Ginkgo biloba*. If you can find that form, I would suggest using 120-160 mg/day, taken in 3 divided doses. Try taking one of those doses before your workout to get the most bang for your buck.

SAW PALMETTO

This is a botanical product that is derived from a small palm tree found in South Carolina and Florida. Over the past couple of years, saw palmetto has gained notoriety for its beneficial effects on a condition called "benign prostatic hyperplasia." In simpler terms, this is also known as enlargement of the prostate; a condition many men over 50 experience. The active constituents in saw palmetto have been found to inhibit the conversion of testosterone into a chemical called DHT or dihydrotestosterone. Apparently, DHT has something to do with causing the prostate to become enlarged.

What might be of interest to bodybuilders is that a double-blind, placebo-controlled study showed that saw palmetto actually has an anti-estrogenic effect, too. Unfortunately, the same study showed that it also blocked testosterone receptor sites.[71]

All in all, it looks like kind of a wash as far as bodybuilding applications go. However, saw palmetto might be effective at helping protect the prostate as men age. If you need this stuff, look for a saw palmetto extract that contains 85-95% fatty acids and sterols.

Dosage: The recommended dose of this extract to help prevent prostate enlargement is 160 mg twice a day.

159

•SPORTS SUPPLEMENT REVIEW, 3RD ISSUE•SPORTS SUPPLEMENT REVIEW, 3RD ISSUE•SPORTS SUPPLEMENT REVIEW, 3RD ISSUE•SPORTS SUPPLEMENT REVIEW, 3RD ISSUE•SPORTS SUPPLEMENT REVIEW, 3RD ISSUE•SPORTS SUPPLEMENT REVIEW, 3RD ISSUE•SPORTS SUPPLEMENT REVIEW, 3RD ISSUE•SPORTS SUPPLEMENT

THE FACTS AND FOLKLORE OF HERBAL SUPPLEMENTS

CHAPTER 7

FACTS AND FOLKLORE OF HERBAL SUPPLEMENTS•THE FACTS AND FOLKLORE OF HERBAL SUPPLEMENTS•THE FACTS AND FOLKLORE OF HERBAL SUPPLEMENTS•THE FACTS AND FOLKLORE OF HERBAL SUPPLEMENTS•THE FACTS AND FOLKLORE OF HERBAL SUPPLEMENTS•THE FACTS AND FOLKLORE OF HERBAL SUPPLEMENTS•THE FACTS AND FOLKLORE OF HERBAL SUPPLEMENTS•

MEXICAN YAM (DIOSCOREA)

This tasty little tuber also contains, as a matter of course, a variety of plant sterols. As I have mentioned, most plant sterols are relatively worthless in the body and don't create the types of changes we are looking for. The Mexican yam's claim to fame is that it supposedly contains a specific plant sterol which is converted in the body to active DHEA. Companies selling products containing this extract advertise it as "a natural form of DHEA."

To my knowledge, there have been no clinical studies looking at this particular plant sterol and its bio-activity in the body. My guess is that if this sterol is indeed converted to DHEA in the body, it is done so in such small percentages that it really wouldn't cause a viable increase of DHEA in your body.

But the real question is why would anybody use a Mexican yam plant sterol that *may* turn into DHEA in the body when you can simply take straight DHEA?

Final analysis: if you want DHEA effects, use DHEA, not Mexican yams.

Dosage: None.

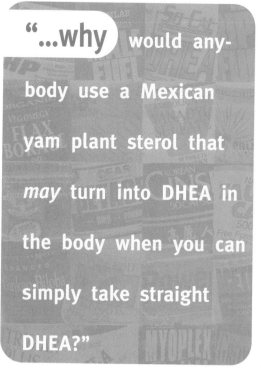

"**...why** would anybody use a Mexican yam plant sterol that *may* turn into DHEA in the body when you can simply take straight DHEA?"

SUMMARY

As I mentioned in the introduction to this chapter, I am not one to really pay attention to herbal extracts and their applications to bodybuilding (or almost anything else for that matter). However, I can't overlook the fact that herbal extracts and chemicals derived from herbs are now classified as dietary supplements, and some are becoming much more popular, as well as more sophisticated.

The overall effects of herbs cover the gamut, from potent diuretics to blood cleansing to testosterone enhancement. Obviously, some of these effects are more relevant to bodybuilders than others.

I think the diuretic effect of dandelion as well as the blood cleansing and organ protective effects of goldenseal and related herbs apply to bodybuilders. Use of guarana, *Gingko biloba,* and ephedra may also be applicable to bodybuilders due to their thermogenic effects, as well as their ability to increase concentration during a hard workout.

If you decide to try any of these compounds, I suggest sticking with reputable, well-known companies that can supply you with documentation of bio-activity and extract concentration. If you choose to venture deep into the realm of herbs, seek a qualified, experienced master herbalist. Many herbal extracts are strong medicine and can do more harm than good if not taken under supervision.

Although I feel herbs and their effects on athletic performance are, for the most part, still undocumented, I think this is going to be a growing field of supplementation. A word of advice to up-and-coming herbalists interested in sports: I see a new professional niche emerging in this industry: namely, "Sports Herbalist." If someone is willing to take the bull by the horns (and I know that some companies are doing it right now) and put the money, time, and effort into testing the purported effects of some of these herbal extracts, I think they can set themselves up with a nice future in this industry.

Personally, I am going to wait until more of the science is developed (or maybe I'll just start developing the science myself) before I jump headfirst into the rampant use of herbal concoctions.

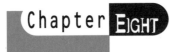

Chapter EIGHT

Amino Acids:
The Building Blocks of
Protein and Muscle Tissue

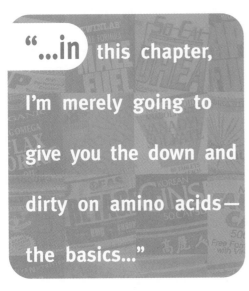

"...in this chapter,

I'm merely going to

give you the down and

dirty on amino acids—

the basics..."

Make no mistake, I could write hundreds of pages about the topic of amino acids alone; however, that is definitely <u>not</u> the purpose of this book. What I hope to accomplish with this bodybuilders' guide to the world of supplements is to assist in the development of your knowledge base—to help you decide which supplements are best for you—which ones might help you build muscle and burn fat faster.

I must admit, putting this book together has been a very big challenge. The primary struggle has not been to come up with a significant amount of scientific information to share with you; my real challenge has been weeding out the things that just aren't relevant.

When I look at the topic of amino acids, I don't think to myself, "Gee... how many dazzling facts about these things can I cram into this book, so I can make it a few pages longer?" In fact, just the opposite is true. I'm sitting here right now thinking, "What do my fellow bodybuilding friends really need to know about amino acids? What really matters?" My better judgment tells me a "crash course" on what amino acids are and what they do would be better than a long, drawn-out, complicated report on the topic. Thus, in this chapter, I'm merely going to give you the down and dirty on amino acids—the basics... with some important observations of my own.

WHAT ARE AMINO ACIDS?

Quite simply, amino acids are the building blocks from which protein molecules are made. Just as a house is made of bricks and this book is "made up" of multiple pages, every type of protein is made of amino acids. Every cell in your body contains amino acids. In fact, about three-quarters of the dry weight

REVIEW•SPORTS SUPPLEMENT REVIEW, 3RD ISSUE•SPORTS SUPPLEMENT REVIEW, 3RD ISSUE•SPORTS SUPPLEMENT REVIEW, 3RD ISSUE•SPORTS SUPPLEMENT REVIEW, 3RD ISSUE•SPORTS SUPPLEMENT

•SPORTS SUPPLEMENT REVIEW, 3RD ISSUE•SPORTS SUPPLEMENT REVIEW, 3RD ISSUE•SPORTS SUPPLEMENT REVIEW, 3RD ISSUE•SPORTS SUPPLEMENT REVIEW, 3RD ISSUE•SPORTS SUPPLEMENT REVIEW, 3RD ISSUE•SPORTS SUPPLEMENT REVIEW, 3RD ISSUE•SPORTS SUPPLEMENT REVIEW, 3RD ISSUE•SPORTS SUPPLEMENT REVIEW, 3RD ISSUE•SPORTS SUPPLEMENT

AMINO ACIDS: THE BUILDING BLOCKS OF PROTEIN AND MUSCLE TISSUE

THE BUILDING BLOCKS OF PROTEIN AND MUSCLE TISSUE•AMINO ACIDS: THE BUILDING BLOCKS OF PROTEIN AND MUSCLE TISSUE•AMINO ACIDS: THE BUILDING BLOCKS OF PROTEIN AND MUSCLE TISSUE•AMINO ACIDS: THE BUILDING BLOCKS OF PROTEIN AND MUSCLE TISSUE•AMINO ACIDS: THE BUILDING BLOCKS OF PROTEIN AND

of most cells is protein, which, of course, is made up of amino acids. As body-builders, when we hear "protein," we think primarily of skeletal muscle—biceps, triceps, quadriceps, etc. Sure, these major contractile muscles do contain a lot of protein, but in actuality, there are thousands of different kinds of protein in your body, including hormones like insulin, growth hormone, IGF-1, enzymes, anti-bodies, etc.

There are 17 amino acids I consider biologically important (and 6 which I don't think bodybuilders should concern themselves with). Each one has a "nitro-gen" part and a "carbon skeleton." The nitrogen part is the same for all amino acids. But the carbon part is different for every amino acid. A protein molecule is nothing more than a large string of these amino acids, connected end to end, much like beads in a necklace.

ESSENTIAL AND NONESSENTIAL AMINO ACIDS

When I was in college, my professors taught me there were eight "essen-tial" amino acids: isoleucine, leucine, lysine, methionine, phenylalanine, threonine, tryptophan, and valine. Hypothetically, if you were to consume a diet rich with these eight amino acids each day, your body would be able to manufacture all of the other amino acids needed for proper muscle growth, hormone and enzyme formation, etc. That's almost true—your body has to have these eight amino acids supplied by the diet—they are essential. But, I'm convinced there are at least four more amino acids which are *essential to bodybuilders: i.e., glutamine, taurine, alanine, and arginine.*

You see, it's my belief (and it's a concept that's shared by several scientific experts who are "in the know") that dividing amino acids into categories of essential (non-dispensability) and nonessential (dispens-ability) is too crude to adequately explain the ways in which amino acids are metabolized under various condi-tions of health, disease, and most importantly for us, under the unique conditions experienced by bodybuilders who are constantly recovering from intense weight-training exercise. I firmly believe the proteins considered to be "complete" by nutritionists and dietitians are actu-ally incomplete proteins for bodybuilders, as they lack the proper amounts of key amino acids which a body subjected to intense weight-training stress requires.

What I'm getting at is that even a diet rich in complete proteins like eggs, chicken, and beef may not

> "...even a diet rich in complete proteins... may not adequately address your body's need for all 'conditionally essential' amino acids."

adequately address your body's need for all "conditionally essential" amino acids. Thus, using supplements, protein powders, or meal-replacement products that are fortified with glutamine and taurine, especially, could be very important to your bodybuilding success.

It's very likely you're familiar with the terms "complete" and "incomplete" proteins. In case you aren't, complete proteins are ones that contain the essential amino acids; complete proteins include things like milk, meats, fish, poultry, as well as eggs. Incomplete proteins, on the other hand, are those that do not contain all the essential amino acids—these are foods which contain some essential amino acids but not all, such as grains and vegetables. For example, corn is deficient in the essential amino acids lysine and tryptophan, and beans lack the essential amino acid methionine.

WHAT HAPPENS TO AMINO ACIDS AND PROTEINS IN YOUR BODY?

When you consume a protein-containing food or supplement, your stomach starts to "cleave" or chop up proteins by subjecting them to an enzyme called *pepsin*. The long chains of amino acids get broken down into shorter chains; then the partially digested protein passes into your small intestine where pancreatic enzymes further break down the protein into either single or short-chain amino acids (polypeptides). Finally, a little further along in your small intestine, another group of enzymes called *peptidases* break down the polypeptides into single amino acids and chains two or three amino acids long (dipeptides and tripeptides, respectively). The single amino acids, along with dipeptides and tripeptides, are absorbed into your bloodstream, which transports them to the liver. From there, one of four things happens—the amino acid can either reenter the bloodstream and circulate through-out the body; it can be converted to a different amino acid; it can be used to form one kind of protein or another; or it can be broken down further into metabolites (for example, the amino acid leucine is broken down to something called KIC and then broken down again into a metabolite called HMB).

Of course, not all the amino acids from the proteins you eat get incorporated into the protein structure of the body. Where they end up depends on what your body needs at that time. As weight trainers, one of our principle concerns is to make sure our bodies have enough protein to rebuild muscle tissue after intense workouts. As I've said before, I think most bodybuilders need at least 1-1.5 grams of protein per pound of bodyweight a day (I weigh around 200 lbs, and I usually try to con-sume around 200-300 grams of protein a day, divided into 5 or 6 feedings).

Once we've satisfied our bodies' need for protein with the amino acids necessary to rebuild muscle tissue and support the rest of our bodies' protein requirements (remember, protein is needed to form hormones, enzymes, even your

165

AMINO ACIDS: THE BUILDING BLOCKS OF PROTEIN AND MUSCLE TISSUE

THE BUILDING BLOCKS OF PROTEIN AND MUSCLE TISSUE•AMINO ACIDS: THE BUILDING BLOCKS OF PROTEIN AND MUSCLE TISSUE•AMINO ACIDS: THE BUILDING BLOCKS OF PROTEIN AND MUSCLE TISSUE•AMINO ACIDS: THE BUILDING BLOCKS OF PROTEIN AND MUSCLE TISSUE•AMINO ACIDS: THE BUILDING BLOCKS OF PROTEIN AND

fingernails), the excess protein is broken up—the nitrogen part gets converted into urea and excreted in the urine, and the carbon part (the carbon skeleton) gets stored as fat. Thus, contrary to what some believe, an excess amount of protein (especially on a high-calorie diet) can be converted to fat.

Protein can also be used as fuel for energy—this is especially true of the branched-chain amino acids (BCAA's) and is one reason many athletes believe supplementing their diets with extra BCAA's will give them greater energy.

Eventually, all amino acids end up being broken down in what's called "protein turnover," which is the continual cycling of protein in the body and includes anabolism (the building up of muscle tissue) and catabolism (the breaking down of tissue).

AMINO ACID FORMS D AND L

Every amino acid comes in two forms, a "right-handed" (D) and a "left-handed" (L) form. These two forms are chemically identical; however, they differ structurally in that one form is a mirror image of the other form. Protein chains cannot be formed from a combination of D and L forms. Almost every protein molecule in our bodies is made exclusively from L forms of amino acids. However, there are D forms, both natural and synthesized, which appear to have some therapeutic value.

FREE-FORM AMINO ACIDS

Free-form amino acid supplements—those that contain the purified or crystalline amino acids, are still quite popular in bodybuilding. These are amino acid supplements that have already been "synthetically digested" or separated. Despite what some experts and marketers claim, consuming free-form amino acids is not the best way to get the protein you need to build new muscle tissue and maintain a healthy body; however, free-form amino acids can be useful under certain circumstances, provided your protein needs are met and you're using the free-form amino acid(s) in an effort to achieve some "special effect." For example, some amino acids, like tryptophan and tyrosine, have a direct effect on neurotransmitters. Consuming free-form amino acids, like glutamine and arginine, may enhance growth hormone secretion (although we're not sure this accelerates muscle growth or fat burning). Here's a quick run through of what the various amino acids are and what they do, as they pertain to bodybuilding.

Essential AMINO ACIDS

METHIONINE

This is an essential amino acid, which, of course, is found in virtually all complete proteins, such as beef, poultry, fish, pork, eggs, soybeans, cottage cheese, and yogurt. This amino acid plays an important role in the formation of RNA and DNA. It's also a pretty powerful antioxidant and is particularly "active" in combating the free radicals released by alcohol. In addition, methionine helps increase the absorption of selenium—a trace mineral that appears to be a powerful antioxidant. It's also one of the three amino acids which is used to form creatine in the body, but despite what some marketers claim, I've found no scientific evidence whatsoever that consuming mega-doses of methionine, with or without creatine, enhances the effects of creatine supplementation. Supplementing the diet with more methionine than you would get in any complete protein doesn't offer any advantage in terms of muscle building or fat loss, either.

"...I've found no scientific evidence whatsoever that consuming mega-doses of methionine... enhances the effects of creatine supplementation."

PHENYLALANINE

This is an essential amino acid found in virtually all complete proteins, as well as nuts, seeds, and lentils.

Phenylalanine, when taken on an empty stomach (200-500 mg), may act as an appetite suppressant in two ways: first, by stimulating noradrenaline and second, phenylalanine can decrease appetite by releasing more "cholecystokinin" (CCK). CCK is released in the small intestine as nutrients pass through and sends a signal to the brain "indicating" enough food has been consumed, so a person would feel satisfied.[251]

The "DL" form of phenylalanine has also been shown to reduce pain by blocking the breakdown of endorphins (natural painkillers) in the body.

A small percentage of the population suffers from a disease called phenylketonuria (PKU) where their systems lack an enzyme in the liver which metabolizes dietary phenylalanine. This is a very serious disease, and it's the reason you see that FDA-mandated warning, "Phenylketonurics: contains phenylalanine" on virtually any aspartame-containing product. Aspartame is made up of three naturally occurring compounds: phenylalanine, aspartic acid, and methanol. It's a virtually nontoxic, very potent sweetener. Nonetheless, people with PKU need to limit their dietary intake of phenylalanine and should therefore avoid the use of aspartame and phenylalanine. Fortunately, PKU is extremely rare. (Just in case you were wondering...)

THREONINE

I'm not exactly sure what the heck this essential amino acid does, but suffice it to say, deficiencies prevent the normal formation of thousands of important

AMINO ACIDS: THE BUILDING BLOCKS OF PROTEIN AND MUSCLE TISSUE

CHAPTER 8

THE BUILDING BLOCKS OF PROTEIN AND MUSCLE TISSUE•AMINO ACIDS: THE BUILDING BLOCKS OF PROTEIN AND MUSCLE TISSUE•AMINO ACIDS: THE BUILDING BLOCKS OF PROTEIN AND MUSCLE TISSUE•AMINO ACIDS: THE BUILDING BLOCKS OF PROTEIN AND MUSCLE TISSUE•AMINO ACIDS: THE BUILDING BLOCKS OF PROTEIN AND

168

protein structures in the body. Of course, threonine can be found in all complete proteins, which, as I'm sure you're aware by now, are dairy products, meats, eggs, etc.

TRYPTOPHAN

This essential amino acid has quite an interesting history. Although, like all essential amino acids, it's critical for muscle building and health, tryptophan was one of the most popular free-form amino acids on the market in the '70's and '80's. However, in 1988, the FDA banned the sale of tryptophan. This was a knee-jerk reaction to a rare blood disease which affected a few tryptophan users in the U.S. Scientists traced the disease to a single contaminated batch of the amino acid produced by the Japanese corporation called Showa Denko. The company had altered the time-honored manufacturing process for tryptophan and introduced a new, untested procedure while abbreviating an important filtering step.

The adverse effects of this tainted batch of tryptophan, which unfortunately included numerous deaths, have never been linked to any other batches of tryptophan. Nevertheless, the FDA has maintained its prohibition, in spite of overwhelming evidence that it is not only unnecessary but may also be forcing people to take more dangerous and expensive tryptophan alternatives.

The main reason tryptophan was so popular was because it was/is a very effective natural sleep aid—consuming a few grams in the late evening works very well for inducing sleep. Remember how I told you some amino acids have almost "drug-like" effects because they influence neurotransmitters (chemicals which basically "run" your brain)? Tryptophan is one of those aminos—when you take tryptophan, it crosses the blood/brain barrier and acts as a precursor to serotonin, a potent neurotransmitter which helps you sleep. (Since tryptophan is no longer widely available in health-food stores, most people have switched to melatonin, which has similar effects.)

> **"The main reason tryptophan was so popular was because it was/is a very effective natural sleep aid..."**

Interestingly enough, most protein foods don't contain all that much tryptophan—but you will find relatively large amounts of this essential amino acid in carbohydrate foods (especially bananas, as well as in sunflower seeds and milk). There's a reason why folks often drink a glass of milk late in the evening to induce sleep—it's because of the tryptophan effect.

There is some evidence tryptophan may be an appetite suppressant—helping to curb cravings for carbohydrates. (However, I've tried tryptophan during a dieting phase, and it didn't really help control my cravings for carbohydrates or any other type of food.)

Strangely, you can buy tryptophan at some health-food stores, but it's labeled for use in animals only (horses, dogs, etc.). Obviously, the companies selling tryptophan for animal use only are just jumping through a legal loophole to get tryptophan back on the market for the millions of insomniacs who relied on tryptophan religiously before it was taken off the market by the FDA. Even though I would personally shy away from any supplement, or drug for that matter, that's labeled for use in animals only (because of concerns about quality and purity), I've heard the tryptophan that's available in health-food stores, labeled for animal use only, is at least 99% pure tryptophan. Nevertheless, I order my tryptophan from a foreign mail-order pharmacy called Inhome Health Services, Suite 401, 302 Regent Street, London, W1R 6HH, England.

The bottom line is, I think tryptophan is a great natural sleep aid, but I don't see any particular reason to use a supplemental form of it for any direct bodybuilding purposes. (Of course, sleep is a very important part of recovery for intensely training athletes, so I guess you might call it an indirect bodybuilding aid.)

VALINE

Valine is one of the branched-chain amino acids (BCAA's). By the way, they're called "branched chain" because of their molecular configuration—I'm not going to bore you with the friggin' details on their "interlocking methyl groups" and all that crap, but suffice it to say, there's a reason they're called branched chain. Then again, who cares?

Valine and the other two BCAA's, isoleucine and leucine, are interesting compounds in that they make up one-third of muscle protein. Of the three branched-chain amino acids, valine is the most mysterious—I don't know exactly why exercise eats up so much of this essential amino acid (neither do scientists). Perhaps it's because, along with the other two BCAA's, it is a vital substrate for two other amino acids, glutamine and alanine, which are released in large quantities during intense exercise. Furthermore, BCAA's are used directly for fuel by muscles, and that spares other amino acids from being catabolized.

There's really no need to use a free-form valine supplement, although the idea of using BCAA supplements is not completely without merit. The good news is, by simply consuming a couple servings of a quality whey-protein supplement each day, you'll be providing gram quantities (high dosages) of all three BCAA's. Unless you've got some major hang-up with using protein powders or meal-replacement products, I don't think supplementing the diet with valine, or any of the BCAA's individually, is going to produce a noticeable effect on your ability to put on new muscle size and gain strength.

AMINO ACIDS: THE BUILDING BLOCKS OF PROTEIN AND MUSCLE TISSUE

THE BUILDING BLOCKS OF PROTEIN AND MUSCLE TISSUE•AMINO ACIDS: THE BUILDING BLOCKS OF PROTEIN AND MUSCLE TISSUE•AMINO ACIDS: THE BUILDING BLOCKS OF PROTEIN AND MUSCLE TISSUE•AMINO ACIDS: THE BUILDING BLOCKS OF PROTEIN AND MUSCLE TISSUE•AMINO ACIDS: THE BUILDING BLOCKS OF PROTEIN AND MUSCLE TISSUE•AMINO ACIDS: THE BUILDING BLOCKS OF PROTEIN AND

CHAPTER 8

AMINO ACIDS: THE BUILDING BLOCKS OF PROTEIN AND MUSCLE TISSUE•AMINO ACIDS: THE BUILDING BLOCKS OF PROTEIN AND MUSCLE TISSUE•AMINO ACIDS:

ISOLEUCINE

In many ways, isoleucine is similar to valine: they're both BCAA's, and neither of them has any specific therapeutic value. Of course, they both serve as precursors for glutamine and alanine, which, as I already mentioned, are used up like crazy during intense weight-training exercise. Also, both valine and isoleucine can be used as fuel by muscle cells, thereby sparing other amino acids from being lost or burned up. Nonetheless, the BCAA's play an important role in protein synthesis, anabolism, and anti-catabolism. Without adequate amounts of BCAA's, muscle cells won't heal as fast, and they won't grow.

As I previously mentioned, using a whey-protein-containing supplement is a great way to make sure your muscles are being loaded up with quality BCAA's.

LEUCINE

This is the third BCAA, and it, along with glutamine, is the most heavily researched amino acid, at least in regards to its effects on protein metabolism and muscle growth. Several scientific studies have shown that supplementing the diet with gram quantities of leucine may improve athletic performance. Other studies have shown that in patients suffering from severe catabolic conditions (such as following an operation or some other type of severe trauma) lose less muscle mass (suffer less proteolysis or muscle catabolism) when they are fed high quantities of leucine.[54, 166] However, there are also studies done with healthy test subjects which show supplementing the diet with extra leucine does not produce a noticeable effect on the muscle-building process or athletic performance.[28]

Of course, like the other BCAA's, leucine is an essential amino acid and is required for the proper formation and function of all kinds of proteins, including muscle tissue.

One researcher who has probably studied the effects of the amino acid leucine as much or more than anyone in the world is Dr. Steve Nissen of Iowa State University. For over ten years, Dr. Nissen tried to unlock the mysteries of leucine's effects. After years of research, he discovered the anabolic and anti-catabolic effects of the amino acid leucine were most likely attributable to a downstream metabolite called beta-hydroxy beta-methylbutyrate (widely known as "HMB"). According to Dr. Nissen's research (which has recently been confirmed by Dr. Vukovich at Wichita State University), HMB seems to exert significantly greater effects than leucine. (For more information about this topic, see the HMB section in Chapter 4.)

I don't believe consuming more leucine than you get from a quality whey-protein supplement or from complete protein sources like meats and dairy products offers any particular advantage. In fact, to really notice the effects of leucine, I think you'd have to take upwards of 20-60 grams of this stuff a day, which would not only be expensive and impractical but would most likely make you very sick to your stomach. Use a few grams of HMB instead.

LYSINE

This essential amino acid is used by the body to form carnitine, another amino acid which plays a key role in transporting fatty acids into muscle cells where they can be used as a source of energy. If carnitine levels are suboptimal, there's a possibility that poor fatty acid metabolism will occur, which may contribute to elevated blood lipid levels and may actually interfere with your efforts to lose bodyfat. But, I have found virtually no evidence that bodybuilders gain any significant fat-burning advantage by supplementing their diets with lysine. If you're consuming a diet rich with quality proteins, you don't need to supplement with lysine.

> "...the anabolic and anti-catabolic effects of the amino acid leucine were most likely attributable to a downstream metabolite called beta-hydroxy beta-methylbutyrate (widely known as 'HMB')."

"Conditionally ESSENTIAL"
Amino Acids for Bodybuilders

GLUTAMINE

This is one of those amino acids I mentioned earlier in this chapter—one that old-school nutrition textbooks tell us is not essential but contemporary science tells us *is* essential. In fact, no amino acid fulfills the criteria of being "conditionally essential" better than glutamine.

Glutamine is involved in a large variety of metabolic processes, including: the regulation of cell volume as a regulator of the balance between anabolism and catabolism of fat, carbohydrate, and protein; as a fuel for the gut and cells of the immune system; and of course, as a component of protein. Over the last 15 years, it has become apparent that there are many situations when the body doesn't get enough glutamine. Although the body actually gets or "borrows" glutamine from many sources (from the diet, from breaking down protein, and/or by depletion of intracellular stores of glutamine), there may not be enough available to satisfy its needs. In such circumstances, glutamine is a conditionally essential amino acid, without which, the body functions suboptimally (which means impaired immunity and crippled muscle metabolism).

I discuss this very interesting amino acid in depth in Chapter 4 of this book. For now, suffice it to say that I am a big, big believer in glutamine supplementation.

AMINO ACIDS: THE BUILDING BLOCKS OF PROTEIN AND MUSCLE TISSUE

THE BUILDING BLOCKS OF PROTEIN AND MUSCLE TISSUE•AMINO ACIDS: THE BUILDING BLOCKS OF PROTEIN AND MUSCLE TISSUE•AMINO ACIDS: THE BUILDING BLOCKS OF PROTEIN AND MUSCLE TISSUE•AMINO ACIDS: THE BUILDING BLOCKS OF PROTEIN AND MUSCLE TISSUE•AMINO ACIDS: THE BUILDING BLOCKS OF PROTEIN AND

I think all bodybuilders should be using a free-form L-glutamine supplement every day or consuming a supplement that is fortified with glutamine, such as many of the popular meal-replacement products and protein powders on the market. I always try to get at least ten extra grams of glutamine a day, above and beyond what I get from whole foods.

ALANINE

This is another amino acid that's not considered essential under old-school theories, but I'm convinced it is essential to bodybuilders. Once you start breaking down muscle tissue and trying to force your body to remodel (to grow), you're creating a whole new metabolic environment—one which has dramatically different nutritional needs than that of the average, sedentary person.

Alanine is one of the amino acids which is broken down and released in massive quantities during intense exercise. Alanine, somewhat similar to glutamine, also plays a role in cell volumizing.[233] And it helps provide a source of glucose to stabilize blood sugar. Fortunately, whey-protein supplements contain a relatively high amount of alanine, and it's also being added to several supplements (including EAS' CytoVol, which I use every day). If you're not using a supplement that contains alanine, consider it—an extra two grams, right after exercise, could make a big difference in your overall bodybuilding endeavors.

TAURINE

This is another amino acid I consider "conditionally essential." Next to glutamine, taurine is the most abundant free amino acid in muscle tissue. (Interestingly enough, it's not part of the actual muscle tissue—it exists primarily in the amino acid "pool" within the muscle cell.) Taurine has a number of interesting bodybuilding applications—it acts as an "insulin mimicker," which means it may enhance glucose and amino acid metabolism. It appears to play a prominent role in cell volumizing, which means it may enhance protein metabolism, and new research shows that taking 3 separate 500-mg doses a day may help decrease protein breakdown, as evidenced by a 20% decrease in something called 3-methylhistidine (3-MH), a muscle breakdown product.[182]

Taurine can be made by the body from the amino acids methionine and cysteine with the assistance of Vitamin B_6, but it's questionable whether or not the

> "...I am a big, big believer in glutamine supplementation. I think all bodybuilders should be using a free-form L-glutamine supplement every day..."

172

body can provide an optimal (remember there's a difference between *normal* and *optimal*) level of taurine—that's why I'm calling it a conditionally essential amino acid.

Intense exercise and other types of stress deplete taurine levels in the body; thus, I'm quite convinced supplementing the body with taurine—at least a gram or two—several times a day is a good idea. (A great time to take a gram of taurine is right after a workout.)

Because of taurine's possible insulin-like effects, a gram of it has also been added to EAS' Phosphagen HP creatine supplement. Taurine can also be found in many multinutrient formulas, including Myoplex Plus.

ARGININE

As with the other conditionally essential amino acids, it's questionable whether or not the body can make enough arginine from other amino acids.

Back in the '80's, supplementing gram quantities of this amino acid was very popular, as some scientific studies showed large doses of arginine increase growth hormone (GH) secretion.[282] Unfortunately, it does not appear the "pulse" of GH that is released by consuming arginine does anything profound in terms of accelerating muscle gains and fat loss. Scientific studies have shown an absence of any positive effect on athletic performance or body composition with arginine supplementation.[236]

Interestingly enough, arginine is now being touted as a pro-sexual supplement—apparently, consuming between 6 and 18 grams helps increase the production of a chemical known as "nitric oxide" (NO), which helps men "get it up" and keep it up, so to speak.

I haven't ruled out large doses (10+ grams per day) of arginine as possibly being anti-catabolic—I've discussed the issue with several scientists who have conducted literally hundreds of studies on protein metabolism, and they believe arginine has some interesting effects. Personally, I believe by supplementing gram quantities of the amino acid glutamine, and by using the leucine metabolite HMB, you will have a significantly greater benefit than you would have by supplementing arginine.

Nonessential AMINO ACIDS

ORNITHINE

Ornithine, along with arginine, was a hot supplement in the '80's—touted as a powerful growth hormone releaser. But, as I mentioned in the section on arginine, I don't think a short-term elevation in growth hormone automatically equates to greater bodybuilding results.

Another supplement that was popular a few years ago combined ornithine with another amino acid compound called alpha-ketoglutarate (AKG). This supplement

AMINO ACIDS: THE BUILDING BLOCKS OF PROTEIN AND MUSCLE TISSUE

THE BUILDING BLOCKS OF PROTEIN AND MUSCLE TISSUE~AMINO ACIDS: THE BUILDING BLOCKS OF PROTEIN AND MUSCLE TISSUE~AMINO ACIDS: THE BUILDING BLOCKS OF PROTEIN AND MUSCLE TISSUE~AMINO ACIDS: THE BUILDING BLOCKS OF PROTEIN AND MUSCLE TISSUE~AMINO ACIDS: THE BUILDING BLOCKS OF PROTEIN AND

CHAPTER 8

was coined "OKG," and in some scientific studies, it did help slow protein breakdown in hospital patients,[67] but the stuff tasted so bad, and you had to take a whopping ten-gram dose all at once to allegedly get the supplement to work. Unfortunately, slamming down ten grams of OKG made most people sick to their stomachs (myself included), so it just wasn't feasible. Thus, the "OKG craze" came and went in a matter of a few months.

Overall, I don't think taking an ornithine supplement will help bodybuilders do much of anything.

CARNITINE

This nonessential amino acid is a very popular "fat-burning" supplement in the sports nutrition market. Research shows that carnitine has a dramatic effect on fat metabolism and the reduction of blood fats, like triglycerides.[220, 221] Carnitine is also responsible for transferring fatty acids across cell membranes to the mitochondria (the furnace of a cell), where they can be used as energy.

Carnitine can be synthesized from the essential amino acid lysine, and deficiencies in this amino acid are rare. But, there are some conditions when carnitine supplementation does seem to offer some benefit. The possible mechanisms by which carnitine could have a positive effect include enhancing oxidation of fatty acids, a critical energy compound during exercise; preserving muscle glycogen during exercise, a factor potentially related to fatigue resistance; shifting fuel use towards glucose, thereby decreasing the oxygen requirement of exercise; improving resistance to muscle fatigue; and increasing the oxidative capacity of skeletal muscle.

Clinical studies looking at carnitine and its effects on exercise performance or metabolism during exercise have usually involved a small number of test subjects and have not been what I would call overwhelmingly convincing. Some evidence suggests it may help athletic performance, but overall, I tend to believe that carnitine, whether administered intravenously or orally, acutely or chronically, has no consistent effects on key metabolic parameters during exercise or on exercise performance. I'm also not convinced it's a potent fat burner, but some experts believe otherwise—they recommend supplementation with two to four grams of L-carnitine (the DL form of carnitine is not recommended, as it may be toxic) taken for two weeks, one hour before exercise. If you want to give it a try, I don't think it would be a really bad idea, but it didn't work for me.

TYROSINE

This amino acid is one of those which is somewhat popular for its "stimulating" effects. You see, tyrosine has the opposite effect of the amino acid tryptophan. Tyrosine actually blocks the absorption of tryptophan across the blood/brain barrier and helps "pick you up." Most protein foods have a relatively high amount of tyrosine in them; thus, it is theorized, and I would say it is true in many cases, if you consume a protein-containing food or even a tyrosine supplement (1-3 grams) 20-30 minutes before consuming a large carbohydrate meal, like pasta, pizza, etc., you may be able to avoid the drowsy, sluggish feeling a large carbohydrate meal can produce.

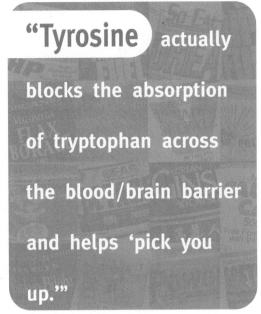

"**Tyrosine** actually blocks the absorption of tryptophan across the blood/brain barrier and helps 'pick you up.'"

Sometimes I'll take a couple grams of tyrosine 30 minutes before I work out as an alternative to using something like caffeine or ephedrine. I am absolutely convinced that using tyrosine in this manner helps increase strength—I've had some of my strongest bench and squat workouts in the past year after loading up on tyrosine. I'm convinced tyrosine supplementation helps increase nerve transmission from the brain to the muscle, exciting more motor units and creating greater strength. I've had several bodybuilding buddies try this, and they've noticed the same thing. Thus, I don't believe it's a placebo effect. When I normally bench press 335 lbs for 2 or 3 reps but can do 4 or 5 after taking tyrosine, it gets my attention! I don't use it before every workout because I suspect there might be some type of down-regulation, or "attenuation" as scientists call it, to its effects.

If you're looking for an interesting, non-nerve-rattling pure workout supplement, I would suggest you stop by a health-food store, pick up some free-form tyrosine, and try popping a couple grams with water or a protein drink (not a carb drink!) about 30 minutes before you train. Also, if you have a problem with an afternoon slump or loss of energy (especially following a carbohydrate meal or snack), I would suggest taking a couple grams of tyrosine 20-30 minutes before you eat lunch. Give it a try—I think there's a good chance you'll be pleased with the results.

GLYCINE

This is an amino acid that may have some interesting bodybuilding effects. For over 50 years, some scientists have believed that glycine may increase athletic performance—exactly how, no one is quite sure. Glycine is one of the three amino acids that leads to the formation of creatine (creatine is naturally formed from the amino acids arginine, glycine, and methionine). Some experts believe glycine may have a positive effect on athletic performance or bodybuilding because it, like several other free-form amino acids that I've discussed in this chapter, acts as a neurotransmitter and may cause an elevation in growth hormone release.

AMINO ACIDS: THE BUILDING BLOCKS OF PROTEIN AND MUSCLE TISSUE

THE BUILDING BLOCKS OF PROTEIN AND MUSCLE TISSUE-AMINO ACIDS: THE BUILDING BLOCKS OF PROTEIN AND MUSCLE TISSUE-AMINO ACIDS: THE BUILDING BLOCKS OF PROTEIN AND MUSCLE TISSUE-AMINO ACIDS: THE BUILDING BLOCKS OF PROTEIN AND MUSCLE TISSUE-AMINO ACIDS: THE BUILDING BLOCKS OF PROTEIN AND

Unfortunately, as with many amino acids, the amount necessary to produce a dramatic increase in growth hormone is impractical (between 10 and 30 grams a day) and may cause a headache and stomachache.

Lately, I've become more interested in glycine because of its effect on cell volume/cellular hydration. According to one of my friends and trusted scientific colleagues, Anthony Almada, glycine—when administered along with glutamine and alanine—may have a synergistic cell-volumizing effect.[286] This is why a very precise dosage has been added to EAS' cell-volumizing formula, CytoVol.

Gamma-Aminobutyric Acid (GABA)

This nonessential amino acid was very popular in bodybuilding in the early '90's; it was billed as a substitute for GHB (back then, touted as a growth hormone releaser, now a "hip" recreational "drug"). Unfortunately, GABA causes some unusual and downright scary side effects in more than a handful of those who experiment with it. After consuming a five-gram dose, it's not uncommon to have a frightening shortness of breath which I attribute to some type of allergic reaction. In some individuals, this sets off a tailspin that often includes hyperventilation, rapid heartbeat, and panic.

Of course, the majority of people who use GABA, or try it, don't have the side effects, but I've experienced it a couple of times myself, and it's very unpleasant, to say the least.

Anyway, those who don't suffer side effects from GABA can actually notice a calming, relaxing, "tryptophan-like" effect. And, like several other amino acids we've discussed in this chapter, GABA is purported to have relatively profound growth hormone releasing effects.[3, 48]

I tried GABA off and on during the early '90's without a lot of success. The feedback from bodybuilders who have used this supplement hasn't been anything remarkable. Thus, I don't recommend it.

Histidine

Now we're really starting to get into the irrelevant amino acid area, and I'll try to shoot through this section as fast as possible. In a nutshell, the amino acid histidine plays a role in the health of nerve cells, blood vessels, etc. All of the histidine your body needs is made from essential amino acids.

Cysteine and Cystine

Metabolically, cysteine and cystine are pretty much interchangeable, and when the rubber hits the road, I don't really give a rat's ass about either. I don't

> "...glycine —when administered along with glutamine and alanine— may have a synergistic cell-volumizing effect."

know of anything unique that either of these nonessential amino acids does that pertains to bodybuilding. Your body's requirements for these amino acids are easily met by consuming adequate quantities of quality protein.

PROLINE

Proline is another amino acid that is nonessential—virtually all you need can be made from other amino acids in the body. This stuff plays a role in the formation of collagen—the protein that supports all other tissues.

ASPARAGINE AND ASPARTIC ACID

Asparagine and aspartic acid play an important role in human metabolism, like virtually all amino acids, but I don't want to bore you with irrelevant details. Suffice it to say, there really aren't any unique bodybuilding applications worth discussing regarding these agents.

CITRULLINE

This is another nonessential amino acid that I really couldn't care less about and one which you don't need to concern yourself with, either.

SERINE

This is yet another nonessential amino acid that I don't even know why I'm listing in this book because there is nothing interesting to say about it.

SUMMARY

All right, let's go back and review this whole issue of amino acids and see what we've learned:

Amino acids are the building blocks of protein—they are the individual components of all the different types of protein in our bodies.

There are 8 amino acids that are considered essential, 4 I classify as conditionally essential, and 11 that are nonessential and can be manufactured, in ample quantities, from essential amino acids.

Generally, consuming 1-1.5 grams of quality protein per pound of bodyweight per day (for me, that's between 200 and 300 grams of protein a day) in 5 or 6 divided doses, from sources such as chicken, fish, red meat, eggs, milk, and quality protein powders, generally provides enough essential amino acids, including the branched-chain amino acids.

Above and beyond that, I think it's especially important to supplement the diet with glutamine, either through a meal-replacement product that's fortified with this very important amino acid, a protein powder, or through a free-form glutamine supplement.

AMINO ACIDS: THE BUILDING BLOCKS OF PROTEIN AND MUSCLE TISSUE

THE BUILDING BLOCKS OF PROTEIN AND MUSCLE TISSUE•AMINO ACIDS: THE BUILDING BLOCKS OF PROTEIN AND MUSCLE TISSUE•AMINO ACIDS: THE BUILDING BLOCKS OF PROTEIN AND MUSCLE TISSUE•AMINO ACIDS: THE BUILDING BLOCKS OF PROTEIN AND MUSCLE TISSUE•AMINO ACIDS: THE BUILDING BLOCKS OF PROTEIN AND

Besides that, specific amino acids can be used for their "drug-like" effects on certain neurotransmitters. For example, tryptophan can be an effective sleep aid, while tyrosine may increase strength and alertness throughout the day. (I especially recommend it before a workout.)

Other amino acids like alanine and glycine may help promote cell volume, which could indirectly enhance muscle growth.

When it's all said and done, this whole topic of amino acids is not really all that complicated. Hopefully, the information in this chapter helped you understand this issue better and gave you some ideas on how to apply the knowledge of this not-so-complex topic to get better results faster from the time you spend in the gym.

Chapter NINE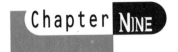

Odds and Ends:
Miscellaneous Supplements with
Possible Bodybuilding Applications

Not every "bodybuilding supplement" is an amino acid, an herb, nor a vitamin or mineral—there are some that fall into a "miscellaneous category." A number of these supplements have unique effects (some are actually "drug like"), while I'd describe the potential of others as "so-so," and a few of them are probably effective only under certain circumstances. In this chapter, I'll review some of these "odds and ends" which I think might be of interest to you.

"...if you have difficulty sleeping, melatonin might be a useful weapon in your bodybuilding supplement arsenal."

MELATONIN

Melatonin is a hormone that occurs naturally in our bodies—it helps set and control the "internal clock" that governs natural rhythms of the body. Each night, the "pineal gland" produces melatonin which helps us fall asleep. Research on this hormone has been going on since it was first discovered in 1958, but its use as a supplement has become popular only over the past few years. Since late 1994, literally millions of people have tried melatonin, and over a thousand articles, in all kinds of media, have been published about the possible effects of melatonin.

Melatonin is an extremely popular "replacement" for the amino acid tryptophan, which was a very popular natural sleep aid before it was taken off the market almost a decade ago. In fact, melatonin is probably more effective for most than tryptophan, as it is one step closer to serotonin—a neurotransmitter which helps one reach a state of slumber (zonk out).

Now, what could melatonin do for bodybuilders? Well, there's no question that good quality sleep, on a consistent basis, is essential to proper recovery—if you didn't already know, your muscles grow when you're *resting*, <u>not</u> when you're

•SPORTS SUPPLEMENT REVIEW, 3RD ISSUE•SPORTS SUPPLEMENT REVIEW, 3RD ISSUE•SPORTS SUPPLEMENT REVIEW, 3RD ISSUE•SPORTS SUPPLEMENT REVIEW, 3RD ISSUE•SPORTS SUPPLEMENT REVIEW, 3RD ISSUE•SPORTS SUPPLEMENT REVIEW, 3RD ISSUE•SPORTS SUPPLEMENT REVIEW, 3RD ISSUE•SPORTS SUPPLEMENT

REVIEW•SPORTS SUPPLEMENT REVIEW, 3RD ISSUE•SPORTS SUPPLEMENT REVIEW, 3RD ISSUE•SPORTS SUPPLEMENT REVIEW, 3RD ISSUE•SPORTS SUPPLEMENT

ODDS AND ENDS: MISCELLANEOUS SUPPLEMENTS WITH POSSIBLE BODYBUILDING APPLICATIONS

SUPPLEMENTS WITH POSSIBLE BODYBUILDING APPLICATIONS–ODDS AND ENDS: MISCELLANEOUS SUPPLEMENTS WITH POSSIBLE BODYBUILDING APPLICATIONS–ODDS AND ENDS: MISCELLANEOUS SUPPLEMENTS WITH POSSIBLE BODYBUILDING APPLICATIONS–ODDS AND ENDS: MISCELLANEOUS SUPPLEMENTS WITH POSSIBLE BODY

training! So, if you have difficulty sleeping, melatonin might be a useful weapon in your bodybuilding supplement arsenal.

Melatonin may also help you beat jet lag—that "out-of-it" feeling you get when traveling from L.A. to New York or across any time zone. In fact, melatonin is *very* effective for this purpose, in my opinion.

Some marketers claim melatonin can help prevent cancer, help you live longer, and boost your sex life. I don't know about all those claims—sometimes marketers take *a little bit* of science and stretch it *a lot*. But, I can vouch for one of the claims marketers make, which is melatonin will give you "more vivid dreams." I don't know how you feel about this, but I don't necessarily want more vivid dreams. I just want to go to sleep and wake up rested seven or eight hours later. I don't need anything remarkable to happen during that period of time.

The first time I took melatonin, I went to sleep all right, but about three hours later, I woke up (or at least I thought I was awake), and I was seeing shit you wouldn't believe. I don't want to get into that right now, but it wasn't pleasant, to say the least. In fact, I've talked to quite a few people who experience bizarre nightmares when they use melatonin, but I'd be joshing you if I said all people get freaked out on this stuff. Some report "pleasant" vivid dreams.

I actually like tryptophan (it produces a healthy state of zzz's without freaking me out in the middle of the night) more than melatonin, but I am definitely in the minority. I know a lot of bodybuilders use melatonin, and that's cool, but I don't think it should be used regularly, as its effects attenuate (downgrade) with continued use. Save it for when you really need it. (If you need it every night, go see your doctor and talk to him/her about possible causes of insomnia as well as possible cures.)

In terms of what dosage people use, it's all over the board, but on average, I'd say most get good effects with 3 mg about 30 minutes before they want to go to sleep.

> "...several new studies have shown that CLA may indeed enhance fat loss and increase lean body mass."

ACETYL-L-CARNITINE (ALC)

This is an interesting and relatively new product that is structurally similar to L-carnitine, but it has significantly different effects. Animal research shows ALC supplementation *might* have a number of positive applications because of its "protective" effects on brain and heart tissue, and it may even lower cholesterol levels.[239]

Of more interest to bodybuilders, ALC may help prevent the reduction in testosterone that can occur with intense training; however, there are no human studies that

I could locate (and I scoured the research), which offer support for claims some marketers of ALC are making—they claim it increases testosterone and works "like steroids" and that it has powerful anti-catabolic effects. These claims are, in my opinion, largely unsubstantiated. But, that doesn't mean ALC is worthless—it's just one of those interesting supplements which might have positive effects for body-builders but one that needs more research in order to make a determination as to just how useful it might be.

CONJUGATED LINOLEIC ACID (CLA)

In last year's *Supplement Review*, I introduced the concept of using CLA as a bodybuilding supplement. Since then, some interesting, new studies have offered further evidence that CLA may indeed be an effective supplement for supporting fat loss and an increase in lean body mass.

Up until a few years ago, CLA was an unrecognized nutrient—it occurs naturally in a wide variety of foods, particularly in beef, turkey, and some dairy products. (Because of this, CLA is not a drug—it's a dietary supplement.) In more than 17 years of research, CLA has been shown to be an anti-carcinogen in several animal models, to reduce the adverse catabolic effects induced by immune stimulation, to enhance growth, and even to improve blood lipid profiles.[23] In the last couple of years, scientists at the University of Wisconsin-Madison, and elsewhere, have begun to study CLA's effects on metabolism and body composition.

In fact, in just the past year, the results of several new studies have shown that CLA may indeed enhance fat loss and increase lean body mass. For example, a study entitled, "Conjugated Linoleic Acid Reduces Body Fat"—conducted by Dr. Michael Pariza and others—showed that CLA-fed laboratory animals exhibited significant bodyfat reductions and increases in lean body mass. This study showed that diets containing at least .5% CLA have a significant effect.

This study, which supports the effects of CLA intake on reductions in body-fat, revealed that it may be effective in very reasonable dosages. After six weeks of feeding, it was found that CLA-fed laboratory animals had a bodyfat percentage of 4.34 versus the control group with a bodyfat percentage of 10.13.[212] Obviously, this is a substantial difference.

One other study looked at the effects of CLA on growth rather than body-fat loss. It was found that CLA fed to lactating laboratory animals improved weight gain. The young animals then continued to ingest CLA in their normal diets and gained significantly more bodyweight than the control group.[53]

It has been postulated from this and other studies that CLA may be a growth factor for at least some species. Whether or not this translates to humans at this

•SPORTS SUPPLEMENT REVIEW, 3RD ISSUE•SPORTS SUPPLEMENT REVIEW, 3RD ISSUE•SPORTS SUPPLEMENT REVIEW, 3RD ISSUE•SPORTS SUPPLEMENT REVIEW, 3RD ISSUE•SPORTS SUPPLEMENT REVIEW, 3RD ISSUE•SPORTS SUPPLEMENT REVIEW, 3RD ISSUE•SPORTS SUPPLEMENT REVIEW, 3RD ISSUE•SPORTS SUPPLEMENT

ODDS AND ENDS: MISCELLANEOUS SUPPLEMENTS WITH POSSIBLE BODYBUILDING APPLICATIONS

SUPPLEMENTS WITH POSSIBLE BODYBUILDING APPLICATIONS–ODDS AND ENDS: MISCELLANEOUS SUPPLEMENTS WITH POSSIBLE BODYBUILDING APPLICATIONS–ODDS AND ENDS: MISCELLANEOUS SUPPLEMENTS WITH POSSIBLE BODYBUILDING APPLICATIONS–ODDS AND ENDS: MISCELLANEOUS SUPPLEMENTS WITH POSSIBLE BODY

182

point is somewhat up in the air, but we should have answers to this question soon, as several university research studies are underway to evaluate the effects of CLA on humans.

Researchers aren't exactly sure how CLA works, but they have several theories—one is that it has a positive effect on chemicals in the immune system known as "cytokines." It's possible that muscle growth and fat loss cannot be optimized when the levels of cytokines and something else, called "prostaglandins," are not in line.

Another theory is that CLA may alter the way nutrients are used by the body—perhaps by enhancing the flow of nutrients at the cell membrane level. Whatever the case, study after study (in a number of different animal species), has shown the same thing—CLA supplementation burns fat and increases lean body mass.

CLA use among athletes and mainstream fitness enthusiasts is increasing at an amazing rate. In fact, the product is being promoted as a fat burner and muscle-tone enhancer in virtually all the muscle magazines, as well as publications like *Shape, Let's Live, Men's Exercise, Health*, and even *Prevention* magazine. You see, if CLA exerts the same positive effects in humans as it does in animals, it is unquestionably going to be a blockbuster supplement. Basically, the stuff could help almost anyone, not just bodybuilders, look and feel better. Another benefit of supplementing with CLA is that it's a potent antioxidant—possibly even more powerful than the "world-famous" antioxidants Vitamin E and beta-carotene, which gives it an even wider appeal.

EAS has been distributing a quality form of CLA for about a year now. Another company, called PharmaNutrients, produces a high-quality form of CLA called Tonalin™, which is also widely available.

CLA is covered by a number of patents which include the use of the compound for fat loss and muscle gain. EAS is licensed by the patent holder (the Wisconsin Alumni Research Foundation) and so is PharmaNutrients.

As is the case with almost all supplements, there are some versions out on the market that are not high quality; in fact, we've tested some supplements that were supposed to contain CLA, and they were nothing but straight vegetable oil. Thus, I'd look for the Tonalin brand name of CLA, or you could just go with EAS', whatever works for you.

One of the lingering questions about CLA use—one that needs to be answered with university research—is exactly what dosage is most effective. Extrapolating the dosages used in animal studies and applying it to humans leads me to believe anywhere between two and six grams per day of CLA might be effective. For the last few months, I've been using four grams per day. I get one gram in each serving of a total-nutrition product I use called Myoplex Plus Deluxe (the *only* meal-replacement/protein powder on the market that is fortified with CLA). That gives me three grams, and I'm guessing I get another gram from my whole-food diet.

The problem with trying to consume the optimal level of CLA from whole foods (as with creatine, HMB, and a number of other nutrients) is that it's impractical, if not impossible, to get enough of this particular micronutrient through regular foods, day in and day out, to experience a positive effect. That's why dietary supplementation of products like this may be important. By consuming a precise amount of this fatty acid every day, you can provide your body with an amount of this stuff that would not be possible to get through a regular whole-food "balanced diet."

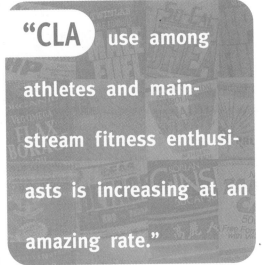

"CLA use among athletes and mainstream fitness enthusiasts is increasing at an amazing rate."

Because CLA seems to exert an effect on fat loss, you might use it while you're dieting. But, using CLA during a bulking phase may work well, too. Studies have shown CLA helps improve what's called "feed efficiency" in animals, which means that the ones receiving CLA and a certain amount of food gained more lean body mass than animals receiving an "inactive" fat, like vegetable oil, and the same amount of feed. This is of great interest to the "meat-producing industry," as they are always looking for drug-free ways to bulk up livestock without spending more money on feed. (Steroid use is banned in animals just like it is in sports.) In fact, CLA was patented in 1994 as a method for increasing the efficiency of feed conversion in animals.

CLA isn't yet "tried and true," so it didn't make my top ten supplements list, but it could easily be classified as an "honorable mention." The animal data on CLA is so compelling and the results are so dramatic that I would be amazed if it doesn't produce good results in human studies. For now, we just have to wait and see. But, I would definitely say it's worth giving it a try.

GLYCEROL

I've received some questions about this supplement from bodybuilders, but I consider it an endurance supplement—in fact, a *long-term* endurance supplement—like for marathoners or triathletes. High-dosage glycerol supplementation, accompanied by massive amounts of water intake, may help enhance performance in endurance athletes by preventing dehydration. There have been some theories thrown around regarding the possible use of glycerol in a pre-contest bodybuilding situation, but it's not something I consider a viable option. So, glycerol isn't worthless altogether, it's just not something that really has any significant bodybuilding applications.

ODDS AND ENDS: MISCELLANEOUS SUPPLEMENTS WITH POSSIBLE BODYBUILDING APPLICATIONS

CHAPTER 9

SUPPLEMENTS WITH POSSIBLE BODYBUILDING APPLICATIONS•ODDS AND ENDS: MISCELLANEOUS SUPPLEMENTS WITH POSSIBLE BODYBUILDING APPLICATIONS•ODDS AND ENDS: MISCELLANEOUS SUPPLEMENTS WITH POSSIBLE BODYBUILDING APPLICATIONS•ODDS AND ENDS: MISCELLANEOUS SUPPLEMENTS WITH POSSIBLE BODY

HYDROXY CITRIC ACID (HCA)

My opinion of HCA hasn't changed much since I wrote the *1996 Supplement Review*. To recap, HCA is a natural compound extracted from the rind of the fruit *Garcinia cambogia*. In clinical studies, with laboratory animals, HCA supplementation acts as an appetite suppressant, and it has shown the ability to inhibit the actions of a specific enzyme in the liver, called ATP-citrate lyase. This particular enzyme is partially responsible for the conversion of dietary carbohydrates to fat.[109] Basically, in animals, HCA can enhance weight loss by influencing the animals to eat less and possibly by modifying the animals' metabolism so they don't convert carbohydrates to fat at the "normal rate."

It looks like it's effective in animals, but there's not a lot (understatement) of solid human data. I think it might work though. Perhaps future research will give us some more conclusive answers. Unfortunately, there haven't been a lot of human studies done on HCA—I suspect the companies that are marketing the product may have reservations about putting this stuff to the test, as it might shoot a hole in their balloon, so to speak.

I think a good way to experiment with HCA is to use it during a dieting or cutting cycle (perhaps during the 2 low-calorie weeks on the Anabolic Burst Cycling System), in a dosage of 500-1,000 mg, taken 30-60 minutes before meals, 3 times a day. You might give it a try—if it doesn't work, don't use it again, but I have received some positive feedback on it, even though I can't honestly say this stuff worked for me. (I've tried it several times.)

> "...fat is not always the enemy and... in certain circumstances, dietary fats may enhance muscle gain."

CHITOSAN

This is a fiber supplement derived from the shells of crustaceans. Some studies have actually shown this particular compound may help block the absorption of fat in the gut. Some marketers claim chitosan "absorbs" up to 12 times its weight in fat when consumed prior to a relatively fatty meal. But, using this stuff may interfere with the absorption of some minerals and fat-soluble vitamins. I've also heard that some people can get a pretty nasty stomachache and/or diarrhea from using it. (In this way, chitosan sounds similar to another "new-to-the-market" fat-blocking compound, which some of the major food companies are experimenting with, called olestra.)

I think chitosan might become popular for those in the mainstream who are seeking something, anything, to help them lose weight, but most bodybuilders have their fat intake under control; in fact, I would say a lot of bodybuilders go off the deep end, in terms of restricting fat, and over the past couple of years, I've had to help "debrainwash" thousands of weight-training athletes—to help convince them fat is not always the enemy and that, in certain circumstances, dietary fats may enhance muscle gain.

I don't see a lot of bodybuilding applications for chitosan, but I don't think it's completely worthless—it may, in fact, help block the absorption of some fat calories, but like I said, it's not something I'm really "rah-rah" about.

BREWER'S YEAST

This stuff has been used by fitness buffs for decades, and today, it's still popular with vegetarians and some athletes who follow what's called a "macrobiotic diet" (which is a very strict vegetarian diet—in its most extreme form, followers of the diet are "allowed" to eat only rice, whole grains, and raw vegetables).

The product is comprised of millions of tiny yeast cells which are grown in culture and then dried. (Boy, that's fascinating stuff, isn't it?!)

Brewer's yeast is far from a "bodybuilding breakthrough," but it is a quality, natural source of Vitamin B_{12}, copper, and iron—all nutrients which strict vegetarian diets may lack. And, it's also rich with chromium, which has important effects on maintaining proper insulin function—something that should be a vital concern to all bodybuilders. I don't use it myself, but one of my friends who is a vegetarian adds a tablespoon to all his meal-replacement drinks, and he gives it the thumbs-up (but then again, he's kind of a flake).

5-HYDROXYTRYPTOPHAN (5-HTP)

This is a novel, relatively interesting compound, which ties into the whole tryptophan, melatonin, sleep-enhancing-supplement thing. This stuff—5-HTP—is what's called an "intermediate" in the conversion process of the amino acid tryptophan to the neurotransmitter serotonin. As I've already discussed in this book, tryptophan is one of those amino acids that has almost "drug-like" effects. It crosses the blood/brain barrier and is converted by 5-HTP to serotonin, which helps set in motion a "cascade" of reactions that make it easier for you to fall asleep.

There is evidence to support the theory that 5-HTP is converted to serotonin in substantial quantities after oral consumption.[270] Another study actually compared tryptophan head to head with 5-HTP and found the latter compound to be superior in helping relieve symptoms of depression. (One cause of depression is a serotonin deficiency. For me, I think depression is caused by pizza—whenever I get around it, I usually binge like crazy, and when I wake up in the morning and look in the mirror, my abs are coated with this "enhanced" layer of fat, and I get very bummed out. Funny how that happens...)

REVIEW•SPORTS SUPPLEMENT REVIEW, 3RD ISSUE•SPORTS SUPPLEMENT REVIEW, 3RD ISSUE•SPORTS SUPPLEMENT REVIEW, 3RD ISSUE•SPORTS SUPPLEMENT REVIEW, 3RD ISSUE•SPORTS SUPPLEMENT REVIEW, 3RD ISSUE•SPORTS SUPPLEMENT REVIEW, 3RD ISSUE•SPORTS SUPPLEMENT REVIEW, 3RD ISSUE•SPORTS SUPPLEMENT

•SPORTS SUPPLEMENT REVIEW, 3RD ISSUE•SPORTS SUPPLEMENT REVIEW, 3RD ISSUE•SPORTS SUPPLEMENT REVIEW, 3RD ISSUE•SPORTS SUPPLEMENT REVIEW, 3RD ISSUE•SPORTS SUPPLEMENT REVIEW, 3RD ISSUE•SPORTS SUPPLEMENT REVIEW, 3RD ISSUE•SPORTS SUPPLEMENT REVIEW, 3RD ISSUE•SPORTS SUPPLEMENT

ODDS AND ENDS: MISCELLANEOUS SUPPLEMENTS WITH POSSIBLE BODYBUILDING APPLICATIONS

SUPPLEMENTS WITH POSSIBLE BODYBUILDING APPLICATIONS•ODDS AND ENDS: MISCELLANEOUS SUPPLEMENTS WITH POSSIBLE BODYBUILDING APPLICATIONS•ODDS AND ENDS: MISCELLANEOUS SUPPLEMENTS WITH POSSIBLE BODYBUILDING APPLICATIONS•ODDS AND ENDS: MISCELLANEOUS SUPPLEMENTS WITH POSSIBLE BODY

Oh... on a related note, 5-HTP has been shown to have some appetite-suppressing effects, but it's really not that potent in this regard.

Products containing 5-HTP are pretty hard to find, but you might ask about them at your local health-food store if you'd like to try an alternative to tryptophan or melatonin. As far as dosage goes, I've heard 200 mg 30-60 minutes before you want to go to sleep gets the job done.

GLUCOSAMINE

This supplement is very popular in the mainstream health and fitness market, and I think it may be effective during certain situations for some bodybuilders. You see, glucosamine, made up of a glucose molecule and an "amine" group (it's actually made when glucose and an amino acid collide), helps stimulate the production of connective tissue, specifically cartilage. Glucosamine has been thoroughly studied in double-blind, placebo-controlled university studies (almost all of them have been done in Europe). The researchers' primary interest is in using glucosamine as a treatment for osteoarthritis—a painful condition in which cartilage slowly degenerates. Studies comparing the effects of glucosamine against the pain reliever/anti-inflammatory ibuprofen showed that glucosamine, although it took a bit longer to take effect (four weeks), worked better than ibuprofen.[271]

Glucosamine not only has anti-inflammatory effects but it may also help treat arthritis by helping regenerate cartilage.[76] This is where I see the possible bodybuilding application—virtually anyone who trains with weights, over a period of years, is bound to experience certain overuse injuries. Eventually, you have to give up certain exercises altogether because your joints just can't take it anymore.

Last year, after I had a nasty motocross accident and completely screwed up my left shoulder and elbow, I took glucosamine every day, for two months, and I suspect that it played an important role in my full recovery.

The bottom line is, research shows glucosamine may help you recover from connective-tissue injuries and may assist in strengthening this tissue. If your shoulders, elbows, or knees ache—if they seem to be crying out for help—you might give glucosamine a try. Of course, you should also see your doctor to make sure you have the situation properly diagnosed. There are many different causes of aches and pains—some are more serious than others.

By the way, some supplements, such as shark cartilage and something called "green lipped muscle" (man, does that sound weird!) do contain glucosamine but in relatively small amounts compared to pure glucosamine supplements.[188, 247]

Here's another tip: if you try glucosamine, stack it with something called "chondroitin sulfate." Chondroitin sulfate is another biological polymer derived from connective tissue. It acts as the flexible connecting matrix between the tough protein filaments in cartilage to help give it both strength and elasticity. In terms of dosage, the research suggests between 500 and 1,000 mg of glucosamine, stacked with 200-300 mg of chondroitin sulfate, 3 times a day with meals, is plenty. There's some evidence to suggest that glucosamine *HCL* is the best form, but I've also heard that the sulfate form is just as good.

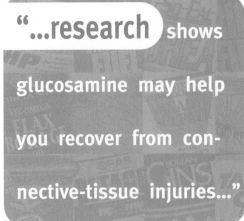

"...**research** shows glucosamine may help you recover from con-nective-tissue injuries..."

PHOSPHATIDYLSERINE (PS)

This supplement, which I reviewed in the last edition of this book, is being promoted as an anti-catabolic agent. PS hit the market in early 1996 after one pretty solid clinical study showed it may reduce cortisol levels (which are often elevated) after exercise.[187] Hypothetically, this might allow the body to avoid some of the catabolic fallout of intense training and could help you recuperate more quickly and, ultimately, build more muscle. The theory behind PS is not unsound and not completely without substantiation, but studies need to be performed (I've offered to help fund research to the company that sells this stuff) to evaluate whether or not chronic PS supplementation may help weight trainers build muscle, lose fat, or improve some aspect of their metabolism and/or health.

Hopefully, in the coming year, we'll learn more about the possible effects of PS and whether it is or isn't a worthwhile bodybuilding supplement. For now, all I can tell you is that the feedback I've been getting from *Muscle Media* readers who've tried this stuff is "very so-so." However, I haven't given up on it yet. By the way, if you do want to give it a try, from what I understand, the best results for cortisol suppression were found with an 800-mg dose in 2 evenly divided doses (400 mg in the morning and 400 mg before workouts or before going to bed, on non-training days) with or between meals.

ALPHA-KETOGLUTARATE (AKG)

Alpha-ketoglutarate is a molecule that plays various intermediate roles in energy metabolism, as well as cellular formation. It functions as a constituent of the "oxidative decarboxylation reaction" involved in generating ATP. Say what? In other words, it's a necessary component for ATP energy production in muscle cells. This is important, but AKG also serves another, probably more important, function for bodybuilders.

AKG acts as a direct precursor to the synthesis of glutamine in the body.[100] You should be aware of the important anabolic and anti-catabolic properties of glutamine. By supplementing with AKG, it's possible to support higher levels of circulating and muscle-bound glutamine. One of the main benefits of consuming AKG with glutamine is that AKG may more efficiently bypass the gut and enter

ODDS AND ENDS: MISCELLANEOUS SUPPLEMENTS WITH POSSIBLE BODYBUILDING APPLICATIONS

SUPPLEMENTS WITH POSSIBLE BODYBUILDING APPLICATIONS–ODDS AND ENDS: MISCELLANEOUS SUPPLEMENTS WITH POSSIBLE BODYBUILDING APPLICATIONS–ODDS AND ENDS: MISCELLANEOUS SUPPLEMENTS WITH POSSIBLE BODYBUILDING APPLICATIONS–ODDS AND ENDS: MISCELLANEOUS SUPPLEMENTS WITH POSSIBLE BODY

the bloodstream. You see, the gut has a great demand for glutamine because of its rapid cellular turnover. When it sees glutamine, it traps much of it for its own use, while AKG slides through "unnoticed." For this reason, AKG may be an effective delivery form of glutamine to muscle cells. I'd suggest consuming between two and four grams of AKG a day. A few extra grams can go a long way. It's good stuff.

PHOSPHATES

This is one supplement which I think is very underrated. Studies show that when athletes supplement their diets with phosphate, it significantly enhances endurance[64, 240, 295] (although it has not been conclusively determined that this translates to an increase in muscle mass). <u>Sodium</u> phosphate (to the best of my knowledge, calcium phosphate is ineffective) is thought to act as a buffering agent—these are compounds that help "squelch" the production of lactic acid during exercise. The theory behind using buffers to enhance athletic performance is to decrease the rate at which lactic acid builds up in muscle tissue. By the way, part of that burning feeling you get when you're training hard is from lactic acid, and if you haven't noticed, shortly after your muscles start to burn, they give out—scientists believe that's from the buildup of lactic acid. Thus, if you can postpone this effect, you can probably get a few more heavy reps in before you hit "failure." And, that could help you and me get better results faster from the time we spend working out.

188

> "...consuming some supplemental phosphate may help you get the most out of your creatine supplementation..."

Another reason phosphates might be important bodybuilding supplements is because they are part of the formation of creatine phosphate or phosphocreatine—the storage form of creatine in muscles. Just about every bodybuilder I know is using creatine on a regular basis, and a lack of phosphates may be a limiting factor in the development of phosphocreatine. Basically, consuming some supplemental phosphate may help you get the most out of your creatine supplementation (that's one reason why phosphate has been added to Phosphagen HP).

Endurance athletes may need as much as four grams of sodium phosphate a day (consumed in four separate one-gram doses with meals), to notice a powerful punch, but I think much lower doses could offer benefits to bodybuilders—possibly preventing lactic-acid buildup and enhancing the effects of the creatine.

Soy Protein

As we discussed earlier in this book, there are all kinds of different protein supplements available. I believe that quality forms of whey protein are the best—egg protein and certain types of milk-protein isolates are also good quality, and then there's soy. Typically, soy is rated relatively low by various measures of protein quality, but in reality, soy is a complete protein, and according to one new measure of protein quality, called the Protein Digestibility Corrected Amino Acid Score (PDCAAS), soy is right up there with the best proteins.[223]

I'm not so sure soy protein is all that great, but there's another reason that you might want to consider using soy protein from time to time. Mounting evidence suggests soy-protein supplementation may help boost thyroid hormone levels or may help maintain them during calorie-restricted diets.[20, 89] In case you don't already know, when you start to diet, your body typically fights back by lowering thyroid hormone levels, making it more difficult to lose fat. Some athletes have tried to circumvent this situation by using thyroid drugs—Cytomel is one of the more popular ones.

Studies have suggested that *isolated soy protein* (not soy-protein concentrate—there is a big difference!) may contain substantial amounts of phytochemicals which may help support natural production of thyroid hormones.

Thus, if you've been dieting, and despite increased exercise and reduced calories, your fat loss is at a standstill, you might try supplementing 50 grams of soy-protein isolate a day—you could add 25 grams to a meal-replacement powder, once in the morning and again at night. It might help get your diet back on track. (By the way, one of the quality products in this category is called Supro™, which is produced by Protein Technologies International.)

Glutathione (GSH)

This is a powerful antioxidant—in fact, it may be the body's most potent naturally occurring free-radical-fighting substrate.

Intense exercise has been shown to decrease the body's natural level of glutathione by 40% in muscle cells and 80% in the liver (which is where muscles derive their supply of glutathione).[224] Some scientists are convinced if we can find a way to offset this decrease in glutathione, it could enhance the positive effects of exercise.

Two popular nutrients which can help increase glutathione levels in your body are N-acetyl-cysteine (NAC) and Vitamin C. Although these two nutrients appear to be very effective in maintaining high glutathione levels, their effects are indirect. The obvious alternative would appear to be using a pure glutathione supplement, but whether or not that works has not been conclusively determined. One animal study, conducted in 1989, showed consuming a glutathione supplement did help protect muscle cells from injury.[278] However, another more recent study, using human

189

ODDS AND ENDS: MISCELLANEOUS SUPPLEMENTS WITH POSSIBLE BODYBUILDING APPLICATIONS

CHAPTER 9

SUPPLEMENTS WITH POSSIBLE BODYBUILDING APPLICATIONS=ODDS AND ENDS: MISCELLANEOUS SUPPLEMENTS WITH POSSIBLE BODYBUILDING APPLICATIONS=ODDS AND ENDS: MISCELLANEOUS SUPPLEMENTS WITH POSSIBLE BODYBUILDING APPLICATIONS=ODDS AND ENDS: MISCELLANEOUS SUPPLEMENTS WITH POSSIBLE BODY

190

test subjects, showed a single dose of 3,000 mg of glutathione did not significantly increase blood levels of this compound. Thus, some scientists have suggested glutathione either does not survive the gut environment well or is not absorbed through the intestinal wall to increase glutathione levels.[298]

I'm convinced using Vitamin C (at least 3 grams/day) and NAC (around 800-1,500 mg/day) significantly elevates your blood levels of glutathione, but if you want to add a glutathione supplement on top of that, go for it.

CYCLO HISTIDYL-PROLINE DIKETOPIPERAZINE (CHP)

One of the biggest challenges in trying to cut up (to lose fat and gain muscularity) is simply trying to control your appetite—to stick with your diet. It's not easy! Scientists and drug companies know this as well; thus, the market for appetite-suppressing pharmaceuticals is enormous. Drugs like Redux (dexfenfluramine) and the popular fen/phen (fenfluramine/phentermine) appetite suppressants are used by hundreds of thousands of folks who are trying to lose fat—their use is even gaining popularity in bodybuilding/fitness. Unfortunately, appetite-suppressing drugs have side effects; in fact, they have some *serious* side effects, which include something called pulmonary hypertension, which is virtually always fatal. Fortunately, this condition occurs in only a small percentage of people who use these drugs, but there is a risk nonetheless. This has caused some researchers to look for more natural, yet effective, appetite suppressants—one of the more interesting ones, which some scientists are very excited about, is called CHP. This naturally occurring compound belongs to a class of nutrients known as "cyclic peptides."

Cyclic peptides are among the simplest peptide (short amino acid chains) derivatives commonly found in nature. Most of these cyclic peptides appear to be byproducts of fermentation and food processing. However, many are natural components of various types of meats and plants. They appear to have a variety of biological effects. For example, animal studies on CHP show that it may alter "food preference." Research carried out by Drs. Chandon Prasad and John F. Wilbur revealed that when blood levels of CHP are increased, voluntary food intake decreases.[10]

Human studies have shown CHP levels are a strong indicator of appetite.[21] Apparently, a high level of CHP correlates strongly with a small appetite and reduced food intake, whereas low levels are associated with increased food intake. Thus, CHP may be a potent appetite suppressant. But, that's not all—apparently, this cyclic peptide may help "turn off" cravings for fatty foods. (By the way, CHP is not one of those "speed-like" appetite suppressants—it does not work in a similar manner to amphetamines.)

At this time, several studies are being designed to evaluate the effects of CHP on healthy subjects who are trying to lose fat. The results from this research should be available later this year.

GELATIN (TYPE II COLLAGEN)

Over the past few years, scientists have been exploring the possibility that supplementing type II collagen (a specific nutrient found in gelatin) may actually help arthritic patients slow the progression of their disease or even halt it. To test this theory, researchers at Harvard Medical School supplemented the diets of arthritic patients with a type of purified type II collagen for three months. What this study seemed to indicate is that collagen supplementation significantly reduced swelling and joint pain.[276] It was further discovered that during the study, collagen appeared to suppress T-cell-mediated autoimmune disease, which, according to U.S. Patent 5,529,786, is one of the mechanisms which might cause the progression of rheumatoid arthritis.

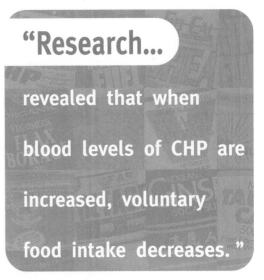

"Research... revealed that when blood levels of CHP are increased, voluntary food intake decreases."

Now, some experts have speculated that type II collagen may also help prevent the degeneration of joints that occurs with weight-training exercise and have suggested that supplementing your diet with gelatin may actually allow you to build healthier joints. In this regard, it seems to act similar to glucosamine.

Purified type II collagen is not on the market yet—for now, the next best thing is simply regular old Knox unflavored gelatin—just add a packet of it to a glass of juice or a protein drink. Stacking it with glucosamine might be a good idea.

ORNITHINE ALPHA-KETOGLUTARATE (OKG)

This is a supplement that I thought was really going to make a big impact on bodybuilding when I discovered it a few years ago. But, for some reason, it just didn't pan out. Some studies show that the use of OKG in hospitalized patients suffering from catabolic conditions, such as burns or severe trauma, may help slow protein loss.[67] This led me to believe that a similar effect might occur in weight trainers, but I tried the stuff, and I've talked to literally dozens of other people who have tried it, and it just doesn't seem to do anything. And, on top of that, it tastes absolutely disgusting, and you have to take ten grams all at once, and that can really upset the stomach. OKG is not worthless, but it's not very popular in bodybuilding either.

KETOISOCAPROIC ACID (KIC)

This supplement is a metabolite of the BCAA leucine which has been extensively studied by doctors and other researchers. KIC has been shown to have some anabolic and protein-sparing properties,[86] but more recently, research has revealed that the positive effects on muscle metabolism seen with leucine and/or KIC use are most likely due to a metabolite of these two compounds called HMB.[94]

KIC, in dosages over 20 grams a day (which could make you sick), may produce a positive effect on muscle growth, although no scientific studies on

ODDS AND ENDS: MISCELLANEOUS SUPPLEMENTS WITH POSSIBLE BODYBUILDING APPLICATIONS

SUPPLEMENTS WITH POSSIBLE BODYBUILDING APPLICATIONS~ODDS AND ENDS: MISCELLANEOUS SUPPLEMENTS WITH POSSIBLE BODYBUILDING APPLICATIONS~ODDS AND ENDS: MISCELLANEOUS SUPPLEMENTS WITH POSSIBLE BODYBUILDING APPLICATIONS~ODDS AND ENDS: MISCELLANEOUS SUPPLEMENTS WITH POSSIBLE BODY

weight-training humans have demonstrated this. KIC isn't trash—HMB is just a lot better and easier to use.

SODIUM BICARBONATE

Scientists have been studying sodium bicarbonate (baking soda) and its effect on exercise performance for over 60 years now. Many studies over the years have concluded that sodium bicarbonate is an effective ergogenic (performance-enhancing) agent,[64, 295] but a number of studies have come to the conclusion that sodium bicarbonate is not an effective ergogenic aid.[148, 213]

It appears the reason for such discrepancy from study to study may be linked to the dosage used in the trials and the amount of time between the delivery of sodium bicarbonate and the start of exercise and testing.

One recent study performed with sodium bicarbonate which did produce positive results used a dosage of 135 mg/lb of bodyweight approximately 90 minutes before exercise. Sodium bicarbonate can be consumed in a capsule form or as a drink by adding sodium bicarbonate powder to a cup of water.

Sodium bicarbonate may help increase performance by acting as a "buffering" agent—neutralizing acid byproducts of exercise and allowing muscles to function at optimal levels for a greater period of time. Another possible mechanism of action that may result in strength increases after sodium-bicarbonate loading is that sodium bicarbonate induces a higher pH level and increases calcium-ion binding to troponin (a chemical involved in muscular contractions).

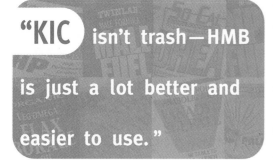

"KIC isn't trash—HMB is just a lot better and easier to use."

The main problem that exists with using an effective dose of sodium bicarbonate (135 mg/lb of bodyweight) is that this solution can often cause stomach discomfort and gastric disturbances. Of course, any ergogenic benefit brought about by using sodium bicarbonate would be nullified if you were forced to work out with a stomachache.

If you want to try sodium bicarbonate to see if you can tolerate it, I'd suggest experimenting with a very small dose at first (20 mg/lb of bodyweight) and gradually increasing the dose. If you start experiencing side effects like stomach pain or nausea, you'll obviously have to discontinue the use of this product. However, if your stomach can tolerate it and you typically work out very intensely, you may indeed notice increased endurance and strength from using sodium bicarbonate.

INOSITOL

This water-soluble chemical is a natural constituent of cellular cytoplasm (fluid)—found inside muscle cells. Inositol is also considered a "hydrophilic compound," which means it grabs hold of water and carries it around with it wherever it goes. For this reason, oral supplementation of inositol may very well have cell-volumizing effects. By increasing blood concentrations of inositol, it may be possible to deliver greater amounts into muscle cells, drawing water and other nutrients in with it, thus, expanding the muscle cell. This is why EAS researchers have added it to the cell-volumizing formula CytoVol.

LYSOPHOSPHATIDYLCHOLINE

This is a compound which was just introduced to the bodybuilding market. It has just recently been approved as a food additive by the FDA due to the lobbying power of the giant food company Archer Daniels Midland, who use a watered-down version in some baking products. (It's used in small amounts to "condition" dough—making it more elastic so it can rise higher and make "fluffier" bread.) It is a natural derivative of lecithin, which is a fatty acid type of substance derived from soy and other natural sources.

Lysophosphatidylcholine is protected under a number of British patents, where it's being used to improve weight gain in livestock. Studies cited in UK Patent 2,269,746 have shown that it causes an expansion of many cells in the stomach and intestinal walls, allowing rapid uptake of some nutrients. This increased permeability and nutrient uptake has apparently increased the feed efficiency in farm animals, allowing them to assimilate more nutrients from the foods they eat.

I think this stuff is a little scary. By opening up cell membranes in the gut, you may be allowing undesirable chemicals to enter your system. I think the science is intriguing, and my guess is further human studies will be done. It may become rather popular in the marketplace as an aid to increasing the effectiveness of some products, such as glutamine.

CHOLINE/PHOSPHATIDYLCHOLINE

Choline is a chemical which is essential for proper neurological function. It's also a functional component of all cell membranes. One other function of choline in the body is to help transport fat out of the liver, thus ensuring proper fat metabolism. Choline can be manufactured in the body from the amino acids methionine and serine, but it's one of those nutrients you might need to consume more of than the body typically produces. It was just recently designated as an essential nutrient—meaning we should consume some in our diets each day.

The most active and beneficial form of choline comes in the form of phosphatidylcholine. This compound has been found to have very strong effects on the liver. It's been used in Germany for many years now to help treat liver disorders, especially those arising from alcohol or other chemical abuse. It's very interesting to note that phosphatidylcholine may possibly help regenerate damaged liver cells.

Phosphatidylcholine supplementation has also been shown to possibly lower cholesterol levels, remove cholesterol from tissue deposits, and inhibit platelet aggregation (which means decrease the stickiness of your blood, preventing it from clogging up your arteries).[41] A recent study showed that patients with elevated cholesterol and triglyceride levels who were treated with phosphatidylcholine for 30 days experienced a 33% reduction in blood cholesterol levels, while triglycerides also fell 33%, and HDL (good) cholesterol levels increased by 46%.[299]

This stuff is quite versatile. It's also been shown to aid Alzheimer's patients suffering from memory loss,[159] as well as to treat certain depressive disorders.[301] The recommended dosage for the treatment of liver disorders (pay attention past and present steroid users) is 350-500 mg; for cholesterol lowering, 500-900 mg should be used. The whole daily dose can be taken at once, with food, or divided up.

PRO-BIOTICS

This is a supplement you've probably never heard of. It's only been tested in animals up to this point. However, some of the data from these animal tests is compelling.

Pro-Biotics are a class of shelf-stable, bio-active bacteria strains that have been shown to help increase feed efficiency in farm animals. Currently unpublished industry studies show that by adding small doses of this bacterial culture to livestock feed, it can help the supplemented animals gain more weight on the same amount of food as control animals. And, it appears that the mass was lean bodyweight and not fat. Pro-Biotics may or may not be of value to bodybuilders. I'll keep you posted if human data becomes available.

RNA

Anytime this ingredient is used in a nutritional supplement, it's typically found in the form of yeast RNA. The theory behind supplementing the body with RNA is to help support the immune system. There have been studies that show, in both humans and animals, supplementation with RNA enhances immune-system function, especially in times of high metabolic stress (such as that inflicted by intense weightlifting). RNA might work well when combined with glutamine and other glutamine-enhancing nutrients. You see, glutamine is a vital precursor to RNA production, and the body has a great demand for RNA synthesis. Supplying RNA in oral form may help spare glutamine in the body, allowing it to be utilized for muscle cell production and repair; hence, it is a component of EAS' glutamine supplements CytoVol and GKG.

SUMMARY

There you have it—a comprehensive list of supplements that are worth a try but didn't fit nicely into any other chapter in this big ole book. What more can I say?

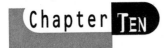

Chapter **Ten**

Brand and
Brand Name Reviews

There are dozens of different companies that sell sports supplements, and there are literally hundreds of different brand names for assorted bodybuilding supplements. Unfortunately, it would be impossible for me to review each and every one of these companies and all their products. It would be boring, too. However, in this chapter, I'll give you my two cents worth on some of the supplement companies <u>and</u> supplements I get asked about most often. As always, my comments are sure to piss a lot of people off, but hey... *that's what I do!*

But First... A Little Background Info

> "**...more** and more bodybuilders... are getting off steroids and seeking natural, safer, legal alternatives to muscle-building drugs."

In recent years, the bodybuilding supplement industry has seen some major changes—former powerhouse companies have gone out of business, or are on their way out, while others have grown by leaps and bounds.

The industry, overall, is growing at a significant rate. I believe there are several reasons for this growth. First, more and more bodybuilders and other athletes are getting off steroids and seeking natural, safer, legal alternatives to muscle-building drugs.

Another reason the market is growing so rapidly is because sports supplements, in general, are getting better and better. It wasn't that long ago when this industry's products were primarily based on hype and hucksterism. But today, there are, <u>in fact</u>, supplements that have been shown in legitimate university studies to produce positive effects, such as: enhanced muscle metabolism, increases in size and strength, accelerated fat loss, and enhanced athletic performance. An increasing number of academic studies on the positive effects of supplements are getting even wider press coverage. For example, last year, literally hundreds of mainstream newspapers and TV news

•SPORTS SUPPLEMENT REVIEW, 3RD ISSUE•SPORTS SUPPLEMENT REVIEW, 3RD ISSUE•SPORTS SUPPLEMENT REVIEW, 3RD ISSUE•SPORTS SUPPLEMENT REVIEW, 3RD ISSUE•SPORTS SUPPLEMENT REVIEW, 3RD ISSUE•SPORTS SUPPLEMENT REVIEW, 3RD ISSUE•SPORTS SUPPLEMENT REVIEW, 3RD ISSUE•SPORTS SUPPLEMENT

REVIEW•SPORTS SUPPLEMENT REVIEW, 3RD ISSUE•SPORTS SUPPLEMENT REVIEW, 3RD ISSUE•SPORTS SUPPLEMENT REVIEW, 3RD ISSUE•SPORTS SUPPLEMENT

BRAND AND BRAND NAME REVIEWS

BRAND NAME REVIEWS~BRAND AND BRAND NAME REVIEWS~BRAND AND BRAND NAME REVIEWS~BRAND AND BRAND NAME REVIEWS~BRAND AND BRAND NAME REVIEWS~BRAND AND BRAND NAME REVIEWS~BRAND AND BRAND NAME REVIEWS~BRAND AND BRAND NAME REVIEWS~BRAND AND BRAND

shows broadcast positive stories on sports supplements like creatine and HMB—introducing millions of people to the concept that it may very well be possible to get better results faster from exercise by supplementing the diet with specific nutrients. As the science of supplements expands, the industry continues to gain credibility and grow.

Another factor in the expansion of the supplement industry is the positive regulatory environment. The passage of the Dietary Supplement Health and Education Act (DSHEA) of 1994 made it more clear what a dietary supplement is and has allowed some claims to be made for supplements that were previously prohibited. This law has also allowed new products to be sold as supplements that were previously in an "undefined" area, such as: DHEA, melatonin, pyruvate, etc. Also, the FDA can no longer "randomly" remove a product from sale; it now needs "proof" the ingredient or product has adverse or toxic effects and can cause harm to users.

Increasingly, fitness buffs are taking a proactive approach to building their bodies and improving their health in general. Sales growth, additional channels of distribution, and Americans' fascination with building a better body have brought about a paradigm shift in the consumer culture in the sports supplement industry; thus, I think the sports supplement market will continue to grow by leaps and bounds (especially if I have anything to do with it).

MISCELLANEOUS SUPPLEMENT COMPANIES

American Bodybuilding® (ABB)

This is a sports supplement company that was started back in 1985 by a guy named Jim Horn. ABB primarily distributes drinks and bars—you might recognize some of their flagship products like Blue Thunder™, High Voltage™, and Inferno™. This is also the company that came out with the Steel Bar™—those huge "bodybuilder candy bars" you'll find on the counters of gyms across the country.

In 1995, ABB was purchased by Weider Nutrition. Prior to Weider's acquisition of ABB, their products had a tendency to be a "bit off" label claims (I tested them back in '94), especially the Steel Bars which had more fat in them than was listed on the label. But since the bigwigs at Weider Nutrition got involved, they've really cleaned up the products—they taste as good as ever, and my recent tests show they meet label claims.

Overall, ABB products aren't bad at all—I occasionally have one of their Steel Bars myself, and though I don't use their drinks, I know quite a few people who like to grab one right after a workout. The products don't taste bad, and in terms of premixed, bottled drinks, ABB has a good reputation in bodybuilding.

The real strength of ABB is their distribution system. This is why Weider acquired them—not so much for their products but for their established system of distribution. They have trucks that deliver pre-made drink products all across the United States.

ABB is a strong brand (not one of the "big boys on the block" in terms of sales but they hold their own), and now that Weider Nutrition is making their supplements, I'm confident of their quality.

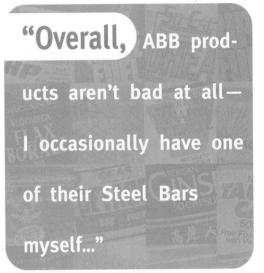

"Overall, ABB products aren't bad at all—I occasionally have one of their Steel Bars myself..."

Beverly International™

This is a sports nutrition company that's been hanging in there for over 20 years now under the leadership of a guy named Jim Heflin (his real name is Earl). In the industry, Heflin is regarded as an honest, hard-working businessman. Beverly International has never sought out the top position in the sports nutrition market—they primarily distribute their products through a tight-knit group of local distributors at the grassroots level. Over the past two decades, Heflin has probably attended more bodybuilding shows than anybody else on the planet—he literally drives around the country, setting up his simple display booth at one show or another, every weekend, and doing his thing.

Although some of the Beverly International products are outdated (they're one of the only sports nutrition companies I know that still carry liver tablets), at least they have a reputation for producing products that contain what their labels claim.

Champion Nutrition™

This is a sports nutrition company that was started back in 1987, and for a while, it was a "big fish." A guy named Michael Zumpano has led the Northern California-based company since its inception a decade ago. In the '80's, Zumpano and Duchaine worked together on the development of a few products. (Tidbit—few bodybuilders realize the infamous *Underground Steroid Handbook* was coauthored by Duchaine <u>and</u> Zumpano.)

Years ago, Champion Nutrition was quite innovative. Their product Metabolol™ was one of the first relatively good quality total-nutrition products—it was billed as a "metabolic optimizer." I used Metabolol myself, back around 1990—the product is still on the market today, but it's not a big seller.

Champion Nutrition also had some success during the mega-calorie mania years (early '90's) with a product called Heavyweight Gainer 900™. But, the high-calorie weight-gain supplement category has pretty much gone down the toilet.

Today, Champion Nutrition's sales are sluggish, and from what I can discern, their profits are not so great. And, as I mentioned, Champion Nutrition, although once a relatively innovative company, has now pretty much been relegated to

BRAND AND BRAND NAME REVIEWS

CHAPTER 10

BRAND NAME REVIEWS-BRAND AND BRAND NAME REVIEWS-BRAND AND BRAND NAME REVIEWS-BRAND AND BRAND NAME REVIEWS-BRAND AND BRAND NAME REVIEWS-BRAND AND BRAND NAME REVIEWS-BRAND AND BRAND NAME REVIEWS-BRAND AND BRAND NAME REVIEWS-BRAND AND BRAND

playing a role similar to that of so many other sports nutrition companies, which is to imitate, not innovate—simply to follow the leader.

Cybergenics®

The story of Cybergenics (originally called L&S Research) is a very interesting one. The New Jersey-based company was founded in 1982 by a guy named Scott Chinery—all he did back then was sell books. A lot of people don't realize Chinery was quite a prolific writer—he penned numerous books, including: *In Quest of Size; Cutting Up: Razor Sharp; Anabolic Steroids in Bodybuilding; Making Money in Bodybuilding;* amongst others. Despite what some people think, Chinery was far from stupid; in fact, in a way, he was/is a genius.

Back in the early '80's, Chinery came up with something he dubbed a "steroid-replacement kit" and called it "Biogenics." In 1984, he changed the name of his product to Cybergenics. The "Cyber" was added after Chinery saw the movie *Terminator*, which came out in 1984. In that killer, sci-fi flick (which I've seen at least 40 times), the Terminator, played by Arnold, of course, was referred to as a "*cyber*netic organism." (Gee... isn't this bodybuilding supplement industry trivia interesting? It's not? Oh.)

Chinery's products were novel—each kit included training and nutrition guides and/or videos and a collection of supplements. Those who followed the training and nutrition recommendations (which were pretty strict and not really easy to stick with), gained muscle and lost fat. Whether the supplements really helped or not is kind of up in the air.

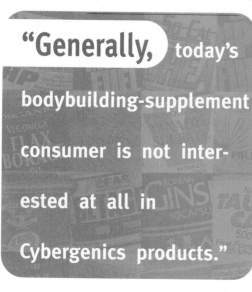

"Generally, today's bodybuilding-supplement consumer is not interested at all in Cybergenics products."

The real "breakthrough" of Cybergenics was their ads—they took the "before and after" concept to a whole new level, featuring amazing physique transformations (that people actually believed!). Chinery knew how to sell.

The company grew and grew. By 1993, Cybergenics was probably the top grossing sports nutrition company in the world—their sales topped $70 million in one particular 12-month period. However, that was as good as it was gonna get. In 1994, the supplement market began to change, and Chinery was burning out. He was smart enough to know it was time to get out. I think Chinery could sense the climate was evolving—consumers were looking for products that were backed by scientific research. In 1994, he decided to "get while the gettin' was good"—he sold the company (reportedly for $60 million in cash), kicked back in his plush, New England country mansion with his beautiful, young family, and basically retired, well before his

40th birthday. Today, I believe Chinery's passion is collecting guitars—he has one of the most elaborate, exotic collections in the world. Now he's writing a book about guitars.

So what happened to Cybergenics after the "key man" bailed? Well, it pretty much went down the toilet. The guy who took over Cybergenics from Chinery, a dude named Matt Chamlan (a "non-industry" guy), couldn't keep it going—in less than two years, this multi-million-dollar supplement giant filed for voluntary bankruptcy.

Anyway, Cybergenics is trying to make a comeback, but I don't think they have a chance—the market has changed so much over the past few years that the once valuable brand name "Cybergenics" is now worthless.

Generally, today's bodybuilding-supplement consumer is not interested at all in Cybergenics products. Did their steroid-replacement kits work like steroids? Of course not. But, if you followed the instructions that came with the kits—did the workouts, followed the diets, and took the vitamins, minerals, and amino acid tablets that came with the kit, you got results. Was it a placebo effect? Or would users have gotten just as good of results with only the training and nutrition program? (Probably a little of both.) Was it a scam, or was it entrepreneurial brilliance? You tell me.

(In a year or two, I'll be able to tell you about the rise and fall of another supplement giant that parallels the Cybergenics saga. Guess which company it is. Here's a hint—I introduced this company's flagship product in 1991. [At least Chinery knew when to get out.])

Experimental and Applied Sciences, Inc. (EAS®)

This company was founded back in late 1992 by a couple of scientists— Anthony Almada and Ed Byrd in Northern California. Almada and Byrd had been involved in the supplement business for a number of years, acting primarily in a research and development capacity. But, they became frustrated with the fact that none of the companies they were working for were making a commitment to advance the "science of supplementation" by funding university research; thus, they started their own company and vowed to contribute a percentage of all product sales to fund independent research grants. The first EAS product was the university-tested Phosphagen™, which set the stage for what would separate EAS from all the other supplement companies. Today, the company has a very focused line—about a dozen products—but each is designed specifically for the serious athlete.

I got involved in EAS back in 1994 after I first tried Phosphagen (and was amazed with the results) and worked with Anthony Almada on some research projects. I knew this company had a lot of potential. Almada and I share a passion for scientific research—a passion that is reflected in the fact that EAS funds more

BRAND AND BRAND NAME REVIEWS

BRAND NAME REVIEWS~BRAND AND BRAND NAME REVIEWS~BRAND AND BRAND NAME REVIEWS~BRAND AND BRAND NAME REVIEWS~BRAND AND BRAND NAME REVIEWS~BRAND AND BRAND NAME REVIEWS~BRAND AND BRAND NAME REVIEWS~BRAND AND BRAND NAME REVIEWS~BRAND AND BRAND NAME REVIEWS~BRAND AND BRAND

independent university research (much more!) than any other bodybuilding supplement company ever. When I look at EAS, I don't just see a company distributing bodybuilding supplements, I see a company which is truly dedicated to research and development and innovation.

In late 1995, I ended up acquiring full ownership of EAS, primarily because of Almada and Byrd's lack of interest in running the day to day operations of a fast-growing, somewhat complicated corporation. Their primary interest is and always has been in forging ahead with research and development—discovering new and better drug-free ways to enhance muscle metabolism and athletic performance. Thus, we worked out a deal where they could dismiss themselves from the day to day complications of business and focus on EAS research.

My ownership of EAS and *Muscle Media* gives me a unique position in the market that allows me to inform and educate, not just "market products." EAS truly is the innovator in this field—determined to introduce the most cutting-edge, effective, university-tested products that enhance the positive effects of exercise.

Over the past three years, EAS has grown rapidly; in fact, last year, EAS took over the spot as the #1 company in the sports nutrition industry. My numbers show EAS is now the most popular sports nutrition brand in the world. TwinLab and Weider are bigger companies overall than EAS, but in terms of sports supplements, EAS is in front by a substantial margin.

SCIENCE sets EAS apart from the other supplement companies (EAS has funded and collaborated on over 25 university studies since 1993). Another reason EAS is the #1 brand is because of our commitment to quality and service. For example, we provide a free technical-support service to anyone (including you!) who wants to learn more about bodybuilding. Even if you don't buy EAS supplements, you can call the EAS technical-support hotline, and we'll do whatever we can to help you. The people who man this hotline are trained nutritionists and bodybuilders themselves. Their sole task is to keep up on the hottest new trends in the industry and share that information with anyone who calls in. (I've included more information about EAS in the back of this book, which you can peruse at your convenience, if you wish, or you can use it to line the bottom of your birdcage—whatever you choose.)

I could go on and on about EAS, but suffice it to say, in my heavily biased opinion, EAS is the company that will lead sports nutrition into a new era, establish greater credibility, and expand the market for all of the companies involved—our goal is not merely to increase our piece of the pie (market share) but also increase the overall size of the pie (market size).

Anyway, expect to see exciting new things from EAS in the future. Our research and development programs are moving forward at a phenomenal pace, and our alliance with world-class sports medicine experts and top universities around the world gets stronger every day. Our investment in research is yielding substantial dividends. I can't give you the details at this time, but we have some awesome new products in the works. Just wait and see!

MLO

This sports nutrition company has been around forever. In fact, I think this is where Fred Flintstone used to get his bodybuilding supplements. The company is owned by a guy named Mel (his real name is Millard) Williamson, and the company's headquarters are in Fairfield, California.

MLO is kind of like Beverly International. They're not one of the "major players," but they hang in there. They don't have any "star products," but a couple of their relatively well-known ones include something called Hard Body™ (a multinutrient powder) and Mus-L-Blast.™ MLO also makes the "Bio" line of products, which include Bio-X™ (formerly Bio-Rx), Bio-Gain™, and some kind of food bar.

In last year's *Supplement Review*, I called one of MLO's products (Bio-Rx) "the Yugo of meal replacements." They didn't like that so much. Maybe I should compare their line with something more sleek, classy, and performance-oriented—how about a 'vette? (A *Chevette*).

MuscleTech™

This is a new supplement company which apparently operates out of Canada—their products are heavily promoted in the bodybuilding publication *MuscleMag International*. Apparently, a young guy named Paul Gardiner (who used to work at a *MuscleMag* retail store in Canada and who is featured in the company's outrageous before and after ads) owns or runs the company. But, I've also heard that's not the case and that the guy's name really isn't Paul Gardiner.

Other rumors are that *MuscleMag* publisher, Bob Kennedy (who is a really good guy), as well as the magazine's Editor-in-Chief, Dennis "Gino" Edwards (who writes under the "tongue-in-cheek" pen name of Johnny Fitness), are somehow involved. But, I haven't found any proof that that's the case, either.

Anyway, MuscleTech is pushing four different products right now through their "articles" in *MuscleMag*: Creatine 6000ES™, Hydroxycut™, Acetabolan™, and something called Meso-Tech™. Make no mistake, these products are being hyped to the max, but aggressive promotions alone are not inherently corrupt. I think that's

> "...EAS is **the** company that will lead sports nutrition into a new era, establish greater credibility, and expand the market for all of the companies involved..."

201

BRAND AND BRAND NAME REVIEWS

CHAPTER 10

BRAND NAME REVIEWS~BRAND AND BRAND NAME REVIEWS~BRAND AND BRAND NAME REVIEWS~BRAND AND BRAND NAME REVIEWS~BRAND AND BRAND NAME REVIEWS~BRAND AND BRAND NAME REVIEWS~BRAND AND BRAND NAME REVIEWS~BRAND AND BRAND NAME REVIEWS~BRAND AND BRAND NAME REVIEWS~BRAND AND BRAND

true whether you sell supplements, gym equipment, cars—whatever. There's nothing wrong with aggressive marketing (if there were, I'd be in big trouble because I pride myself on being a very aggressive, creative, *yet straightforward* promoter). But, is the MuscleTech campaign straightforward? What's the *whole* story? Unfortunately, I really can't tell you the "whole story" behind MuscleTech because I simply don't know it.

Why *MuscleMag* runs pages and pages of editorial plugs for MuscleTech products, if they aren't getting paid something besides regular advertising rates, I have no idea. Eventually, somebody's gonna have to "come clean." What I've learned over the years is that the more honest you are, the better off you'll be—the truth always comes out.

MuscleTech is definitely one of the most talked about new sports nutrition companies, and one of the most controversial. Their products aren't bad, but they are definitely "pushing the envelope" in terms of making claims. My advice to whomever is behind MuscleTech is to get a good FTC attorney <u>now</u> (instead of waiting until they have to), and consider promoting the products in a little bit more of a straightforward manner. Certainly, there's nothing wrong with fair competition between companies. It's good for the consumer, as it forces companies to offer greater value and service. No one can dispute the fact that MuscleTech has every right to compete in the sports supplement market. It will be interesting to see where this campaign is in a year—MuscleTech could crash and burn (big time), or they might turn out to be a success story. Only time will tell...

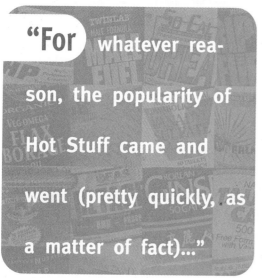

"**For** whatever reason, the popularity of Hot Stuff came and went (pretty quickly, as a matter of fact)..."

National Health Products®

This company was somewhat famous back in the early '90's when their product, Hot Stuff®, became *the* most popular bodybuilding supplement on the market (by a long shot!). Hot Stuff put National Health on the map, so to speak, but the company has actually been around since 1970. It was founded by a guy named Tom Ciola. I believe the company was originally headquartered in Utica, New York, before Tom set up shop in Orlando, Florida.

For whatever reason, the popularity of Hot Stuff came and went (pretty quickly, as a matter of fact), and today, National Health Products' sales aren't nearly what they were back in the early '90's. A recent effort to "jump start" sales with a massive advertising campaign for an enhanced version of their Hot Stuff product, called Hot Stuff Super X™, may have missed the mark—I don't think it worked.

Ciola is a clever marketer and has withstood many ups and downs over the years; he may find himself back in the thick of things somehow, someway, someday, but for now, it seems like bodybuilding supplement consumers no longer "perceive a need" for Hot Stuff, and once consumers decide they no longer need a product, it will be relegated to back-shelf space, collecting dust at health-food retailers, along with countless jugs of weight-gain powder, Cybergenics bodybuilding kits, and dozens of other "has-been" sports supplements.

Natrol

This is a supplement company that doesn't specialize in bodybuilding products, but they put out a pretty high-quality line of various herbs and other "odds and ends" that you might be interested in, such as glucosamine, guarana, and melatonin, as well as a whole slew of vitamins and minerals. The company was started in 1980—their headquarters are in Chatsworth, California. They're a solid, reputable company, and their products are available at health-food stores everywhere.

Next Nutrition®

This company, located in Carlsbad, California, was started back in 1986 by a friend of mine named David Jenkins. (Did you know he won a silver medal in the 4 x 400-meter relay? He was in three Olympic games: 1972 in Munich; 1976 in Montreal; and 1980 in Moscow. Jenkins was on the United Kingdom's team.) Next Nutrition is a reputable supplement company, for certain. Dan Duchaine has formulated several products for Next Nutrition. Their flagship (most popular) product is Designer Protein™. Another one of their relatively popular products is called Ultimate Orange™.

Next Nutrition is not one of the sports supplement industry's biggest companies, and I don't think they want to be—their strategy seems to be to stay focused on a very small line of high-quality sports supplements—it's a strategy which seems to be working. Their supplements are very popular with bodybuilders and can be found at GNC and health-food stores everywhere.

Schiff™

This supplement company is not typically considered a distributor of bodybuilding supplements—they carry a wide spectrum of different supplements, including: melatonin, DHEA, glucosamine, as well as a whole slew of antioxidants and vitamins and minerals. Schiff is another subsidiary of Weider Nutrition. Schiff is a big supplement company and produces quality products which are competitively priced. I get a lot of questions about which brands of vitamins and other supplement odds and ends are reputable—this is one brand I think you can trust. Schiff supplements can be found at health-food stores all over the place.

SportPharma®

This is a bodybuilding supplement company that was founded eight years ago by a guy named Mike Walls who, back in the late '80's, worked for Champion Nutrition. This is one of the "medium-sized" sports supplement companies. Their product line is really not very innovative, but it's popular with some bodybuilders. The company appears to be sound. Their products are available at gyms and health-food stores.

Strength Systems/AmeriFit™

This company was founded back in 1980 by a guy named Zak Nathan who was a pretty wiley cat—he was a hustler—an entrepreneur to be certain. Despite some on-again/off-again problems with products not meeting label claims (which I reported in my publications back in 1990—some of the Strength Systems' protein powders were *way off*), the company's products (and they have hundreds of them) have continued to sell over the years. However, in August of 1995, Zak Nathan pulled "a Chinery" (he sold the company for a number I believe was in the low eight-figure range) and said farewell to the bodybuilding supplement scene. Now, a guy named Marty Herman runs Strength Systems—he's renamed it AmeriFit. Herman worked for Chinery at Cybergenics from 1990-1992.

Anyway, Strength Systems/AmeriFit continues to chug along—I think their strategy is to try to compete with Weider on the mass-market level at places like Walgreen, Wal-Mart, Kmart, and Target. I don't think their products sell very well at health-food stores.

TwinLab®

This is one of the big boys. TwinLab was started back in 1968 by David and Jean Blechman and is now run by their sons—the five Blechman brothers: Brian, Neil, Ross, Steve and Dean. (Brian and Neil are twins, as are Ross and Steve—hence, "*Twin*Lab.")

TwinLab originally distributed primarily predigested liquid protein supplements to health-food stores. Over the years, the company has had its ups and downs, but in the last decade, they've really come on strong. Now TwinLab distributes over 800 different supplements, including everything you can imagine: vitamins, minerals, amino acids, fish oils, specialty formulas, and sports nutrition products. They also distribute herbal supplements and teas under the brand names Nature's Herbs™ and Alvita™.

TwinLab also publishes the bodybuilding magazine *Muscular Development®*, which they acquired from York Barbell founder Bob Hoffman's publishing company in August of 1988. (The magazine was first published in 1964. Hoffman also published a magazine called *Strength and Health*, which he founded back in 1932.

Hoffman passed away in 1985; *Strength and Health* was discontinued in May of 1986.) Steve Blechman pretty much runs *Muscular Development* magazine and is also heavily involved in the development and marketing of TwinLab products.

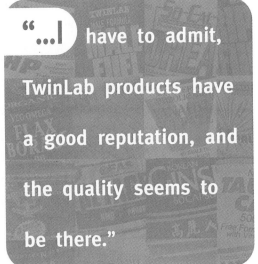

"...I have to admit, TwinLab products have a good reputation, and the quality seems to be there."

TwinLab's sports nutrition line (their bodybuilding supplements) make up about 33% of their sales; vitamins, minerals, and amino acid formulas make up about 22%; specialty formulas make up about 25%; and their herbal lines make up a majority of the remainder. I think probably their most popular sports nutrition products, which are actually herbal "fat burners," are Diet Fuel™ and Ripped Fuel™. Overall, I think their sports nutrition line is pretty good. Their products, Rx Fuel™, Creatine Fuel™, Creatine Fuel Plus™, Creatine Fuel Cocktail™, Whey Fuel™, etc., are competitive in their catagories. Back in early 1993, Steve Blechman declined an offer from Almada and Byrd that would have made TwinLab the first company to launch creatine monohydrate as a sports supplement. (Tip: *first* to the market is always *first* in the minds of consumers.) Blechman ended up adding creatine to their "Fuel line" later.

TwinLab was privately owned (by the Blechman family) up until last year when, through a series of complicated financial transactions, they sold 55% of the company for $212.5 million (yes, the decimal point *is* in the right place!) in cash—outside investors and partners now own most of the company, while the five Blechman brothers each own 9%. Since their Initial Public Offering (IPO) on October 24, 1996, TwinLab stock has been traded on NASDAQ National Market System under the symbol "TWLB."

Even though Steve Blechman (who is a great businessman) probably hopes I get hit by a flying chunk of blue ice—even though we are fierce competitors (there have been "issues" between some of the writers for his magazine, *Muscular Development*, and myself), I have to admit, TwinLab products have a good reputation, and the quality seems to be there. TwinLab supplements are distributed at health-food and grocery stores.

Ultimate Nutrition

This is another one of the relatively small sports nutrition companies that has "staying power" (it was founded in 1979). The Stamford, Connecticut, based business hasn't grown a lot in recent years, but it has a reputation for putting out a pretty good quality line of supplements (although they're certainly not an innovator). Some of their product line is a bit "stale." (For example, their once popular amino acid tablets and weight gainers could probably be dropped and no one would

205

REVIEW•SPORTS SUPPLEMENT REVIEW, 3RD ISSUE•SPORTS SUPPLEMENT REVIEW, 3RD ISSUE•SPORTS SUPPLEMENT

•SPORTS SUPPLEMENT REVIEW, 3RD ISSUE•SPORTS SUPPLEMENT REVIEW, 3RD ISSUE•SPORTS SUPPLEMENT REVIEW, 3RD ISSUE•SPORTS SUPPLEMENT REVIEW, 3RD ISSUE•SPORTS SUPPLEMENT REVIEW, 3RD ISSUE•SPORTS SUPPLEMENT REVIEW, 3RD ISSUE•SPORTS SUPPLEMENT REVIEW, 3RD ISSUE•SPORTS SUPPLEMENT

BRAND AND BRAND NAME REVIEWS

BRAND NAME REVIEWS~BRAND AND BRAND NAME REVIEWS~BRAND AND BRAND NAME REVIEWS~BRAND AND BRAND NAME REVIEWS~BRAND AND BRAND NAME REVIEWS~BRAND AND BRAND NAME REVIEWS~BRAND AND BRAND NAME REVIEWS~BRAND AND BRAND NAME REVIEWS~BRAND AND BRAND NAME REVIEWS~BRAND AND BRAND

miss them.) But they also carry some of the more popular new products, and they have a good vitamin supplement called Super Complete Capsules™. Ultimate Nutrition products are available at some gyms, health-food stores, and a few GNC's.

Unipro®

This is another California-based supplement company which was founded in the early '80's. Unipro used to be one of the more popular lines with bodybuilders—I remember using their amino acid tablets and carbohydrate supplement Carboplex™ back when I was bodybuilding in Venice around 1985-1986. Those were probably Unipro's strongest years—they never really "made a move" in the market. They were acquired by Metagenics/Ethical Nutrients, a Southern California supplement company. They're dead in the water, you might say.

Weider Nutrition

You might think the Weider companies, with their numerous, BIG circulation fitness magazines and decades at the forefront of bodybuilding, would "own" the sports supplement category. But that's not the case. Even though it was Joe and Ben Weider who brought bodybuilding out of subculture obscurity and developed it into an industry, Weider sports supplements aren't that popular with bodybuilders—not nearly as popular as they could/should be (in my opinion, of course).

"The Weider Nutrition philosophy seems to be just to go with the market trends."

Those of you who've been around bodybuilding a while, like I have, have probably used at least a few Weider supplements over the years—a protein powder, some aminos, or even those infamous Anabolic Mega-paks™ that were popular back when I was bodybuilding in high school.

Of course, I know what Weider's bodybuilding supplement sales are (I know every company's numbers), and although they are way ahead of most companies, like Beverly International™, SportPharma®, Ultimate Nutrition, etc., they are not at the head of the pack.

So why don't you (and so many other bodybuilding supplement consumers) buy Weider supplements? Here's my guess (pay attention, Richard, because I'm a pretty good guesser): part of the problem is the way the products are marketed, which usually involves an endorsement from a top professional bodybuilder—guys who are absolutely ENORMOUS. The typical bodybuilding supplement consumer can't relate to these super-huge muscle freaks. The endorsements lack credibility. (Sorry, but it's true.)

Another reason Weider bodybuilding supplements are not "the rage" still has to do with problems Weider products had years ago with the ingredients not quite measuring up to label claims. I believe this was a problem that had to do with an independent manufacturer of Weider supplements.

Here's another problem—Weider's very popular, high-quality bodybuilding magazines, *Flex®* and *Muscle & Fitness®* (headquartered in Woodland Hills, California) aren't working closely with the Weider Nutrition Group (based in Salt Lake City, Utah). In fact, even though you might think these companies are "one," they are actually completely separate corporations; each has its own agenda.

But, even though Weider's bodybuilding nutrition product sales are "so-so," that didn't keep a guy named Richard Bizzaro, who's the President and CEO of Weider Nutrition (he took over in 1990), from growing this company into a multi-multi-million-dollar enterprise. Bizzaro's strategy has been to grow Weider Nutrition by acquiring other companies and streamlining them. For example, Weider Nutrition now owns a number of subsidiaries, including: Schiff, American Bodybuilding®, Tiger's Milk Food Bars™, Excel Sports Drinks™, Fi-Bar™, Great American Nutrition, as well as Victory™, MegaMass™, and the Joe Weider signature line. And, Weider Nutrition just recently shelled out a few million bucks to pick up another bodybuilding supplement company called Science Foods™, which also distributes energy/carbohydrate drinks at gyms. In all, Weider Nutrition manufactures and distributes over 1,300 products. (Their brand new state-of-the-art manufacturing facility, in Utah, is the size of several aircraft hangers—it's over 400,000 square feet!)

One of Weider Nutrition's greatest strengths is their distribution capabilities—they can place products in literally tens of thousands of retail outlets, including: Sam's Club, Walgreen, Thrifty/Pay Less, Kmart, Wal-Mart, grocery stores, drug stores, as well as health-food stores like GNC. They're everywhere!

The Weider Nutrition philosophy seems to be just to go with the market trends. When melatonin and DHEA became hot sellers, Weider Nutrition had their versions of those supplements out on the market, at low prices, *fast*. From time to time, certain vitamins and minerals (selenium is the hot one now) "catch fire," and to capitalize, you've got to be where the action is—where the people are, which, when you're talking mass marketing, is Wal-Mart, Kmart, and the supermarkets. Basically, what Weider Nutrition lacks in terms of popularity in bodybuilding, they more than make up for in the <u>mass market</u>, which is where Bizzaro wants to go and grow. (By the way, Weider Nutrition, previously a private corporation owned by the family, just went public—they're selling stock to outside investors.)

It seems fitting that the Weider companies are now major players in the mainstream supplement market. When you think about it, Joe Weider really was ahead of his time—over 50 years ago he was promoting the use of vitamins, minerals, and protein supplements and praising the benefits of weight-training exercise. He was doing this in a day and age when it was very out of vogue; in fact, he was considered an extremist. But there's no question he was a visionary. I

BRAND AND BRAND NAME REVIEWS

BRAND NAME REVIEWS~BRAND AND BRAND NAME REVIEWS~BRAND AND BRAND NAME REVIEWS~BRAND AND BRAND NAME REVIEWS~BRAND AND BRAND NAME REVIEWS~BRAND AND BRAND NAME REVIEWS~BRAND AND BRAND NAME REVIEWS~BRAND AND BRAND NAME REVIEWS~BRAND AND BRAND NAME REVIEWS~BRAND AND BRAND

CHAPTER 10

actually have a lot of respect for the guy. I know that in bodybuilding, it's "cool" to rip on Joe—even I used to do it—but in reality, he deserves a lot of credit. Joe Weider is a man who, throughout his life, has done everything he can to promote bodybuilding—even today, well into his 70's, and despite recent heart surgery, he is working hard every day to do what he thinks is right to promote bodybuilding. He pretty much lets Richard Bizzaro handle the nutrition company—Joe likes to work on the magazines and deal with the athletes. (He spoils the pro bodybuilders he has under contract—he treats them so well; I hope they appreciate it.)

Anyway, now that Weider Nutrition handles virtually all its own manufacturing, they produce quality products. It would be way too easy to knock a big competitor like Weider and try to make you think there's something wrong with their line so you are more likely to buy my brand, but the truth is, there's nothing wrong with Weider products. They are a force to be reckoned with.

MISCELLANEOUS BRAND-NAME SUPPLEMENTS

Okay, now that I've given you a quick review of some of the supplement companies that I get asked about, I'll review a number of the particular brand-name supplements that I'm frequently asked about. Here goes...

Acetabolan™

This is one of MuscleTech's formulas. The product contains ALC, glutamine, BCAA's, OKG, zinc, and taurine. MuscleTech claims Acetabolan increases testosterone and growth hormone production and has anti-catabolic effects, but I don't know if that's very accurate. As I mentioned previously in this book, the main ingredient in this formula that they are hyping, ALC, is not worthless—it just hasn't been tested in athletes or weight trainers. I'm under the impression, after reviewing all the ALC studies referenced in the Acetabolan ads (most of which were conducted on rats or *in vitro* [test tubes]), that an "effective dose" of ALC might be upwards of five to ten grams a day. The recommended daily dose of Acetabolan contains one gram of ALC. Until some type of solid research comes out, I'd have to say Acetabolan is one of the many new products on the market that may or may not work. It's too early to tell.

Androstene 50™

This is the first product on the market which contains androstenedione, that interesting testosterone precursor I reviewed in Chapter 3. (If the FDA clamps down on this stuff, it will not be around for long.) Androstene 50 also contains lysophosphatidylcholine, which has been shown to help increase uptake of various nutrients in the gut. The creators of this product have also thrown in some zinc, which is a micronutrient necessary in the production of testosterone. The product is put out by a company called Osmo™, out of San Francisco, and distributed by Duchaine's company GURUetc (601-376-0495 [Ext. #500]). It's pretty pricey—$60 for 60 capsules (each capsule contains 50 mg of androstenedione), and from what I understand, there isn't a whole lot of it around. If other companies start to carry the product, the prices could go down.

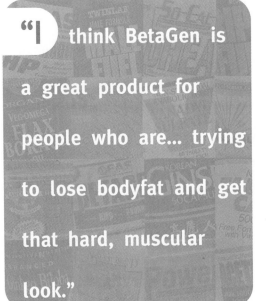

"I think BetaGen is a great product for people who are... trying to lose bodyfat and get that hard, muscular look."

BetaGen™

This new EAS supplement is very popular. The concept behind BetaGen is rather simple—it didn't take any Nobel Prize winners to come up with this one, but sometimes the simplest ideas are the best ones. The BetaGen formula contains the two powerful nutrients creatine and HMB, which have both been shown to produce dramatic results in the laboratory and the real world, and it also contains glutamine and taurine, the two most abundant amino acids in muscle tissue.

BetaGen is very convenient as well as being a super value. A 30-serving supply of BetaGen costs only $3 more than a 30-serving supply of HMB capsules (which, of course, doesn't contain creatine, glutamine, nor taurine). And, with BetaGen, you just take a small scoop of this orange-flavored drink mix and pour it in four ounces of water, stir it up, and drink it down. Or you can add it to a protein drink, a milk shake, or a meal-replacement powder. This is much more convenient (for me at least) than taking all those capsules.

I think BetaGen is a great product for people who are working out hard and are trying to lose bodyfat and get that hard, muscular look. (Studies have now shown HMB may support fat loss that occurs secondary to exercise.[204, 206]) I use BetaGen three times a day. Sometimes I mix it with water; sometimes I put it in my Myoplex Plus shake. BetaGen was not designed for creatine loading, which you should do the first week you take creatine. Phosphagen HP is better for creatine loading. BetaGen, however, contains an effective maintenance dose of creatine.

Blue Thunder™

This is one of ABB's drink products that is popular at gyms. Each 22-oz bottle contains a hefty dose of protein, carbohydrates, and calories, as well as a lot of other "bells and whistles." Blue Thunder tastes okay, and I think it's a pretty good post-workout drink—remember, consuming an ample dose of protein and carbs within one hour after you work out works wonders!

REVIEW•SPORTS SUPPLEMENT REVIEW, 3RD ISSUE•SPORTS SUPPLEMENT REVIEW, 3RD ISSUE•SPORTS SUPPLEMENT REVIEW, 3RD ISSUE•SPORTS SUPPLEMENT

•SPORTS SUPPLEMENT REVIEW, 3RD ISSUE•SPORTS SUPPLEMENT REVIEW, 3RD ISSUE•SPORTS SUPPLEMENT REVIEW, 3RD ISSUE•SPORTS SUPPLEMENT REVIEW, 3RD ISSUE•SPORTS SUPPLEMENT REVIEW, 3RD ISSUE•SPORTS SUPPLEMENT REVIEW, 3RD ISSUE•SPORTS SUPPLEMENT REVIEW, 3RD ISSUE•SPORTS SUPPLEMENT

BRAND AND BRAND NAME REVIEWS

BRAND NAME REVIEWS~BRAND AND BRAND NAME REVIEWS~BRAND AND BRAND NAME REVIEWS~BRAND AND BRAND NAME REVIEWS~BRAND AND BRAND NAME REVIEWS~BRAND AND BRAND NAME REVIEWS~BRAND AND BRAND NAME REVIEWS~BRAND AND BRAND NAME REVIEWS~BRAND AND BRAND NAME REVIEWS~BRAND AND BRAND

CHAPTER 10

BRAND AND BRAND NAME REVIEWS~BRAND AND BRAND NAME REVIEWS~BRAND AND BRAND NAME REVIEWS~BRAND AND BRAND NAME REVIEWS~BRAND AND BRAND NAME REVIEWS~BRAND AND BRAND

210

Citrimax™

This is a brand of HCA (hydroxy citric acid) distributed by Natrol. As I mentioned in my review of this product in Chapter 9, I think it might be worth a try, especially during a dieting phase.

Cort Bloc™

This is a product put out under the brand name Muscle Linc™, which is *Ironman* magazine's supplement line. The primary active ingredient in this stuff is called phosphatidylserine (PS). PS has been reported to help suppress cortisol production. Not a lot of new information has come in about this supplement over the past year—although I've heard that a university study is currently underway. I think it might be worth a try, but the feedback I'm getting on it is inconclusive.

Creatine 6000ES™

This is MuscleTech's allegedly "enhanced" creatine product. It contains creatine monohydrate, in addition to the amino acids methionine, arginine, and glycine. According to MuscleTech's ad/article claims, creatine works better when it's taken with these amino acids. I try not to be hypercritical or excessively rip on other companies' products because it's just so easy; however, I have to take a stand against Creatine 6000ES because they have positioned this product against Phosphagen HP—claiming Creatine 6000ES works better and that they've got studies that show this. This is absolutely, positively ridiculous. The fact is, Phosphagen HP is the only enhanced creatine supplement that has been tested in university studies and shown to produce better results than regular creatine. I challenge anyone to prove that this is not the case.

> **"I try not to be hypercritical or excessively rip on other companies' products because it's just so easy..."**

CytoVol™

In 1993, EAS introduced a product called GKG®, the Glutamine Preservation System®. This supplement was designed to reinforce your body's "glutamine pool" not only by providing that amino acid directly but also by providing precursors to glutamine such as alpha-ketoglutarate (AKG). CytoVol takes this concept a step further by combining the ingredients in GKG with nutrients like L-alanine, glycine, and inositol, which seem to have cell-volumizing effects, too.

I use one serving of CytoVol every night combined with a serving of BetaGen right before I go to sleep. The next day, I can really feel the difference—when I get up, my muscles feel full or "pumped."

CytoVol is available in a lemon-flavored powdered drink mix which you simply stir in a small amount of water or juice and consume. You can also add CytoVol to a meal-replacement powder, a protein drink, yogurt, a milk shake, etc. It's very convenient—much better than taking 12 capsules of GKG at once which I never was too crazy about.

Designer Protein™

This is the original whey-protein supplement that started all the excitement back in 1993. It contains whey peptides, whey-protein concentrate, ion-exchanged whey, and a whey/glutamine peptide blend. It tastes great and mixes easily. I think it's the best pure protein product on the market.

Diet Fuel™

This is one of TwinLab's best products if you ask me—it's a formulation that's designed to mimic the powerful fat-burning and appetite-suppressing effects of the caffeine/ephedrine stack. TwinLab uses standardized ma huang and guarana extracts in an effort to hit a 10:1 ratio of caffeine to ephedrine. Three capsules provide about 200 mg of the herbal equivalent of caffeine and around 20 mg of ephedrine. A serving also includes 500 mg of HCA and 200 mcg of chromium, as well as 100 mg of L-carnitine, and green tea.

Endo-Pro™

This stuff has developed a cult following among some bodybuilders. Some who take it say it makes them "hard all over." The strange thing is the ingredients on the bottle list only amino acids and willow bark (a botanical form of aspirin). My guess is that Endo-Pro actually contains the herb *Tribulus terrestris*. If it does contain *Tribulus terrestris*, I'm unsure of its potency.

Endurox™ (Ciwujia)

This new product is being marketed mainly to endurance athletes. It contains the Chinese herb commonly called ciwujia (*Eleutherococcus senticosus*). Currently distributed by Pacific Health Laboratories, Endurox has been getting some pretty strong exposure in such publications as *Triathlete Magazine* and *Runner's World*. Marketing material makes claims that studies using this substance show suppression of lactic-acid accumulation and decreased heart rate during exercise, as well as increased fat utilization during training by 43% and increases in aerobic and anaerobic endurance.[129]

The two studies which these claims are based on were funded by Pacific Health Laboratories. I really don't have a problem with "house studies" as long as they are well designed, double blind, and placebo controlled. Unfortunately, neither of these studies met those requirements. There were no placebo groups, and study administrators knew exactly what they were giving participants—it was not "blind."

Animal research on ciwujia is contradictory. Some shows effective increases in aerobic endurance in mice (albeit with doses higher than those used in humans),[203] while others show no effect.[167]

EAS recently funded a study at a prestigious university by unbiased investigators. The results of this study indicated that Endurox, at 800 mg/day (the recommended dose) in trained athletes, had no significant effects on aerobic nor anaerobic endurance.[263] But who knows, maybe Endurox works under certain conditions and not others.

First Strike™

This is another phosphatidylserine (PS) product that's distributed by a company called Atletika. The overall effectiveness of this product is unknown. I haven't received much positive feedback on it, but I also haven't received an indication that many people have even tried it.

Gainers Fuel 1000™

This is one of TwinLab's weight-gain powders. Each serving of this multi-nutrient formula contains 1,000 calories. Today, weight gainers aren't nearly as popular as they used to be, and Gainers Fuel is a slow mover.

Gatorade®

This really isn't a bodybuilding supplement, but it's such a world-famous "sports drink," I thought I'd review it. Gatorade is the market leader in this category of products that are really being sold more as "beverages" than sports supplements. Gatorade is really a simple product—it's a combination of simple sugars and electrolytes. It does help rehydrate your body if you're working out hard, especially in a hot, humid climate; in fact, that's exactly what it was developed for. You see, Gatorade was "invented" back in 1965 by researchers at the University of Florida. (Their mascot is a "Gator," hence *Gatorade*.) The Exercise Physiology Department at the university that developed the supplement was simply evaluating different ways to replenish the body of lost fluids. When Gatorade was tested head to head against water, it actually enhanced recovery and performance.[194] In fact, the "Gators" became widely known, way back when, as "the second half" team, due primarily to their use of Gatorade at half-time to help replenish energy stores as well as rehydrate. Gatorade is now distributed by Quaker Foods, and sales are in the hundreds of millions of dollars a year.

Grow Hard™

This is a homeopathic supplement distributed by a company called American Nutriceuticals. As I've already explained in this book, I don't believe that homeopathic bodybuilding supplements do much of anything, but believe it or not, this Grow Hard supplement is pretty popular—I have no idea why.

Growth Factor 1™

This supplement sucks. It contains a combination of sterols. It's supposed to increase the level of anabolic hormones in your blood and give you increased strength and greater muscle growth. This stuff is a total joke; I wouldn't recommend it to anyone.

> **"When** Gatorade was tested head to head against water, it actually enhanced recovery and performance."

Hydroxycut™

This is yet another MuscleTech product (that I get a lot of questions about). It's probably their best formula—a pretty potent combination of HCA, ma huang extract (for the ephedrine), guarana extract (for the caffeine), and willow bark (for the salicin, or aspirin). Hydroxycut is similar to Diet Fuel by TwinLab. I've had the product tested, and although it doesn't match label claims exactly, it's pretty close—the truth is, none of these herbal supplements that are designed to mimic the effects of caffeine/ephedrine and/or aspirin are exact. (That's why a lot of lifters just take caffeine, ephedrine, and aspirin instead of the herbal blends.)

IGF-1A™

This is one of those products that I just have to call a scam. As far as I'm concerned, it's meant to confuse consumers—it's obviously named after the drug/hormone IGF-1. And, what really yanks my chain is that this company quoted things that *Muscle Media* writers wrote about the actual hormone, IGF-1, and made it sound like we endorsed their product.

Here's another sleazy trick these guys use—they say the product is manufactured by "Squib Labs"—a lot of you will recognize that Squibb Labs (spelled with *two b's*) is a drug company that makes anabolic steroids.

Anybody who might be considering trying this stuff should be well aware that IGF-1A is not the same as, or even similar to, IGF-1.

Ironman PR* Bar®

I think this sports nutrition bar, distributed by PR* Nutrition, is great. It comes in several awesome flavors. Each PR* bar contains 16 grams of protein, 24

BRAND AND BRAND NAME REVIEWS

BRAND NAME REVIEWS~BRAND AND BRAND NAME REVIEWS~BRAND AND BRAND NAME REVIEWS~BRAND AND BRAND NAME REVIEWS~BRAND AND BRAND NAME REVIEWS~BRAND AND BRAND NAME REVIEWS~BRAND AND BRAND NAME REVIEWS~BRAND AND BRAND NAME REVIEWS~BRAND AND BRAND NAME REVIEWS~BRAND AND BRAND

CHAPTER 10

BRAND AND BRAND NAME REVIEWS~BRAND AND BRAND NAME REVIEWS~BRAND AND BRAND NAME REVIEWS~BRAND AND BRAND NAME REVIEWS~BRAND AND

grams of carbs and 8 grams of fat—it's designed along this new 40/30/30 macro-nutrient philosophy (40% carbs, 30% protein, 30% fat) that's gaining popularity with athletes.

Not very many bodybuilders use the Ironman PR* Bar, but I think it's a good snack. It contains a variety of vitamins and minerals, the fat content (although pretty high) is made up of "good" fats, and it even has whey protein in it. This bar is not bad at all.

Male Fuel™

This is a product TwinLab came out with about a year ago that is billed as a male-potency formula. The product contains a blend of yohimbe bark, L-arginine, *Ginkgo biloba*, Vitamin E, zinc, B vitamins, saw palmetto, as well as various plant sterols.

What do each of these supplements have to do with "getting it up" or "getting it on"? Well, yohimbe is converted by the body to yohimbine, a potent vasodilator which increases blood flow to your extremities, so to speak. L-arginine may promote the production of nitric oxide (NO), which has been reported to help potency, and saw palmetto is widely heralded for its beneficial effects on minimizing or treating prostate enlargement. Standardized *Ginkgo biloba* extract is probably added because one study showed men (who were impotent) had a very good response to *Ginkgo biloba* extract. This study was not a double-blind study, but because *Ginkgo biloba* extract can improve blood flow, it *may* work.

It seems the other ingredients have been included for a logical reason as well: zinc plays an important role in the formation and production of testosterone, and so on. I've talked to a few people who say Male Fuel actually works pretty well.

> "The taste, the convenience, everything about Myoplex Plus Deluxe is just great."

Metabolol™

This is the original "metabolic optimizer" put out by Champion Nutrition. It's a pretty decent supplement, but I think it's a bit outdated at this point. The whole metabolic-optimizer craze has pretty much come and gone. I don't know many bodybuilders who still use this product.

Metaform™

This is a meal-replacement powder put out by Great American Nutrition—one of the Weider Nutrition companies. It's a decent supplement, although I don't believe it's the best in its category.

Myoplex Plus Deluxe™

This is a new meal-replacement product distributed by EAS. It's a combination of five of the most popular supplements on the market—a high-quality meal-replacement powder, whey protein, V2G™, GKG®, and CLA.

I actually came up with the idea for Myoplex Plus Deluxe myself (thank you... thank you very much). I've been having this formula custom made especially for me by one of our manufacturing plants in California, for months. (But we just recently released it to the market.) I just don't have time to screw around with all those capsules and whatnot. I've got 6 capsules of CLA over here, 12 capsules of GKG over there, V2G capsules, vitamins and minerals, and so on. It's a royal pain. So, I told our manufacturer to take all these supplements and just combine them into one.

The taste, the convenience, everything about Myoplex Plus Deluxe is just great. I guess the only thing about this supplement that's not so great is that it costs so damn much to manufacture that there's very little room for profit. As a matter of fact, there was quite a bit of discussion among managers in the sales division about whether this product should even be brought to the market because putting all of these supplements into one was just so expensive. After checking out the numbers myself, I told them to go for it and not worry about the low profit margin because it's so convenient and so high in nutrition that I knew bodybuilders would like it and repurchase it, and over the long term, the profits would be there.

This truly is one of the best values on the supplement market today—especially when you're talking high-quality products—the type EAS is famous for.

Myoplex Plus Deluxe Bar™

This is a new bodybuilding <u>bar</u> that also includes V2G, GKG, CLA, and whey protein. It's available in chocolate and chocolate-peanut butter flavors which taste great. They're super high in nutrition, convenient, and contain much less fat than found in traditional candy bars.

Nutrimet™

This is a new meal-replacement powder put out by Champion Nutrition that has a good nutritional profile, but I think it tastes awful. I've been ribbing Champion Nutrition for a while now, encouraging them to improve the taste of their powdered products. I think they've been trying, but whoever's making these powders for them needs to get a new "taste tester" because they're not good.

Perfect Rx™

This is a meal-replacement powder put out by Nature's Best®. It's supposed to contain the same ingredients as the more expensive products in this category. I

BRAND AND BRAND NAME REVIEWS

CHAPTER 10

BRAND NAME REVIEWS~BRAND AND BRAND NAME REVIEWS~BRAND AND BRAND NAME REVIEWS~BRAND AND BRAND NAME REVIEWS~BRAND AND BRAND NAME REVIEWS~BRAND AND BRAND NAME REVIEWS~BRAND AND BRAND NAME REVIEWS~BRAND AND BRAND NAME REVIEWS~BRAND AND BRAND

have tried this stuff, but I have the same problem as I do with most powders in this market—it doesn't taste very good, and it upsets my stomach.

Phosphagain 2™

This is EAS' new "lean-mass stimulator" which is gaining popularity in body-building. While other companies have been frantically trying to keep up with EAS' creatine research and product development, EAS has been moving forward—expanding and improving our creatine product line. This commitment to research helps us stay ahead of the pack. For example, a recent university study showed Phosphagain 2 produced results that are significantly better (up to 142% better) than our original Phosphagain formula which is one of the best-selling and most-popular body-building supplements on the market.[150]

Phosphagain 2 contains higher levels of key cell-volumizing amino acids, creatine, and protein than the original formula. It also has an improved carbohydrate matrix which causes a rapid, natural rise in insulin levels to help shuttle creatine and other nutrients to their ultimate destination in muscle tissue.

Phosphagain 2 is an excellent supplement for bodybuilders who want to bulk up but don't want to put on additional bodyfat. It, like all EAS supplements, is available at health-food stores everywhere, including GNC.

PhosphaGems™

This novel EAS product is basically "creatine candy." Typically, candy and other "sweet snacks" are the first things you want to abandon when you start a strict bodybuilding program because these foods are nothing more than empty calories—they contain virtually no nutrition. What bodybuilders want to do is consume the greatest amount of nutrition through their whole foods and supplements without taking in so many calories they get fat.

Well, PhosphaGems are not your ordinary candy. This supplement actually contains a special high-energy carbohydrate blend and over five grams of creatine per serving. When you eat PhosphaGems, the special blend of carbs causes a rapid release of the anabolic hormone insulin which helps carry creatine into muscle tissue. The concept behind this "transport system" is similar to our Phosphagen HP formula, which was developed after researchers discovered insulin significantly increases the uptake of creatine and glycogen by muscle tissue. This, in turn, may cause an increase in lean mass and strength above and beyond using creatine by itself.[103]

One of the great things about PhosphaGems is that you can take them with you anywhere—in your gym bag, briefcase, your car, when you travel, etc. I sometimes nibble on PhosphaGems throughout the day and even during a workout. And, if I don't feel like having a serving of Phosphagen HP when I get done training, I'll just have a serving of PhosphaGems along with a protein-rich drink. I think

PhosphaGems are great for athletes looking for both convenience and effectiveness in a creatine product—which leads to extra energy and strength.

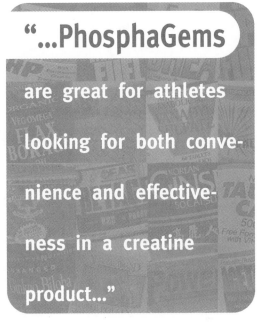

Phosphagen HP™

As many of you know, Phosphagen HP was recently shown in a university study to work significantly better (up to 160% better!) than the extremely popular and effective bodybuilding supplement creatine monohydrate.[265] The doctor who did the statistical analysis of the data from one of the recent university studies on Phosphagen HP remarked that he couldn't believe the incredible results which the test subjects using Phosphagen HP experienced. In fact, he stated he's never seen anything produce gains like this except anabolic steroids! (But, despite rumors you might see on the Internet or hear at your gym, Phosphagen HP does not contain steroids!) The HP formula is drug free. I think this could be the best bodybuilding supplement on the market right now.

PowerBar®

PowerBar is *the* sports nutrition bar—it outsells all other food bars put together, by a long shot, simply because it was first to the market, has great name recognition, and the company has a reputation for supporting athletes and athletic events. Each PowerBar contains around 230 calories with 45 grams of simple and complex carbs, around 10 grams of protein, and only 2 grams of fat. This is a good supplement for endurance athletes and a decent snack for bodybuilders.

Probestan™

This is another one of those homeopathic formulas put out by American Nutriceuticals. It's supposed to contain chrysin (a supplement I reviewed in Chapter 3). We had a sample of Probestan tested a few months ago; the lab analysis showed that if it contains any chrysin at all, it's less than .03%. Not good.

Pure Protein Bar™

This is a nutrition bar put out by a company called Worldwide Sport Nutrition—a company I definitely won't be getting any Christmas gifts from. In a recent issue of my magazine, *Muscle Media*, I revealed lab reports that showed the product's contents didn't match the label claim. The reports offered evidence the "Pure Protein Bar" was not as low in carbohydrates and fat as the label claimed. A lot of the vitamins and minerals were off as well. Apparently, they're trying to fix the

BRAND AND BRAND NAME REVIEWS

BRAND NAME REVIEWS•BRAND AND BRAND NAME REVIEWS•BRAND AND BRAND NAME REVIEWS•BRAND AND BRAND NAME REVIEWS•BRAND AND BRAND NAME REVIEWS•BRAND AND BRAND NAME REVIEWS•BRAND AND BRAND NAME REVIEWS•BRAND AND BRAND NAME REVIEWS•BRAND AND BRAND NAME REVIEWS•BRAND AND BRAND

problem, and I hope they do, because their bar actually tastes good, and a lot of bodybuilders would like to have access to a bar that contains 33 grams of protein, only 7 grams of carbs, and 7 grams of fat (which is what the Pure Protein Bar is *supposed to* contain).

Ripped Fuel™

This TwinLab supplement is basically Diet Fuel without the HCA and green tea. And, you have to take only two caps, instead of three, to get an effective dose. This is a popular product with bodybuilders, as are many other "speed-like" fat burners.

Steel Bar™

This is my favorite ABB product—it's a huge candy-bar-like supplement, with 16 grams of protein per bar, 5 grams of fat, and 68 grams of carbohydrates. And, like most other "sports bars," it contains a wide range of vitamins and minerals. Once in a while, I'll pick one of these up at the gym and promise myself I'm going to eat only half of it, but I invariably eat the whole thing and feel guilty. But then I rationalize, "It's <u>not</u> a candy bar... it's a *bodybuilding bar!*" (Am I kidding myself?)

> "I have to imagine that Vanadyl pH is pretty decent stuff even though I've never tried it."

SuperGlu™

This is a new glutamine supplement designed by Dan Duchaine and distributed by his company called GURUetc. It's high-grade, pure glutamine combined with lysophosphatidylcholine. As I mentioned in the Odds & Ends chapter, lysophosphatidylcholine may help increase gut absorption of some nutrients, including glutamine. It's possible that SuperGlu will help the body absorb more glutamine, thus giving you a greater bang for your buck. Duchaine also contends that taking SuperGlu with other nutrients, such as creatine monohydrate, may help increase the efficiency of these compounds as well. SuperGlu isn't cheap, at $.20 a gram, but if it can help you substantially increase absorption rates, it may be worth it. I don't think you can get it at health-food stores yet. If you want to check it out, you can call GURUetc at 601-376-0495 (Ext. #500).

T3-FX™

This is a supplement that is distributed by a company called So Cal Sports Supplements in Southern California. The product contains ALC, glutamine, and phosphatidylserine (PS). T3-FX is supposed to help enhance the testosterone to cortisol ratio and support anti-catabolism. Overall, I don't think it's a bad theory, but as with many of the new products that are available on the market, more research is needed to discover how effective it is.

Tonalin™

This is a quality brand name of the supplement CLA, which is put out by PharmaNutrients, Inc. PharmaNutrients® is a relatively new company, headquartered in Illinois. One of the things I like about this company is they aren't afraid to spend money on real research; in fact, even though EAS was the first supplement company to license the patent rights to CLA for bodybuilding purposes, PharmaNutrients and EAS are working together to fund university research. It would be good for the whole industry if more companies collaborated in this manner.

Tribestan®

This is a product which contains the herb *Tribulus terrestris*, which I reviewed in depth in Chapter 3. It's apparently imported from Bulgaria. I've had Tribestan tested—laboratory analysis shows it does meet label claims for *Tribulus terrestris*. (It contains right around 250 mg/tablet.) It's a bit expensive, but if you want to check it out and your health-food store doesn't carry it, you might want to call a company called Euthenics, which is run by a couple of guys I know and trust. Their number is 1-800-468-5931 (Ext. #250).

Tribestrone™

This is another *Tribulus terrestris* product which contains a couple of other Ayurvedic herbs: namely, ashwagandha (an Indian herb with "ginseng-like" effects) and something called mucuna. This product is similar to Tribestan but has not gained the same popularity in the marketplace. I'm not sure about the quality of the *Tribulus terrestris* in this product.

Ultimate Orange™

This is an energy/thermogenic supplement put out by Next Nutrition and designed by Dan Duchaine. It's a good product for people who are looking for an energy boost before their workouts. If you're looking for a "jolt" to help propel you through a workout, I recommend giving Ultimate Orange a try.

Vanadyl pH™

This is a vanadyl sulfate supplement put out by SportPharma USA. It's supposed to have a special delivery system that increases the uptake of vanadyl

BRAND AND BRAND NAME REVIEWS

CHAPTER 10

BRAND NAME REVIEWS~BRAND AND BRAND NAME REVIEWS~BRAND AND BRAND NAME REVIEWS~BRAND AND BRAND NAME REVIEWS~BRAND AND BRAND NAME REVIEWS~BRAND AND BRAND NAME REVIEWS~BRAND AND BRAND NAME REVIEWS~BRAND AND BRAND NAME REVIEWS~BRAND AND BRAND NAME REVIEWS~BRAND AND BRAND

sulfate. I'm not sure if it's absorbed any better than regular vanadyl sulfate, but it's a relatively inexpensive supplement, and I do recommend vanadyl sulfate. I have to imagine that Vanadyl pH is pretty decent stuff even though I've never tried it.

Victory Super Mega Mass 2000™

This is a Weider Nutrition product that was fairly popular a few years ago in the era of mega-calorie mania, and I think the product is still used by some teenagers and young athletes who are looking to pack on weight (muscle and fat).

X-Plode™

This is a product which is produced by USA Sports Labs™—a company which I think is having a problem with their quality control. We've tested a number of their supplements, and there seems to be a wide discrepancy between label claims and what's actually in some of their products. This is not a supplement I recommend.

SUMMARY

What I hope I'll accomplish with this book is to help you become a body-building supplement *expert*, so you can make intelligent, informed decisions about which supplements might work best for you. Thus, even though I might not have offered you my "two cents worth" on each and every supplement company and supplement that you might have questions about (a task that would be almost impossible), by the time you get done reading this book, I think you'll know precisely which supplements might benefit you and how they should be used. In fact, if you read this entire *Sports Supplement Review*, you're going to know more about body-building supplements than 99% of the people who ever picked up a weight—you are, at this very moment, earning your "Masters Degree" in sports supplementation, and that's *bad news* for companies that have flourished in an uninformed, ignorant marketplace. Your best way to fight back is with knowledge. And that, my friends, you now have.

Chapter ELEVEN

How to Prioritize Your Supplement Choices with the "Supplement Pyramid"

You see the exaggerated headlines all the time in most magazines: "Gain 20 lbs of Muscle," "Lose 50 lbs of Fat," or "Increase Strength Overnight." It's true: certain supplements will help you gain muscle, lose fat, and increase strength, but as most people have found out the hard way, the majority of supplements will do none of the above. When it comes to training and dieting, the average bodybuilder has somewhat of a blueprint or plan to follow. However, when it comes to supplements, there's more of a "hit-or-miss" mentality with unrelated products being mixed together with the hope that something—anything—will happen to improve lean mass or cut bodyfat levels. This tends to be a rather expensive and confusing process which generally leaves people frustrated and just plain sour on the prospect of trying new supplements.

> "...when it comes to supplements, there's more of a 'hit-or-miss' mentality... with the hope that something—anything—will happen..."

For example, you have Bob who is taking boron, Vitamin A, and L-carnitine; and then, there's his partner Joe, who is taking L-arginine, yohimbe, and MCT oil. Joe's girlfriend Mary takes HMB and chromium picolinate, and Mary's friend Lisa takes DHEA, dibencozide, and wild yam extract.

People will often ask me about a certain supplement and look dissatisfied when they don't get the particular answer they want to hear. There are supplements that are good for a specific application but bad for another. There are supplements which are good to take at specific times but not so effective at other times. There are supplements that should be taken all year, and of course, there are supplements that just plain suck all the time! A person will ask me, "What do you think of this supplement called Mega Grow Testosterone Builder 9000?" I often can't give them a straight "It's good" or "It bites the big one" answer. Bottom line? There are few black-and-white areas in the field of nutrient supplementation and an abundance of gray areas. In an effort to clear up some of the confusion, I'd like to propose a way of viewing and organizing supplement needs: the "Supplement Pyramid."

HOW TO PRIORITIZE YOUR SUPPLEMENT CHOICES WITH THE "SUPPLEMENT PYRAMID"

THE SUPPLEMENT PYRAMID-THE SUPPLEMENT PYRAMID-THE SUPPLEMENT PYRAMID-THE SUPPLEMENT PYRAMID-THE SUPPLEMENT PYRAMID-THE SUPPLEMENT PYRAMID-THE SUPPLEMENT PYRAMID-THE SUPPLEMENT PYRAMID-THE SUPPLEMENT PYRAMID-THE SUPPLEMENT PYRAMID-THE SUPPLEMENT

SPECIFIC-APPLICATION SUPPLEMENTS

WORTHLESS SUPPLEMENTS

SUPPLEMENTS WORTH TRYING

PERFORMANCE AND HEALTH-ENHANCING CONVENIENT SUPPLEMENTS
whey protein or products that have whey protein in them, creatine, antioxidants

FOUNDATION SUPPLEMENTS
multivitamins, multiminerals, essential fatty acids

Take a look at the pyramid above. In my opinion, there are supplements, such as multivitamins, multiminerals, and essential fatty acids, which should be staples—you should take them all the time. This group forms the base or foundation of the pyramid. Then there are the convenient supplements you can take regularly to improve performance and/or health, such as creatine and whey protein or products which contain whey. They form the middle level of the pyramid. You can cycle these products or change them because they aren't necessarily essential to your health. Finally, there are the supplements that may or may not work for you but are worth trying.

There are also two specific categories that have to be added to the top of the supplement pyramid. One is the huge category of "crap supplements," which are those not worth bothering with, regardless of the alleged application. The other category contains those supplements that are useful only at specific times or for defined periods of time.

FOUNDATION SUPPLEMENTS—

multivitamins, multiminerals, essential fatty acids

(Base of the Pyramid)

A foundation supplement is something you take all year and is usually an essential nutrient such as a vitamin, mineral, fatty acid, etc. Essential nutrients are just that—essential to life itself. The basic definition of an essential nutrient is "any nutrient which is essential to maintain proper bodily function and which the body cannot manufacture itself and therefore must be obtained from the diet." Without essential nutrients, people get sick and sometimes perish. We know there are approximately a dozen essential and "conditionally essential" amino acids, a multitude of vitamins and minerals, and two essential fatty acids that must be obtained from the diet on a regular basis and in adequate amounts, or we can't function at optimal capacity. (There are roughly 45 essential nutrients identified so far: 20 or 21 minerals, 13 vitamins, 8-12 amino acids, and 2 fatty acids.) You should be aware that there's no such thing as an "essential carbohydrate," but that's another story.

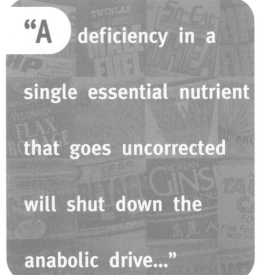

"A deficiency in a single essential nutrient that goes uncorrected will shut down the anabolic drive..."

When a lifter asks my opinion of some new supplement, the conversation usually goes something like: "What do you think of this new product called Super Bull-Gonad Testomax? Should I take it?" My answer is always something like, "Do you take a good multivitamin and multimineral? Are you taking flax oil or other oil blends and a good protein powder?" The bodybuilder will usually look at me confused and say, "Well, no, I'm not, but what does that have to do with the product I asked about?"

The above is the equivalent of asking me if I like leg extensions for training quads. I would ask, "Do you squat?" The point is, why should you do leg extensions if you don't do a foundation exercise such as squats? There is no reason—unless your goal is to have legs that look like Olive Oyl's!

What reason is there to even bother with a fancy new supplement if all your essential-nutrient needs are not being met? Every single cell in your body relies on some vitamin, mineral, or other essential molecule to function at peak levels. A deficiency in a single essential nutrient that goes uncorrected will shut down the anabolic drive faster than a centerfold of Monica Brant gives the average guy a... well, you get the point! Why spend your hard-earned cash on a new supplement that promises "30 lbs in 30 days" if your body is shunting what little essential nutrients it gets away from building muscle to keep you alive and well?

How about that ongoing argument by mainstream nutritionists and doctors who say, "You get all the vitamins you need from your food" or "Supplements just give you expensive urine"? If you're reading this book, you probably know that those statements are false. If you do believe that crap, then I have a bridge in Brooklyn and some waterfront property in Florida I think you might be interested in. Bottom line? The chances of strength-training athletes getting optimal (as opposed to adequate) amounts of vitamins, minerals, and

HOW TO PRIORITIZE YOUR SUPPLEMENT CHOICES WITH THE "SUPPLEMENT PYRAMID"

THE SUPPLEMENT PYRAMID•THE SUPPLEMENT PYRAMID•THE SUPPLEMENT PYRAMID•THE SUPPLEMENT PYRAMID•THE SUPPLEMENT PYRAMID•THE SUPPLEMENT PYRAMID•THE SUPPLEMENT PYRAMID•THE SUPPLEMENT PYRAMID•THE SUPPLEMENT PYRAMID•THE SUPPLEMENT PYRAMID•THE SUPPLEMENT PYRAMID•THE SUPPLEMENT

essential fatty acids from our nutrient-deficient, processed-food supply is zero, zip, *nada*, ain't gonna happen!

And while we're on the topic of expensive urine, the last time I checked, chemotherapy, cholesterol medications, heart-bypass operations, and countless other somewhat avoidable medical treatments are considerably more expensive than the average multivitamin and mineral supplement. *Don't get me started...!*

I realize it has taken a bit of time just to get to the point of this section, which is that you should be taking a good multivitamin and multimineral supplement every day of your life. Although this seems like common sense, you would be amazed at how many bodybuilders don't take them because they assume they'll get all they need from those nine chicken breasts and three boxes of white rice they eat every day.

Okay, there are two more related nutrients that should be considered part of the foundation products: the two unprocessed and unaltered essential fatty acids. As with most vitamins and minerals, it's virtually impossible to get optimal amounts of unprocessed essential fatty acids (especially the omega-3 fatty acids) from our heavily processed food supply. The two essential fatty acids we need are linoleic acid, which is an omega-6 fatty acid, and alpha-linolenic acid, which is an omega-3 fatty acid.

Although early research told us we need a bit more linoleic acid than alpha-linolenic acid, I find, in practice, a diet higher in alpha-linolenic acid causes the best results in terms of bodyfat levels, health, and muscle-mass increases. Americans tend to get their fats from saturated fats, rancid fats, and highly processed fats (which contain byproducts such as trans-fatty acids). However, the essential fatty acids—in particular, the omega-3 fatty acids—are anti-lipogenic (block fat storage), are anti-catabolic and anti-inflammatory, increase beta oxidation (fat burning!), improve insulin sensitivity, and a whole lot more. Unless you've been living in a cave for the past few years, you know Dan Duchaine, Anthony Almada, Dr. Mauro Di Pasquale, Dr. Michael Colgan, and just about every other bodybuilding expert "in the know" have been singing the praises of these amazing fatty acids for some time now.

> **"...you should be taking a good multivitamin and multimineral supplement every day of your life."**

The best known source of the alpha-linolenic acid is flax oil, which also contains a small amount of linoleic acid. (It has a 4:1 ratio of alpha-linolenic acid to linoleic acid.) One to three tablespoons of a mixture of flaxseed and safflower oils, in a 1:1 ratio each day over a salad, in a protein drink, or taken straight will do the trick. A great source of the omega-3 fatty acids can be found in fish such as salmon, mackerel, and sardines, and I advise people to eat at least one serving of these fish several times a week. (For more information on the many benefits of the essential fatty acids, read *Fats that Heal, Fats that Kill* by Dr. Udo Erasmus. You can order it from Alive Books at 1-800-661-0303.)

PERFORMANCE AND HEALTH-ENHANCING CONVENIENT SUPPLEMENTS

whey protein or products that use whey protein in them, creatine, antioxidants

(Middle of the Pyramid)
Whey Protein

The astute person will have noticed that although certain amino acids are considered essential nutrients, I didn't mention them with foundation supplements. Unlike vitamins, minerals, and essential fatty acids, adequate amounts of essential and nonessential amino acids can be obtained from our foods. However, getting all the amino acids we need from our food isn't very convenient, and it's arguable whether or not we can get optimal (or even adequate) amounts for growth. Several protein supplements have the specific amino acids and other properties we want. For example, whey protein has the highest biological value (BV) of any protein, which leads to greater nitrogen retention. It's roughly 25% branched-chain amino acids and is moderately high in glutamine (though some companies add even more glutamine). Besides being a great protein for growing muscle, whey protein may also improve immunity and raise levels of glutathione (an antioxidant). Knowing this, it's a given that a good protein supplement or high-quality meal-replacement product which includes whey protein is an important part of any supplement program, but you don't need it to survive. Two to three servings a day of a whey protein supplement such as Designer Protein or a product that includes whey protein such as Myoplex Plus will do the trick.

Antioxidants

Without going into a long (and boring) biochemical explanation, antioxidants are a special class of vitamins and other non-vitamin compounds which neutralize free radicals. (Certain antioxidants are essential nutrients but not all.) Free-radical pathology has been implicated in a broad range of diseases such as cancer, atherosclerosis, immune deficiency, and diabetes. More important to bodybuilders, free radicals cause inflammation, damage to muscle fibers, fatigue, and possibly immune-system suppression. Intense exercise causes a dramatic rise in free radicals with a simultaneous reduction of antioxidant systems within the body to fight them. If left unchecked, free radicals will lead to the breakdown of muscle tissue and cause various other problems. Antioxidants just aren't all that sexy and don't get much attention these days in the bodybuilding magazines, but I can assure you they are

225

•SPORTS SUPPLEMENT REVIEW, 3RD ISSUE•SPORTS SUPPLEMENT REVIEW, 3RD ISSUE•SPORTS SUPPLEMENT REVIEW, 3RD ISSUE•SPORTS SUPPLEMENT REVIEW, 3RD ISSUE•SPORTS SUPPLEMENT REVIEW, 3RD ISSUE•SPORTS SUPPLEMENT REVIEW, 3RD ISSUE•SPORTS SUPPLEMENT REVIEW, 3RD ISSUE•SPORTS SUPPLEMENT

HOW TO PRIORITIZE YOUR SUPPLEMENT CHOICES WITH THE "SUPPLEMENT PYRAMID"

THE SUPPLEMENT PYRAMID–THE SUPPLEMENT PYRAMID–THE SUPPLEMENT PYRAMID–THE SUPPLEMENT PYRAMID–THE SUPPLEMENT PYRAMID–THE SUPPLEMENT PYRAMID–THE SUPPLEMENT PYRAMID–THE SUPPLEMENT PYRAMID–THE SUPPLEMENT PYRAMID–THE SUPPLEMENT PYRAMID–THE SUPPLEMENT PYRAMID–THE SUPPLEMENT

very important nutrients for long-term health and continued progress in muscle gains. No one ever exploded with new muscle from the simple addition of antioxidants to his or her diet, but in the long run, antioxidants will help build muscle and improve immunity. (You can't build muscle if you're sick in bed.)

Ah yes, for you drug-using athletes—and you know who you are—antioxidants have also been shown to protect the liver from damage caused by the use of oral steroids.

Antioxidants such as Vitamins E and C, selenium, N-acetyl-cysteine (NAC), proanthocyanidins (derived from grape seed extract), various bio-flavonoids, and many others can be found in a good antioxidant formula. They should be used year-round by all hard-training bodybuilders and other athletes of both the natural and non-natural variety. In the December 1996 issue of *Muscle Media* (pages 92-97), Michael Mooney has an informative rundown on the antioxidants with the recommended dosages. You can also check out this article on the *Muscle Media* home page at www.mm2k.com.

Creatine Monohydrate

Though it may be the best performance-enhancing supplement around, creatine isn't an essential nutrient. Certain foods (like red meat) are moderately high in creatine, and the body can synthesize it from the amino acids arginine, glycine, and methionine. Regardless, supplementing with creatine in far greater amounts than could ever be found in food or synthesized in the body has been verified by real research to put lean mass on people and increase strength. It's affordable, it works, and it's safe, so this is definitely a year-round staple supplement, but it's not an essential nutrient, so it goes in the middle of the pyramid.

SUPPLEMENTS WORTH TRYING

WORTHLESS SUPPLEMENTS

SPECIFIC-APPLICATION
SUPPLEMENTS

(Top of the Pyramid)

Now, we must divide the tip of the pyramid into three subsections.

Supplements Worth Trying:

This category contains those supplements that might a) have some good research behind them, b) seem to work for some people but not for others, c) be relatively expensive, or d) be all of the above! DHEA, HMB, CLA, flavones, androstenedione, *Tribulus terrestris*, and vanadyl sulfate, are supplements I would lump in this broad category. I won't discuss all their effects here, but the main point of this section is this: although they might be worth trying, and some of them *definitely* are, I would never recommend giving up any of the supplements in the first two levels of the pyramid for these products.

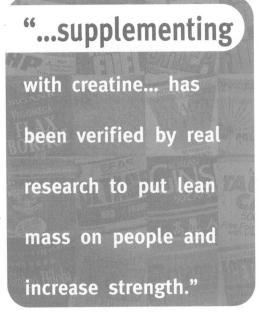

"...supplementing with creatine... has been verified by real research to put lean mass on people and increase strength."

The first two levels contain supplements that should be taken year-round and should not be cycled or exchanged for another type of product. For example, you should never stop taking antioxidants to start taking vanadyl sulfate, or you shouldn't stop taking whey protein to start taking DHEA. You might change brands of antioxidants, protein powders, or essential fatty acids, but you would exchange them for a related product (e.g., exchanging one brand of multivitamin for another or one brand of flax oil for another). Of course, any one of the above products might become a staple of your personal supplement program if it works for you, but none of them should ever replace anything from the lower two levels of the pyramid.

Worthless Supplements

From bug-molting hormones (beta-ecdysterone) to smilax, this is a long, long list! Hmmm, where do we start? Boron? Colostrum? Plant sterols? Ground bull gonads? What can I say? There are a lot of worthless supplements out there. Read Chapter 5 for a complete list of supplements that are a total waste of time.

Specific-Application Supplements

The supplements in this category can't be classified as either "good" or "bad" because they're useful at specific times and for specific purposes. Ephedrine comes to mind as the perfect example of a product in this category. Ephedrine is not something that should be taken year-round in my view. Taken occasionally before a workout for an energy boost, the stuff works great. If taken for a defined period of time, mixed with caffeine and aspirin, it's a fantastic and fairly safe (unless you have cardiac problems) way to reduce bodyfat. Say you want to get lean for the summer. You clean up your diet a little; add some aerobics; and take an ephedrine, caffeine, and aspirin mixture for a few weeks. *Voilà!* You're ripped and ready for summer. However, taking ephedrine year-round is hard on the system, can

HOW TO PRIORITIZE YOUR SUPPLEMENT CHOICES WITH THE "SUPPLEMENT PYRAMID"

THE SUPPLEMENT PYRAMID~THE SUPPLEMENT PYRAMID~THE SUPPLEMENT PYRAMID~THE SUPPLEMENT PYRAMID~THE SUPPLEMENT PYRAMID~THE SUPPLEMENT PYRAMID~THE SUPPLEMENT PYRAMID~THE SUPPLEMENT PYRAMID~THE SUPPLEMENT PYRAMID~THE SUPPLEMENT PYRAMID~THE SUPPLEMENT

have side effects, and will ultimately be counterproductive to adding muscle. The problem is, I see people popping handfuls of the stuff every time they train throughout the year. That's a mistake. The best way to use ephedrine is maybe two to three days per week for workouts and for five to eight weeks a year continuously (with caffeine and aspirin) to lose some fat for a contest, the beach, or whatever other reason you might have.

Hydroxycitrate (HCA) is another product that comes to mind in this category. Though it works through very different mechanisms than ephedrine, it's best suited for specific periods of dieting. If you just yelled, "I'm always dieting!" then you need to get a life!

SUMMARY

Obviously, I didn't tell you everything to stay away from in this chapter, but at least I've given you some ideas of what you should be taking on a regular basis, and that's half the battle, right? As far as this chapter is concerned, I hope it helps clear up *some* of the confusion faced by those of you who don't know what to take all the time, what to take most of the time, and what is worth an honest try.

Chapter TWELVE

New Theories on Stacking and Cycling
Bodybuilding Supplements

Each week, the readers of my books and magazine, *Muscle Media*, send me literally hundreds of questions. One of the topics that bodybuilders ask me about most frequently is how to stack and cycle supplements. It seems everyone is aware of the fact that there are more than a handful of good bodybuilding supplements on the market now, but unfortunately, there's not a lot of information available on exactly how to combine these supplements with one another. In this chapter, I'm going to answer the most frequently asked questions I get about stacking and cycling supplements and give you some new ideas which I think will allow you to maximize the muscle-building and fat-burning effects of various supplements, as well as help you save money. Here goes...

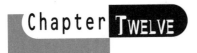

"...I'm going to answer the most frequently asked questions I get about... the muscle-building and fat-burning effects of various supplements..."

Q What do "stacking" and "cycling" mean?

A This jargon, as it relates to bodybuilding, was once used only by steroid-enhanced muscle men. "Stacking" meant taking two or more steroids at the same time. The rationale behind this practice is that the user could saturate multiple steroid-receptor populations—more than if only one androgen were used. Thus, better results could be achieved at lower dosages.

As far as supplements go, stacking basically means the same thing—taking two or more bodybuilding supplements at once in an effort to get better results faster.

The term "cycling" was also popularized by steroid users and simply refers to going on and off anabolic steroids in an effort to maximize results while minimizing side effects.

Cycling supplements means pretty much the same thing—using them for a certain period of time for a specific purpose. Fortunately, "minimizing side effects"

NEW THEORIES ON STACKING AND CYCLING BODYBUILDING SUPPLEMENTS

NEW THEORIES ON STACKING AND CYCLING BODYBUILDING SUPPLEMENTS•NEW THEORIES ON STACKING AND CYCLING BODYBUILDING SUPPLEMENTS•NEW THEORIES ON STACKING AND CYCLING BODYBUILDING SUPPLEMENTS•NEW THEORIES ON STACKING AND CYCLING BODYBUILDING SUPPLEMENTS•NEW THEORIES ON STACKING

CHAPTER 12

NEW THEORIES ON STACKING AND CYCLING BODYBUILDING SUPPLEMENTS•NEW THEORIES ON STACKING AND CYCLING BODYBUILDING SUPPLEMENTS•NEW THEORIES ON STACKING AND CYCLING BODYBUILDING SUPPLEMENTS•NEW THEORIES ON STACKING AND CYCLING

230

when using nutritional supplements isn't really an issue, but cycling may indeed help maximize results and save you money.

Q Is there a reason why I should stack or cycle supplements?

A Yes, I believe there is. In fact, I think there are several good reasons to stack and cycle some (but not all) supplements. I don't think supplements which are being used to guard against nutrient deficiencies need to be cycled. For example, if you're using a vitamin and mineral supplement, a protein supplement, a meal-replacement powder, etc., these really fall into the category of food—they're not being used to produce any supraphysiological or "drug-like" effect. They're merely being employed to improve the diet and to make sure you're getting the proper nutrients, day in and day out, that your body needs to respond adequately to exercise.

On the other hand, many of the supplements bodybuilders favor, which I review in this book, are being used for a reason other than to improve a nutrition program. For example, DHEA, *Tribulus terrestris*, melatonin, and androstenedione seem to exert "drug-like" effects, as do fat-burning herbs like guarana and ephedra (the herbal equivalents of caffeine and ephedrine). If you take these compounds over an extended period of time, it's likely your body will attenuate or down-regulate its response; thus, the supplements will no longer exert their full effects. Cycling these products may prevent down-regulation, boost their effects, and save you money.

Supplements that are not being used to make up for deficiencies nor to boost hormone levels—ones like HMB, CLA, and creatine—may or may not need to be cycled. The scientific rationale behind using these products is that providing supplemental amounts of them to the diet will enable you to up-regulate your ability to burn fat and build muscle size and strength in response to intense exercise. The best reason I can think of for cycling these supplements is simply to save money. Some of these products are expensive, and you might want to save them for certain periods of training, especially HMB. Studies show HMB might be more effective when it's used during intense training periods and/or when you are switching over to a new program. For example, if you've been following one training strategy/program for a couple of months and are going to switch over to a new program, it might be a good idea to take HMB for the first month on that new program—especially if you're working out very hard and doing a lot of eccentric (negative) contractions.

Q I want to get maximum results. Is there a right way and a wrong way to stack and cycle supplements?

A Unfortunately, there's no 100% absolute, ironclad right or wrong way to use supplements. There's not a lot of scientific data available to tell us the best ways to stack and cycle supplements. In fact, designing scientific studies to test every supplement combination you can come up with would be virtually impossible. Drug companies, which spend over $11 billion a year on research, don't even know the answers to questions like this—they couldn't tell you if there's an advantage or disadvantage to stacking various antibiotics, pain relievers, ulcer medications, etc. It's an imperfect area of science, and because of this, bodybuilding supplement theorists, like myself, must make decisions based on the available scientific literature (which as I said, is not all that extensive in this area), combined with something called empirical data (real-world evidence). This, meshed with personal experience (which I have a great deal of as I try virtually every new supplement that comes out on the market, in many different combinations and various cycling strategies), is how I develop my theories.

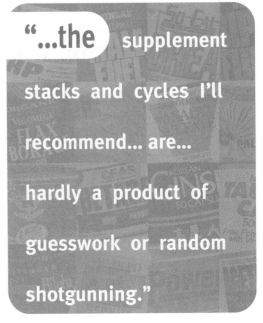

"...the supplement stacks and cycles I'll recommend... are... hardly a product of guesswork or random shotgunning."

Even though the supplement stacks and cycles I'll recommend in this chapter are not based on rock-solid science, they're hardly a product of guesswork or random shotgunning.

Q How do I decide which supplements I should be stacking or cycling?

A After reading about all the various supplements discussed in this book, you'll have a much better idea which products might work and which ones are probably a waste of time and money. That's the first thing you want to do—get informed and educated about all of these supplements.

Then, decide what your goals are. If you want to build muscle and lose fat (which is what my goal is), then you want to develop a precise strategy for accomplishing this. It can't just be a supplement cycle—you have to plan a training, nutrition, *and* supplementation program.

One of the things that is very basic, yet important, is making sure your nutrition and supplement program provides your body with a constant supply of all essential nutrients. I'm not going to go into a long and tedious explanation about what every one of these nutrients is, but in a nutshell, your body requires about 45 basic nutrients, most of which are vitamins and minerals, and a lesser number

NEW THEORIES ON STACKING AND CYCLING BODYBUILDING SUPPLEMENTS

NEW THEORIES ON STACKING AND CYCLING BODYBUILDING SUPPLEMENTS•NEW THEORIES ON STACKING AND CYCLING BODYBUILDING SUPPLEMENTS•NEW THEORIES ON STACKING AND CYCLING BODYBUILDING SUPPLEMENTS•NEW THEORIES ON STACKING AND CYCLING BODYBUILDING SUPPLEMENTS•NEW THEORIES ON STACKING

CHAPTER 12

232

are essential amino acids, and 2 of these nutrients are fatty acids. If your nutrition and supplement program doesn't provide enough of these basic nutrients each and every day, then you won't be able to maximize the effects of other supplements you might be taking, much less get the most out of the time you spend training. Don't be an idiot—make sure you're getting all of the essential vitamins and minerals you need. This can easily be accomplished by taking a daily vitamin and mineral supplement or by consuming a total-nutrition supplement/meal-replacement powder that's fortified with vitamins and minerals. Also, if you're consuming a very low-fat diet, you should use an essential fatty acid supplement—one that provides at least 10 grams (a little less than 1 Tbsp) each of linolenic and linoleic acid per day. And, of course, don't forget protein. Virtually all bodybuilding experts agree that without the proper amount of protein (I recommend at least one gram per pound of bodyweight per day), you'll never be able to maximize your muscle-building potential.

This is very basic stuff, but don't make the assumption that it's so basic it's not important—it's actually a vital part of achieving bodybuilding success.

After you've mastered the basics, you should consider what your goals are and pick supplements which might help you in that area. If your objective is to gain muscle size and strength, I think using creatine monohydrate is an absolute must, as it has been shown in numerous clinical studies to boost gains in mass and power. If you're trying to lose bodyfat, stacking supplements like HCA, ephedrine, and caffeine makes sense.

> "If your objective is to gain muscle size and strength, I think using creatine monohydrate is an absolute must..."

Q I want to put on about 10 lbs of solid muscle and increase my bench press by 25 lbs. What's a good supplement stack to help me accomplish this?

A Once again, I think it's important to look at your entire program, not just your supplement stack. If your primary goal is to gain muscle and strength, you'll want to be following a training and nutrition program that will help you accomplish these objectives and then add supplements to it that might help you get better results faster. The program I'm highly recommending for getting big, *fast*, is the Anabolic Burst Cycling System, which is outlined in Chapters 15 and 16. I'm convinced it's among the most effective bodybuilding systems I've ever reviewed. You should give it a try.

Q   What's a good supplement to stack with DHEA? I'm looking for something to boost my testosterone levels.

A   Remember, DHEA is a precursor to several hormones, including testosterone. Taking a DHEA supplement may help increase your testosterone levels, but some of this depends on what your pituitary gland (which produces something called luteinizing hormone [LH]) is "telling" your body to do.

Now, if you take DHEA by itself, it may or may not get converted to testosterone by the body, but if you combine it with a supplement called *Tribulus terrestris*, which may help increase the production of LH, you could end up with a synergistic effect. And, if you throw in another new supplement, which *Muscle Media* writer and bodybuilding guru Dan Duchaine told me about—something called androstenedione—you'll have, in my opinion, a potent "dietary-supplement" stack that produces mild steroid-like effects. (If you could get chrysin, it might be a good supplement in this stack too.)

An example of how I might stack and cycle these supplements is shown in the chart on the next page. As you can see, I recommend starting out with a dosage that's higher and then tapering off. This is in sync with the most up-to-date theories on androgen (anabolic steroid) use by bodybuilders and medical professionals who are "in the know." The theory is that you blast the system with a high dose of these compounds to take advantage of the wide-open receptor sites. When you taper off, your body will get the "signal" that the dosage levels are going down, and it won't shut off its natural production of these hormones nor develop the "expertise" to convert these substances into something else nor dismantle them.

As I explained in Chapter 3, androstenedione produces a rapid increase in testosterone levels. Adding DHEA could produce an additive effect if your body is getting the proper signal from the pituitary to produce LH (which it could be if you're taking *Tribulus terrestris*). A good time to take a dose of androstenedione is one hour prior to training—it may significantly boost strength and workout intensity. Another option is to take one dose in the morning and another at night.

I think the full effects of this three-way supplement stack will be realized in about six weeks. After that, I think the effects may subside, and it would be a good idea to take a few weeks off before starting this cycle again.

Make no mistake, this is a serious supplement stack, and it should not be used by women nor anyone under the age of 18. It should also be avoided by anyone with any medical conditions, such as an enlarged prostate, high blood pressure, heart disease, etc. It may also aggravate gynecomastia in steroid users.

A person could combine this testosterone-boosting cycle with other supplements, too. For example, using this testosterone-blitz stack with Phosphagen HP, a meal-replacement powder, flaxseed oil, and/or vitamins and minerals is what some bodybuilders would do. I don't think these testosterone-enhancing supplements would help or hinder the effects of the other supplements.

Cycle #1
DESCENDING TESTOSTERONE-BLITZ CYCLE

Week of Cycle	DHEA	Androstenedione	Tribulus terrestris
1	200 mg/day	200 mg/day	1,000 mg/day
2	150 mg/day	150 mg/day	1,000 mg/day
3	100 mg/day	100 mg/day	750 mg/day
4	100 mg/day	100 mg/day	750 mg/day
5	50 mg/day	50 mg/day	500 mg/day
6	50 mg/day	50 mg/day	250 mg/day

(Take at least three weeks off before repeating.)

As you'll surmise, there are an endless number of stacks, and what I'll recommend in this chapter are just some of the ones I think work. You can mix and match and create your own stacks and cycles. It's quite likely the ideas I share with you in this chapter will spawn some creative theories of your own. The point I think needs to be underscored is that some supplements are synergistic and should be used together, and others can be used together but don't necessarily enhance the effects of the other supplements in the stack.

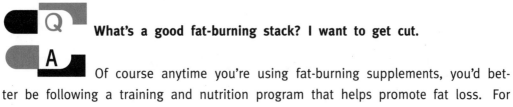

Q What's a good fat-burning stack? I want to get cut.

A   Of course anytime you're using fat-burning supplements, you'd better be following a training and nutrition program that helps promote fat loss. For example, I think it's a great idea to do aerobic exercise first thing in the morning on an empty stomach if you're trying to burn fat. (Studies show this may accelerate fat burning by up to 300% versus exercising later in the day after eating.)

Also, there's simply no way to lose fat unless you're consuming fewer calories than your body is burning. Using fat-burning supplements may help increase your metabolic rate, but if you're consuming too many calories, even the best ones won't help you get cut.

If you're restricting your calorie intake, doing aerobic exercise, and training with weights, I would recommend the fat-burning stack in the chart on the next page. This five-week program could significantly accelerate the rate at which your body burns fat.

You'll notice this program involves the use of the powerful combination of caffeine, ephedrine, and aspirin, which I believe is the best fat-burning stack legally available. There are many supplements on the market which contain the herbal equivalents of caffeine, ephedrine, and aspirin, but I don't believe they are quite as effective as using the actual over-the-counter drugs. (Do not use this stack if you have any medical conditions, and never exceed the recommended dosages!) This stack also helps suppress the appetite, while giving your central nervous system a boost, which can be very advantageous on a low-calorie diet.[77]

However, I have discovered that the continual use of caffeine, ephedrine, and aspirin, or their herbal equivalents, can cause rapid attenuation (the body becomes "immune" to the effects). To help prevent this, I think it is a very good idea to take this potent stack only every other day. Be sure not to take this stack late in the day as it can cause insomnia. And try to take a dose 30-60 minutes before exercise as it can enhance the intensity of your workout and help you burn more fat during exercise.

On the days you don't take this stuff, I recommend using yohimbe, which may give you a bit of a "lift" while also stimulating fat loss, although through a different mode of action. A recent clinical study showed that oral intakes of ten milligrams of yohimbine (the prescription form of yohimbe) a day in healthy test subjects significantly increased plasma catecholamine levels.[195] Epinephrine—which is very closely related to ephedrine but even more potent—was one of the catecholamines measured. Therefore, it appears that yohimbine (or the herbal yohimbe) may actually increase your body's internal production of fat-burning agents. A daily dose of around 200 mg of yohimbe bark extract standardized to 3% yohimbine

NEW THEORIES ON STACKING AND CYCLING BODYBUILDING SUPPLEMENTS

CHAPTER 12

NEW THEORIES ON STACKING AND CYCLING BODYBUILDING SUPPLEMENTS~NEW THEORIES ON STACKING AND CYCLING BODYBUILDING SUPPLEMENTS~NEW THEORIES ON STACKING AND CYCLING BODYBUILDING SUPPLEMENTS~NEW THEORIES ON STACKING AND CYCLING BODYBUILDING SUPPLEMENTS~NEW THEORIES ON STACKING

Cycle #2
FIVE-WEEK FAT-BURNING CYCLE

Week	Day of Cycle	Caffeine (200 mg) Ephedrine (20 mg) Aspirin (300 mg) Stack	Yohimbe (1,000 mg)	Soy Protein (25 grams)
1	1	3 times/day	—	
	2	—	2 times/day	
	3	3 times/day	—	
	4	—	2 times/day	
	5	3 times/day	—	
	6	—	2 times/day	
	7	3 times/day	—	
2	8	—	2 times/day	
	9	3 times/day	—	
	10	—	2 times/day	
	11	3 times/day	—	
	12	—	2 times/day	
	13	3 times/day	—	
	14	—	2 times/day	
3	15	3 times/day	—	
	16	—	2 times/day	
	17	3 times/day	—	
	18	—	2 times/day	2 times/day
	19	3 times/day	—	2 times/day
	20	—	2 times/day	2 times/day
	21	3 times/day	—	2 times/day
4	22	—	2 times/day	2 times/day
	23	3 times/day	—	2 times/day
	24	—	2 times/day	2 times/day
	25	3 times/day	—	2 times/day
	26	—	2 times/day	2 times/day
	27	3 times/day	—	2 times/day
	28	—	2 times/day	2 times/day
5	29	3 times/day	—	2 times/day
	30	—	2 times/day	2 times/day
	31	3 times/day	—	2 times/day
	32	—	2 times/day	2 times/day
	33	3 times/day	—	2 times/day
	34	—	2 times/day	2 times/day
	35	3 times/day	—	2 times/day

(Take at least four weeks off before repeating.)

(which is a typical standardization level) would contain about 6 mg of active yohimbine. However, due to various other chemical and structural components of the whole herb, all of that active yohimbine chemical will probably not be absorbed into the body. As a matter of fact, scientists I have spoken with estimate that maybe only 20% of the total yohimbine actually makes it into your bloodstream. Therefore, to obtain a viable 6-mg dose of yohimbine, it may be necessary to consume about 1,000 mg of the yohimbe herb. Obviously, if you could find a more potent version of yohimbe, you could get by with less. However, I am not aware of any at this time. Therefore, I suggest taking about 1,000 mg in the morning with solid food (the longer yohimbe stays in your gut, the more yohimbine that might be extracted) and another 1,000 mg at night.

Towards the later part of this stack, I recommend using 50 grams a day (25 grams in the morning with breakfast and 25 grams in the evening with another meal) of soy protein, which may have an interesting effect on thyroid hormone levels. It appears that soy-protein isolate, taken in this quantity, may actually stimulate thyroid hormone production. This effect is supported by a study done in seven elite female gymnasts. It showed that supplementation of isolated soy protein during heavy training not only increased thyroxine levels but lean body mass as well. The control group showed a decrease in thyroxine levels.[266] One very recent animal study also found that soy-protein isolate increased both total thyroxine (T_4) and free thyroxin (FT_4) by 23% and 36%, respectively, over and above the same amount of a casein protein. This type of boost to internal thyroid production is very important in helping to maintain a strong thermogenic metabolism because during periods of dieting, thyroid hormone levels drop, making fat loss even more difficult.[160]

This stack should work very well for about five weeks; after that, your body will probably adjust and override the effects. Save this cycle for your most intense dieting phase.

Q **I can't use any stimulants. What's a good fat-loss stack for me?**

A Another example of a good cutting cycle appears on the next page (Cycle #3). Notice, in this program, we are not using any central-nervous-system stimulants—some people just can't tolerate these compounds. In this cycle, we're utilizing supplements like BetaGen, which is a powerful combination of creatine and HMB. The creatine may support muscle cell volume and, in turn, could prevent excess catabolism or loss of muscle mass during a dieting phase. Scientific studies on HMB have shown that it may in fact stimulate fat loss and, at the same time, help preserve muscle tissue.[205, 206] HMB has also been shown to increase the amount of fat used as fuel by muscle cells.[2] Thus, it may help preserve glycogen stores (for energy) and muscle protein during a low calorie diet.

In this cycle, I've also included CytoVol—EAS' glutamine preservation supplement. This supplement may also prevent a loss of muscle tissue during an intense dieting program, which is always a concern.

I've also added HCA to this stack. This supplement might help prevent the conversion of carbohydrate calories to fat. It's best to use this supplement before meals. (I take 1 gram 30-60 minutes before lunch and 1 gram an hour before dinner.) Taking HCA after meals does not appear to work.

This stack also includes a high-quality total-nutrition supplement, Myoplex Plus, which provides 29 vitamins and minerals, a high dose of quality protein, while being very low in fat.

You'll notice in Cycle #3, shown below, I start off with a "loading dose" of BetaGen and CytoVol. (I think this can be very helpful—I'll tell you all about it in the next Q&A.)

Cycle #3
"STIMULANT-FREE" FAT-LOSS CYCLE

Week of Cycle	HCA	BetaGen	CytoVol	Myoplex Plus
1	2 grams/day	5 servings/day	4 servings/day	2 servings/day
2	2 grams/day	3 servings/day	1-2 servings/day	2 servings/day
3	2 grams/day	3 servings/day	1-2 servings/day	2 servings/day
4	2 grams/day	3 servings/day	1-2 servings/day	2 servings/day
5	2 grams/day	3 servings/day	1-2 servings/day	2 servings/day
6	2 grams/day	3 servings/day	1-2 servings/day	2 servings/day
7	2 grams/day	3 servings/day	1-2 servings/day	2 servings/day
8	2 grams/day	3 servings/day	1-2 servings/day	2 servings/day

(After completing this cycle, you can repeat it or switch to a bulking program.)

Q What's a good cycle for bulking up? I'm using creatine, HMB, and glutamine. How should I combine these?

A Cycle #4 on the following page gives you an example of how I might use these supplements. The first week, I recommend loading up on Phosphagain 2—a mass-building supplement which has been shown, in clinical studies, to produce effects above and beyond creatine, which is a very good supplement itself.[150] Almost all experts agree that loading up with creatine the first week you take it is a great way to put on size and strength fast. After the first week, you can cut back the dosage.

I also recommend loading up on HMB, in the form of BetaGen, and glutamine in the form of CytoVol. There is a new and seemingly valid theory that loading up on supplements like glutamine and HMB may be as important as loading up on creatine. The theory is that when you first start taking a supplement, it's possible to super-saturate muscle tissue with it. And, there's another important developing theory that insulin, which very efficiently carries nutrients into muscle tissue, may also enhance the uptake of supplements like HMB and glutamine. Studies have already shown that using an insulin-releasing carbohydrate like dextrose, along with a dose of creatine, substantially enhances the muscle's ability to take in that supplement. Future studies will be needed to confirm whether or not insulin exerts a powerful effect on the uptake of amino acids like glutamine and/or the leucine metabolite HMB. But, it's logical to believe this might be the case.

Thus, loading up on creatine, HMB, and glutamine for five to seven days—using each supplement in conjunction with a high-glycemic carbohydrate drink (one that causes a rapid and natural release of insulin)—may produce extraordinary results.

What I recommend is taking one serving of vanilla Phosphagain 2 (blended with juice) and mixing it with a serving of BetaGen and a serving of CytoVol. Consume this three times a day for seven days (in divided doses throughout the day, with or between meals). Then cut back to a regular dose of all supplements the second week. This is an awesome stack. Try this for seven days, and I think you'll be utterly amazed by how pumped your muscles get! I believe you'll also see a significant increase in strength and weight. "Reloading" every six weeks may offer additional advantages.

Remember, if you are trying to "bulk up," you need to be consuming more calories each day than your body burns. A bulking cycle isn't going to produce maximum results unless you are eating enough and training heavy.

NEW THEORIES ON STACKING AND CYCLING BODYBUILDING SUPPLEMENTS

NEW THEORIES ON STACKING AND CYCLING BODYBUILDING SUPPLEMENTS~NEW THEORIES ON STACKING AND CYCLING BODYBUILDING SUPPLEMENTS~NEW THEORIES ON STACKING AND CYCLING BODYBUILDING SUPPLEMENTS~NEW THEORIES ON STACKING AND CYCLING BODYBUILDING SUPPLEMENTS~NEW THEORIES ON STACKING

CHAPTER 12

Cycle #4
BULKING CYCLE

Week of Cycle	Phosphagain 2	BetaGen	CytoVol
1	3 servings/day	5 servings/day	5 servings/day
2	1-2 servings/day	3 servings/day	1-2 servings/day
3	1-2 servings/day	3 servings/day	1-2 servings/day
4	1-2 servings/day	3 servings/day	1-2 servings/day
5	1-2 servings/day	3 servings/day	1-2 servings/day
6	1-2 servings/day	3 servings/day	1-2 servings/day

(After completing this cycle, you can repeat it or switch to a cutting program.)

Q I'm a college student, and I'm on a very tight budget. Keeping in mind that I don't have a lot of money, but am very into bodybuilding, what supplementation would you recommend?

A A very popular, economical, and simple way to cycle supplements is to take just one supplement for one week and then switch to another. In Cycle #5, you'll see a supplement cycle that involves using Phosphagen HP for a week, CytoVol for one week, and then the vanadyl-sulfate-containing supplement V2G for a week.

Some studies show that after your muscles are loaded up with creatine, they'll maintain an elevated concentration (albeit a diminishing one) of that important nutrient for two to four weeks before these levels return to normal. And, vanadyl sulfate has been shown to continue to produce an effect for about two weeks after you stop taking it. Thus, by cycling these supplements, you may be able to save a lot of money and still enjoy good results.

A supplement cycle doesn't have to be complicated or expensive. I know many bodybuilders who don't have a lot of money and just use one supplement at a time, such as BetaGen. This is one of the best supplements for gaining muscle and accelerating fat loss. Simply using three servings of BetaGen a day (after loading up on creatine at 20-30 grams/day for a week) seems to produce tremendous results, and it's not complicated nor expensive. Simply eating right, training hard, and using BetaGen every day could offer a tremendous advantage.

Likewise, using a supplement like Phosphagain 2, three servings a day for one week and then one serving a day from then on, is a very economical way to boost your gains. Phosphagain 2 is rich with vitamins and minerals, quality protein, glutamine, creatine, and other important nutrients.

Cycle #5
REPEAT 3-WEEK-BLITZ SIZE AND STRENGTH CYCLE

Week of Cycle	Phosphagen HP	CytoVol	V2G
1	4 servings/day		
2		4 servings/day	
3			3 capsules 3 times/day
4	4 servings/day		
5		4 servings/day	
6			3 capsules 3 times/day

Repeat Program

Q **Should I take my supplements all at once, or do I have to take them throughout the day?**

A Typically, most supplements—such as vitamins (with the exception of Vitamins A, D, E, and K), HMB, glutamine, and DHEA—have a very short half-life in the blood. This means they're in and out of your system pretty quickly. Creatine is the exception. Once it is stored in muscle tissue, it can't escape until it's used to produce energy. Generally, you want to take your supplements in divided doses throughout the day to produce an optimal effect.

NEW THEORIES ON STACKING AND CYCLING BODYBUILDING SUPPLEMENTS

NEW THEORIES ON STACKING AND CYCLING BODYBUILDING SUPPLEMENTS–NEW THEORIES ON STACKING AND CYCLING BODYBUILDING SUPPLEMENTS–NEW THEORIES ON STACKING AND CYCLING BODYBUILDING SUPPLEMENTS–NEW THEORIES ON STACKING AND CYCLING BODYBUILDING SUPPLEMENTS–NEW THEORIES ON STACKING

Which supplements work synergistically?

Synergy means that two things in combination add up to something greater than the sum of their parts. In simple math, it's 1+1=3. An additive effect is when taking one supplement in combination with another provides an effect that is similar to 1+1=2.

Scientific studies have shown that using caffeine, ephedrine, and aspirin is synergistic.[122] Using creatine along with a simple carbohydrate has also been shown to be synergistic.[264, 265]

Likewise, using an insulin-releasing carbohydrate along with supplements such as glutamine and HMB may also produce a synergistic effect.

Stacking creatine with HMB is likely to produce just an additive effect because I believe they work through different mechanisms or pathways in the body.

Are there any specific times to take certain supplements that are best?

> "After training is an excellent time to consume an abundance of protein and carbohydrates, as well as important supplements like creatine, HMB, and glutamine."

I believe you can increase the effects of supplements by taking them at certain times. For example, a great time to use a protein supplement is right before you go to bed at night, since during sleep, your body builds up protein for the first few hours and then ends up recycling and breaking down protein for several hours. If you're the type of person who gets up in the middle of the night to use the bathroom or whatever, you might slam a whey protein supplement, with about 30-40 grams of protein in it. This is something a lot of great bodybuilders do, and it's a very effective way to help improve anabolic drive and muscle metabolism. (I sometimes mix a serving of chocolate Designer Whey Protein with 8 oz of skim milk and drink it around 4:00 a.m. Good stuff!) Likewise, consuming a glutamine supplement with simple carbs in the middle of the night and/or right before you go to bed may also work well. But, I wouldn't wake up on purpose to have a protein or glutamine supplement at night—sleep is also a very important part of bodybuilding.

A great time to take a testosterone booster or a testosterone-boosting stack, like androstenedione, DHEA, and *Tribulus terrestris*, is about an hour before training, as testosterone levels are significantly elevated during an intense workout, thus further potentiating the "spike."

After training is an excellent time to consume an abundance of protein and carbohydrates, as well as important supplements like creatine, HMB, and glutamine. After you finish working out, your body's metabolism is primed to feed muscle tissue. And a fast acting protein/carb drink right after exercise may even suppress exercise-induced cortisol production. Some experts recommend that 20-30% of your total calorie intake for the day be consumed within an hour or two after training (especially if you're working out hard and trying to gain muscle size and strength).

Q **If I'm using a supplement stack and it's working, why should I stop taking it?**

A Eventually, almost all supplement stacks that involve the use of these "drug-like" supplements will stop working. It's very similar to training programs, in that variety is important. If a supplement stack works for you, make sure you keep detailed notes about what you were taking, when, and what type of results you experienced. Then, take a few weeks off from using these supplements and maybe try some others. Come back to the stacks and cycles that worked for you and learn from the ones that didn't—don't repeat them. Not every supplement works for every person, and some trial and error on your part is needed to develop the best program for you.

SUMMARY

I hope this information gives you some fresh, new ideas about how to stack and cycle supplements. I wish I could tell you there's one absolutely right or wrong way to go about this, but there really isn't. Just don't make things too complicated. If you develop a program that's too complex, you won't be able to follow it. Consistency in supplement use, just like in training, is very important.

In future issues of *Muscle Media*, we'll explore the latest ideas about how to stack and cycle various supplements. Be sure to check it out so you can stay on the cutting edge. Also, if you give one of the programs that I outlined in this chapter a try, send me a letter or fax, and let me know how it works for you, so I can pass your feedback along to other bodybuilders.

243

SPORTS SUPPLEMENT REVIEW, 3RD ISSUE•SPORTS SUPPLEMENT REVIEW, 3RD ISSUE•SPORTS SUPPLEMENT REVIEW, 3RD ISSUE•SPORTS SUPPLEMENT REVIEW, 3RD ISSUE•SPORTS SUPPLEMENT REVIEW, 3RD ISSUE•SPORTS SUPPLEMENT REVIEW, 3RD ISSUE•SPORTS SUPPLEMENT REVIEW, 3RD ISSUE•SPORTS SUPPLEMENT

SPORTS SUPPLEMENT REVIEW, 3RD ISSUE–SPORTS SUPPLEMENT REVIEW, 3RD ISSUE–SPORTS SUPPLEMENT REVIEW, 3RD ISSUE–SPORTS SUPPLEMENT REVIEW, 3RD ISSUE–SPORTS

244

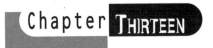

Chapter THIRTEEN

Buyer Beware! How to Buy Supplements Without Getting Ripped Off!

Now that we have an idea which supplements work and which ones don't, we need to decide which brands to go with and where to buy our supplements so we get a fair deal. In this chapter, I'm going to share some very valuable information with you that could help you make those important decisions.

First things first, I must warn you that some bodybuilding supplement companies are quite deceptive: they look for any and every opportunity to rip you off—to literally steal your money. In Chapter 5, you'll recall, I warned you about supplements that are deceptively marketed with ridiculous claims like, "This stuff is as effective as anabolic steroids." I told you about how these claims are often based on no valid science whatsoever. So we already know about those things. But, now I need to warn (or rewarn) you about some of the other sneaky tricks unscrupulous supplement manufacturers will use to try to get you to fork over your money.

"...far too many supplements you find on the shelves of your local health-food store... DO NOT contain the ingredients listed on the label!"

BEWARE OF PRODUCTS THAT DON'T CONTAIN WHAT THEIR LABELS CLAIM!

One of the very disturbing things I have documented, with dozens and dozens of independent laboratory studies, is that far too many supplements you find on the shelves of your local health-food store, or for sale from discount mail-order houses, DO NOT contain the ingredients listed on the label! (Obviously, this allows them to sell these products for a very low price—if they don't contain what's on the label, they usually contain something that costs virtually nothing to manufacture. It's a pure profit deal for them.)

I can provide strong evidence that some companies' products contain as little as ten percent of the protein they claim and sometimes <u>no</u> traces of the "active

•SPORTS SUPPLEMENT REVIEW, 3RD ISSUE•SPORTS SUPPLEMENT REVIEW, 3RD ISSUE•SPORTS SUPPLEMENT REVIEW, 3RD ISSUE•SPORTS SUPPLEMENT REVIEW, 3RD ISSUE•SPORTS SUPPLEMENT REVIEW, 3RD ISSUE•SPORTS SUPPLEMENT REVIEW, 3RD ISSUE•SPORTS SUPPLEMENT REVIEW, 3RD ISSUE•SPORTS SUPPLEMENT

REVIEW•SPORTS SUPPLEMENT REVIEW, 3RD ISSUE•SPORTS SUPPLEMENT REVIEW, 3RD ISSUE•SPORTS SUPPLEMENT REVIEW, 3RD ISSUE•SPORTS SUPPLEMENT

BUYER BEWARE! HOW TO BUY SUPPLEMENTS WITHOUT GETTING RIPPED OFF!

OFF!~BUYER BEWARE! HOW TO BUY SUPPLEMENTS WITHOUT GETTING RIPPED OFF!~BUYER BEWARE! HOW TO BUY SUPPLEMENTS WITHOUT GETTING RIPPED OFF!~BUYER BEWARE! HOW TO BUY SUPPLEMENTS WITHOUT GETTING RIPPED OFF!~BUYER BEWARE! HOW TO BUY SUPPLEMENTS WITHOUT GETTING RIPPED OFF!~BUYER BEWARE!

CHAPTER 13

BUYER BEWARE! HOW TO BUY SUPPLEMENTS WITHOUT GETTING RIPPED OFF!~BUYER BEWARE! HOW TO BUY SUPPLEMENTS WITHOUT GETTING RIPPED OFF!

ingredients" that are supposed to be in the formula! Other products I've tested contain more than twice as much fat and sugar as listed on the label.

Over the last year, it seems like there have been more mislabeled supplements than ever before. For example, in recent months, we've had six different companies' "HMB supplements" tested, and none contained any beta-hydroxy beta-methylbutyrate (the *real* HMB). One of these products was sold by Dexter Sports Supplements under the brand name Power Star, another by a company called Twenty First Century Products; another was put out by Castlewood Nutrition Systems and yet another by the Conan Corporation.

And, just recently, I tested a creatine monohydrate supplement distributed by USA Sports Labs (Lot #84310) which contained virtually no creatine at all! We retested the supplement (Lot #85450) to make sure this wasn't a fluke, and again, it contained virtually <u>no</u> creatine! And, get this, the product was called "Creatine <u>Plus</u>"! (Plus what?)

I have been warning consumers about this for many years now, but I'm still amazed at the number of people who get ripped off every day because they don't heed my advice—they don't listen when I say if you buy a "discount brand" of a popular supplement, like whey protein, a meal-replacement powder, creatine, HMB, ephedra-containing fat burners, etc., there's a chance you're throwing your money away. More often than you might imagine, companies that promise you the same high-quality products the reputable companies do but at much lower prices are up to no good.

As you know, I'm in the supplement business, so it's my job to know what the competition is doing, and it's also my job to get people to buy my company's products, but I'll make a very honest confession—even though supplement companies like TwinLab, Next Nutrition, and Weider Nutrition are direct competitors of mine, I would rather see you go into a health-food store and walk out with one of these companies' products (if you decided not to buy EAS supplements, of course), than leave with one of those alleged "bargain brands." You see, I've tested supplements put out by TwinLab, Next Nutrition, Weider Nutrition, and so on, and I've seen very consistent results: the lab tests show these products are pretty high quality.

Of course, every single batch of all EAS supplements are tested for purity and potency by independent analytical laboratories. These labs use sophisticated scientific methods, such as high-performance liquid chromatography (HPLC), which is used to separate and very accurately quantify organic compounds such as hormones, vitamins, etc. by injecting the product into a flowing stream of an ionic solvent; and high-performance capillary electrophoresis (HPCE), which is used to separate and quantify mainly water-soluble biomolecules such as amino acids, creatine, HMB, etc. by separating molecules by their unique polar charges as well as their atomic weight; and gas chromatography (GC), which is used for fatty acid analysis; this method changes compounds into a gas form and then runs them through an ionic capillary column for analysis.

EAS has always produced quality supplements; we have an excellent reputation in the industry for having first-rate products. But, like I said, if you choose not to buy EAS, that's fine—I would just encourage you not to take a chance of getting ripped off by buying one of these bargain-basement products. I feel *very* strongly about this for two primary reasons: first of all, I just hate to see people not get what they paid hard-earned money for. And secondly, I am proud of my reputation for providing accurate, cutting-edge information on how to use bodybuilding supplements to gain new muscle size and strength. And, you know what? If you go buy a brand of creatine that *doesn't contain any real creatine* and try it for several weeks, you know what you'll probably think? I do. You'll think I'm full of B.S.—you'll think to yourself, and maybe even say to your friends, "I tried that creatine stuff for a few weeks, and it doesn't even work—no size, no strength, no new muscle... nothing! That Phillips guy doesn't know what he's talking about!"

> **"There** are several good brands on the market, but there are *many* more supplement companies I don't trust..."

Believe me, that's *the last thing I want you to say!* If I give you a tip on some new supplements that might help you with your bodybuilding efforts, *I want you to get great results*. Quite literally, I'm staking my reputation on my recommendations.

Basically, the point I really want to get across to you is that you don't have to buy just one brand of supplements. There are several good brands on the market, but there are *many* more supplement companies I don't trust than ones I have faith in.

WATCH OUT FOR "FALSE GUARANTEES"

What could be worse than not putting the ingredients in the products that are listed on the labels? Well, how about promising to give customers their money back if they're not satisfied and then reneging? That seems to be the latest unscrupulous practice to get you to fork over your money.

I've heard from several people who tried supplements sold by a new outfit in Canada, and when they tried to get their money back, the company sent them a letter which explained why they weren't eligible to receive a refund, even though this company's ads offer an "unconditional money-back guarantee." Once again, you've got to be extremely careful. There's no pretty way to paint this picture; the

BUYER BEWARE! HOW TO BUY SUPPLEMENTS WITHOUT GETTING RIPPED OFF!

OFF!•BUYER BEWARE! HOW TO BUY SUPPLEMENTS WITHOUT GETTING RIPPED OFF!•BUYER BEWARE! HOW TO BUY SUPPLEMENTS WITHOUT GETTING RIPPED OFF!•BUYER BEWARE! HOW TO BUY SUPPLEMENTS WITHOUT GETTING RIPPED OFF!•BUYER BEWARE! HOW TO BUY SUPPLEMENTS WITHOUT GETTING RIPPED OFF!•BUYER BEWARE!

CHAPTER 13

people behind these companies are liars—they cheat, steal, and deceive for a living. Perhaps you've already been robbed by one of these companies and can confirm what I'm saying. Unfortunately, far too many of you will fall into that category. It's my objective to keep you from getting ripped off again.

A company with neither reputation nor brand recognition has nothing to lose by ripping you off. This is yet another reason to stick with a well-known brand.

HOW TO EVALUATE AN AD

Before you respond to an advertisement you see in a muscle magazine or a sales letter you get in the mail, stop and think about what you're doing. Ask yourself some questions, such as: "Is there a scientific basis for this supplement to help with my bodybuilding efforts?" Were any specific studies mentioned in the advertising material? If so, call up the company trying to sell you the product and ask for copies of the studies. If they send you a copy (which they rarely do), review it and see if it really supports the claims being made in the advertisement. A lot of times, supplement companies will totally misrepresent what the study really says. You've got to be extremely careful.

Also, take a look at who's selling the supplement. Is it a company that has a reputation for producing quality products in the market, or is it some unknown "fly-by-night" outfit which is probably being run out of the basement of some con-man's house? Ask yourself who's sending you the sales letter or who's making the promises in the advertisement. Often times, rip-off artists will hide out—they'll use someone else as a "puppet" or "front man," or sometimes they use a fake name. Con men will do almost anything to hide their true identity or their involvement in a campaign/scam.

> **"Reputable** businesspeople have no reason to hide—they put themselves in full view of their buying public."

Reputable businesspeople have no reason to hide—they put themselves in full view of their buying public. For example, Lee Iacocca, a world-famous businessman who completely rebuilt the Chrysler Corporation, was so confident in the quality of his corporation's products, he appeared in advertisements for the company. Many businesspeople who are selling their products with straightforward advertising do the same. Believe me, it takes a lot of confidence and pride in your company and products to put yourself right in front of the consumer and basically say, "Hey... if this product isn't everything this advertisement says it is, you have me to blame." Keep an eye out for this kind of thing—very few owners or operators of supplement companies don't "hide out," so to speak.

Next, review the advertisement and see if a lot of "absolute" claims are made. For example, does it say, "This supplement produces mind-boggling muscle growth in *every person* who uses it…"? Statements like that are never true. Even the best supplements, *even steroids*, don't work for *every* person. "All-or-nothing" statements are usually a sign that someone's trying to pull one over on you. It's just not accurate nor honest.

Another thing that piques my suspicion about whether a supplement company, or an advertisement, is reputable or not is, as we've already discussed, the price of the product. For example, if almost every company is selling a 2-lb container of whey protein for $30-$40 and you find a company that's offering it for $15, you should be concerned. You shouldn't be excited you're going to get a great deal. You should be suspicious that you're going to get ripped off.

Another thing I'm usually skeptical about is "celebrity-bodybuilder" endorsements. Typically, top-level amateur bodybuilders and pros will accept money to endorse anything. There are a few exceptions, but generally, this is just another marketing tactic that is nonsense.

My main problem with endorsements from big bodybuilders is that they're usually lies. I know they almost all use *a lot* of anabolic steroids to build their bodies. It's not that they don't use supplements; in fact, every single top bodybuilder I know uses some supplements, but because they're also taking high doses of anabolic steroids, it's impossible to tell how much of an effect the supplements are having and how much of an effect the drugs are having. Thus, I think it's hypocritical for top bodybuilders to endorse supplements with the direct or implied claim that those products significantly contributed to their present conditions.

Any bodybuilder who's endorsing a supplement should be subject to random steroid testing. This is what we do with the EAS bodybuilding spokespersons we have under contract. For example, one of our endorsers is a guy named Danny Hester. Every few weeks, Danny gets called in for random steroid testing with no advance notice whatsoever. He's been tested six times so far, and all of his tests have come back clean. In fact, all of our spokespersons are tested before they're even signed. If I find out any of our spokespersons are using steroids or any other bodybuilding drugs, there's a clause in the contract that says that spokesperson will be fired—the contract will be revoked.

The bodybuilders we have under contract, who do compete, are not penalized if they don't place in the top of the contests they enter. I think that would put too much pressure on them to use bodybuilding drugs. Their job is to train hard, eat right, use EAS supplements, and just do the best they can. It doesn't matter if they finish first or last; as long as they do the best they can with what they've got, they have fulfilled their obligation.

I think the other supplement companies are making a big mistake by letting their bodybuilding spokespersons use drugs while endorsing their supplements. Consumers are too smart today to fall for that kind of thing.

Here's something else you should watch for—ridiculous-looking before and after pictures. Some of these pictures are computer enhanced, and others are deliberately set up—a person will bulk up for a couple of weeks and get all bloated, then go on a strict training and nutrition program, and maybe even use the supplement he/she gives a testimonial for in the ad, and then represent that taking the supplement caused miracles to happen and he/she lost 30 lbs in 30 days or something equally ridiculous. Use your brain—the people who sell supplements in this manner aren't stupid; *the people who buy them are!*

An honest company that uses before and after pictures will make it *perfectly clear* the subject trained and fed his/her body correctly, in addition to using the supplement(s). And, they will note that the photos offer <u>evidence</u> (not proof!) of what can happen and that different people will get different results.

Unfortunately, the FDA (Food and Drug Administration) and FTC (Federal Trade Commission), and other government regulatory agencies, like Better Business Bureaus, that are supposed to protect consumers, are simply way too busy to keep track of everything that's going on in the bodybuilding supplement business. Believe me, the things that some of these supplement companies are getting away with are very wrong.

POSITIVE THINGS TO LOOK FOR

Here are some things you should look for that are good signs: watch for a reputable brand, like EAS, TwinLab, Weider, Next Nutrition, etc. Even then, use as much common sense as you can in your decision process. Ask yourself, "Is this supplement backed by science—*real science*?" A reputable supplement company will send you copies of studies that support the claims being made for their products.

Ask people at your gym what supplements they've used or what brands they trust. Typically, these people will have no reason to mislead you—if they've used a supplement that's worked for them, it's usually their pleasure to share that information with you.

LOOK FOR A STRONG GUARANTEE

Another thing you should look for is a company that stands behind its products—one that offers a *real guarantee*. For example, my company offers a rock-solid, ironclad LIFETIME MONEY-BACK GUARANTEE on any product we sell—books, magazine subscriptions, and supplements. We're the only company in the industry that offers an authentic lifetime money-back guarantee. Other supplement companies think it's a crazy thing to do because people could rip us off—they could use the product, get great results, then lie and get their money back. Does this happen on occasion? Well, yes, sometimes it does. (Not every consumer is honest either!) Sometimes people run a "con" on us and rip us off, but fortunately, the majority of bodybuilders we work with are very honest people. They're looking for nothing more than a fair deal, and that's what my company offers. Perhaps that's why EAS is the most popular line of bodybuilding supplements in America today.

Those of you who know me understand that I'm a pretty controversial figure in the bodybuilding supplement world—a lot of folks (especially my competitors) have an "intense disliking" for me, to put it politely. Sometimes they'll accuse me of the most outrageous things, but one thing no one can ever say about me or any of my companies is that I've ever ripped anyone off in any way, shape, or form. I'm in business to make a profit, just like every other businessperson, but I recognize the only way for a company to be successful in this

> "I perceive it as my responsibility to help you with your body-building efforts—to help you discover effective, new training and nutrition programs..."

market over the long term is to provide extremely high-quality products, tremendous service, and to do everything possible to satisfy customers' wants and needs. For example, if you were to buy an EAS supplement, like Phosphagen HP, and for some strange reason you weren't absolutely thrilled with the results you got from using this product, you would be entitled to 100% of your purchase price back on that product. That's a simple, straightforward deal, with no fine print. In fact, it's a promise from me to every one of my customers. I've always run my businesses this way, and it's the only way I would think of doing it.

WHERE TO BUY SUPPLEMENTS

Okay, let's talk more about just exactly where you should buy supplements and how you can get the best ones at the lowest prices. Well, one thing that's very popular with a lot of bodybuilders is picking up their supplements every month at a General Nutrition Center (GNC) store. GNC has a fantastic selection of bodybuilding supplements, and they have a great "Gold Card" program where members save 20% on high-quality bodybuilding supplements if they buy them on the first Tuesday of every month. (It costs only $15 a year to get your GNC Gold Card!) For example, if you wanted to stock up on Myoplex Plus Deluxe (a great total-nutrition product), typically, you'd pay $62 for 20 servings. But, on Super Tuesday (the first Tuesday of every month), at GNC you can buy that same supplement for $49! If you make out a list of the products you want to stock up on and buy them the first Tuesday of every month, you could easily save well over $100 a month on your

BUYER BEWARE! HOW TO BUY SUPPLEMENTS WITHOUT GETTING RIPPED OFF!

OFF!•BUYER BEWARE! HOW TO BUY SUPPLEMENTS WITHOUT GETTING RIPPED OFF!•BUYER BEWARE! HOW TO BUY SUPPLEMENTS WITHOUT GETTING RIPPED OFF!•BUYER BEWARE! HOW TO BUY SUPPLEMENTS WITHOUT GETTING RIPPED OFF!•BUYER BEWARE! HOW TO BUY SUPPLEMENTS WITHOUT GETTING RIPPED OFF!•BUYER BEWARE!

supplement bill and have the confidence of knowing you're dealing with a reputable establishment.

You can also find a variety of quality bodybuilding supplements at many gyms and independent health-food stores. But, you should use caution here, too—be sure to deal with a reputable outfit. Some of these discount health-food stores follow some pretty shady business practices; in fact, dozens of them go out of business every week.

Good health-food retailers will not only stand behind their products and give you a fair deal, they'll also be able to help you decide which supplements are best for you. We keep an up-to-date list of literally hundreds of them in our database, and one of our representatives checks up on them virtually every month. We have the names, addresses, and phone numbers of reputable health-food retailers in virtually every city across the country. It would be our pleasure to help you locate the store nearest you—just call my Customer Care Department at 1-800-297-9776 (ask for Dept. #4055) and give us your zip code, and we'll tell you where the best health-food retailers in your area are located. Alternatively, you can access this information on the Internet by visiting our home page at www.eas.com. This could be very valuable information for you. We have gone to great lengths to screen these retailers and eliminate all the bad seeds.

If you prefer to buy your supplements through mail order, please review the info in the back of this book. I've included a listing of quality products, where to call to order them, how to save up to 25%, and so on.

FOOD FOR THOUGHT

Now, I want to make something perfectly clear—this book was not written simply to promote EAS products. If my sole objective were to try to get you to buy an EAS supplement, I would have done what everybody else in this industry does and just sent you a pushy sales letter or a fancy flyer that some advertising agency came up with. Believe me, that would have been a lot easier than spending 5 months wracking my brain, putting together this 350+ page book. Do you know why I wrote this book and why I continue to dig deep into the supplement industry to try to bring you accurate information on what works and what doesn't? It's because... THAT'S MY JOB! I perceive it as my responsibility to help you with your bodybuilding efforts—to help you discover effective, new training and nutrition programs, as well as teaching you about the ins and outs of bodybuilding supplements.

"Nothing bums me out more than seeing a fellow bodybuilder get ripped off while an undeserving con man puts another buck in his pocket."

CHAPTER 13

BUYER BEWARE! HOW TO BUY SUPPLEMENTS WITHOUT GETTING RIPPED OFF!•BUYER BEWARE! HOW TO BUY SUPPLEMENTS WITHOUT GETTING RIPPED OFF!

If I can help you build a better body, to get better results faster from the time you spend working out, then I'll be satisfied that I've done my job. And you know what? If I continue to do this—if I continue to do the right thing and put the wants and needs of bodybuilders like you ahead of what I want for my company—then in the long run, we'll all be winners. I believe that only by helping other people get what they want will I be able to get what I want—to have more people read my magazine, use EAS supplements, and buy my books. This is a pretty bizarre business approach, for this industry especially, but it's one I believe in and one I'll stick with to the end. Make no mistake, it's not a "get-rich-quick" philosophy. It's a *long-term* strategy for success—a commitment not just to get customers but to *keep* them. You see, in the bodybuilding supplement business, the market is only so big, and if you burn bridges by selling products that don't work and if you run advertisements that are filled with misleading information or downright lies and you don't honor your guarantees or don't treat your customers right, you will never achieve success in the long run. Those of you who have been around this industry a while have probably seen some very big supplement companies come and go over the past few years; they had the wrong philosophy about business and greatly underestimated *your* intelligence and *your* power. Today, these companies are going out of business left and right.

EAS Is About Quality and Service

My goal is to go above and beyond your expectations. I'm not going to be satisfied by merely providing you with quality information and effective products. My mission is to go to a higher level, and part of that commitment is service. For example, if you've got a question about something you read in this book, all you have to do is phone or fax us, and we'll help you out. Ask us anything—we'll do whatever we can to get you an accurate, straightforward answer right away.

At EAS, you can place your order 24 hours a day, 365 days a year, using any major credit card. And, we ship your order by two-day Federal Express service at no premium charge. That means if you place your order with us on Wednesday, it could be sitting on your doorstep Friday morning. And, on top of all this, in the back of this book, you'll find a full page of money-saving coupons towards the purchase of products we sell.

I feel very confident in saying EAS is the best place to buy supplements, by phone or mail order. We have what I truly believe are the best products. (Remember, EAS supplements are scientifically designed and evaluated. They are also convenient, our powders taste great, and EAS supplements are a tremendous value!) We have a full staff of bodybuilding experts who are always delighted to help you in any way they can; we're open 24 hours a day; we have the most convenient payment options available; we offer a lifetime money-back guarantee, which basically allows you to try any supplement *without risk*; and we do whatever we can to treat our customers like royalty! What more could you ask for?

An Unprecedented Commitment to Research

Here's something else you might want to consider: EAS is the only bodybuilding supplement company that allocates a portion of every dollar of our supplement sales to support university research to advance the science of drug-free muscle building and performance. Last year alone, we allocated over one million dollars to fund research grants at prestigious institutions, including: Kent State University, Iowa State University, State University of New York at Stony Brook, Wichita State University, the University of Memphis, Creighton University, Wisconsin University, the University of Nebraska at Omaha, and Nottingham University in England. This massive and unprecedented commitment to research has already led to several powerful, new drug-free supplement discoveries. Basically, when you buy EAS products, you are supporting university research programs, which will undoubtedly help all of us who want to build muscle without resorting to steroids. (Keep this in mind, *please!*)

Summary

Okay, that's the end of my sales pitch. Seriously, even if you decide not to buy EAS supplements, or if you buy some products from us and some from another company, I want you to know that I'll always do whatever I can to help you out—you can call our technical support line (even if you buy supplements from another company and want to ask us what the best way to use them might be), and you can also fax or write to me. You'll find our address, phone, and fax numbers in the back of this book. I will always do whatever I can to get you the answers you're looking for and help you out... fair enough?

And finally, please give the tips I gave you in this chapter some serious consideration. Nothing bums me out more than seeing a fellow bodybuilder get ripped off while an undeserving con man puts another buck in his pocket.

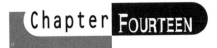

Chapter FOURTEEN

How to Maximize Your Gains, and Prevent Overtraining, with Proper Nutrition

During all the years I've been studying and practicing bodybuilding, I don't recall meeting anyone with a great physique who didn't train at least three, four, or five days a week. Yet, whenever I open many of today's popular bodybuilding magazines, there always seems to be some story about how people should cut back on their training—the argument is that "overtraining" is keeping us from growing. The source of overtraining can be difficult to pinpoint because there are so many variables that can cause it. These variables include a person's age, genetics, muscle-fiber ratio, training level, intensity, recuperative abilities, and how he/she eats. Many articles focus on and point to the number of sets and reps which can contribute to an overtrained state. And while those aspects are very important, I would also like you to consider another perspective on overtraining.

I contend that most overtrained states stem from an inadequate diet, <u>not</u> from too much exercise. Without adequate nutritional support for your muscles, there's no way in hell they'll grow! Imagine a long-distance runner eating one meal a day. How long and how far do you think he or she would last? Do you think you could reach peak performance eating only one, two, or even three meals a day? Too many bodybuilders focus all their attention on the importance of not overtraining, yet they ignore their nutrition programs. In this chapter, I'm going to give you some very important advice on what I believe constitutes a sound nutritional program for serious bodybuilders. If you do not master the fundamentals of proper bodybuilding nutrition, you

"**In** this chapter, I'm going to give you some very important advice on what I believe constitutes a sound nutritional program for serious bodybuilders."

255

HOW TO MAXIMIZE YOUR GAINS, AND PREVENT OVERTRAINING, WITH PROPER NUTRITION

OVERTRAINING, WITH PROPER NUTRITION•HOW TO MAXIMIZE YOUR GAINS, AND PREVENT OVERTRAINING, WITH PROPER NUTRITION•HOW TO MAXIMIZE YOUR GAINS, AND PREVENT OVERTRAINING, WITH PROPER NUTRITION•HOW TO MAXIMIZE YOUR GAINS, AND PREVENT OVERTRAINING, WITH PROPER NUTRITION•HOW TO MAXIMIZE

CHAPTER 14

will <u>not</u> get optimal results from your workouts, even if you train correctly <u>and</u> use great supplements, like creatine and others. So pay close attention... Okay!?

Protein Intake

One dietary factor which could cause you to become more susceptible to overtraining is inadequate protein intake. This is a key component in retaining muscle and providing adequate amino acids to the amino-acid pool within your body. If you are concerned that too much protein is bad for you, you needn't be. It's not uncommon for many young bodybuilders to be led astray by a doctor or dietitian stating that too much protein can cause kidney damage. There has never been, to my knowledge, any study that proves protein causes any type of kidney damage in healthy individuals. And keep in mind that the Recommended Daily Allowance (RDA) for protein is based on inactive people, not athletes.

Protein is the most important nutrient for bodybuilders. I'm also a big believer in spreading protein intake out over six meals. People who ingest the right amount of protein for their bodyweight but do it over the course of only three meals will invariably hit plateaus in their lean body mass gains. I've personally witnessed and documented the dramatic changes in bodybuilders' physiques when they went from eating four balanced meals per day to six. But keep in mind, the protein has to be from a low-fat, high-quality source, like chicken or turkey breast, egg whites, fish, or a high-quality protein supplement.

In order to induce muscles to respond, you have to maximally stress them with weight resistance. Secondly, amino acids must then be present to aid in the tissue repair. If your diet is lacking in protein, you can basically train as hard and as intensely as you want and spend as many days pounding the weights as you desire, and I'll guarantee you won't see any growth. One of the criteria people use to gauge whether they're overtrained or not is their ability to recuperate. If protein intake is inadequate, recuperation is affected, so it's easy to see how some people could mistakenly think their weight training, and not their diet, is the cause of overtraining.

Water Intake

A little-known fact about water is that the less you drink, the more likely you are to become overtrained. There's a direct correlation here. Muscle is comprised of over 70% water. A higher protein intake requires more water. Sweating from intense workouts causes you to dehydrate and lose body water. And water is an essential transport mechanism for a vast array of nutrients like vitamins and minerals and even carbohydrates. It serves an important role in all cellular activity. If your water intake is too low, your ability to transport nutrients becomes compromised, muscle fullness decreases, and a toxic buildup of ammonia, urea, uric acid, and other junk begins to accumulate in your body. As the entire row of dominoes begins to fall, your body's not capable of pushing water into the muscle because too much is pulled out to handle the demands and stresses being placed on it.

To stay adequately hydrated, take your bodyweight and multiply it by .55—that's about how much water you should drink in ounces every day. For example, I currently weigh 202 lbs; therefore, I try to drink 111 oz (202 x .55) of water every day. If you are a long-distance runner or are exercising in extreme heat, multiply your bodyweight by .66.

COMPLEX CARBOHYDRATES

Carbohydrates provide a "protein-sparing" effect. Under normal circumstances, protein serves a vital role in the maintenance, repair, and growth of body tissues. When carbohydrate reserves are reduced, the body will convert protein into glucose for energy. This process is called "glyconeogenesis." Carbohydrates are very important because if your body doesn't have enough, it has to metabolize more protein. The price paid is a reduction in the body's protein stores; in other words, muscle is depleted!

Also, eating too few carbohydrates can leave your muscles feeling and looking flat. Muscle fullness depends, to a large extent, on the glycogen stores within them. Likewise, your vascularity also depends on your carbohydrate intake. Have you ever noticed while dieting that your veins disappear between meals and reappear shortly after you eat? Competitive bodybuilders often note that drinking a glass of wine or ingesting some simple sugars before a competition brings out their vascularity.

A lot of the weight you drop while on a low-carbohydrate diet is water weight. For every gram of carbohydrate that gets stored in muscle tissue, around three grams of water usually accompany it. By decreasing your carbohydrate intake, you naturally drop body water. Although this may sound like a good idea, when you resume eating carbohydrates, you may find that your body rebounds and retains *excess* water. The water retention will dissipate after several days, but it can wreak havoc on the dieter's mental state. Keep this in mind: if your carbohydrate intake is too low, your energy will also be low. And one common complaint from people who feel overtrained is less energy and loss of muscle fullness.

> "...eating too few carbohydrates can leave your muscles feeling and looking flat. Muscle fullness depends, to a large extent, on the glycogen stores within them."

257

HOW TO MAXIMIZE YOUR GAINS, AND PREVENT OVERTRAINING WITH PROPER NUTRITION

OVERTRAINING, WITH PROPER NUTRITION•HOW TO MAXIMIZE YOUR GAINS, AND PREVENT OVERTRAINING, WITH PROPER NUTRITION•HOW TO MAXIMIZE YOUR GAINS, AND PREVENT OVERTRAINING, WITH PROPER NUTRITION•HOW TO MAXIMIZE YOUR GAINS, AND PREVENT OVERTRAINING, WITH PROPER NUTRITION•HOW TO MAXIMIZE YOUR GAINS, AND PREVENT OVERTRAINING, WITH PROPER NUTRITION•HOW TO MAXIMIZE

CALORIE INTAKE

It's very easy to place yourself in an overtrained state by undereating. We walk a very fine line between losing bodyfat and losing muscle while dieting. It is necessary to ingest less calories in an attempt to drop bodyfat, but by dropping calories too low, you cause your muscles to give up precious nutrients to make up for the lacking diet. And, to top it off, the more cardio you do while restricting your calories, the more likely you are to notice a loss of lean body mass. Of course, the stress hormones are always lurking in the background ready to wreak havoc on your muscle tissue as well.

If you're ingesting too few calories, you'll not only lose muscle, you'll also lose energy and endurance. Naturally, you won't have the energy to get through the workout, and your strength will suffer as well. It's easy to see how some people who are undereating could attribute the loss of energy and strength to overtraining.

MEAL FREQUENCY

Consider the exponential benefits eating more meals would have on your ability to recuperate from intense workouts. If you currently eat four evenly spaced meals, each balanced with protein and complex carbohydrates, think of the impact that adding two more meals would have on increasing your energy by adding additional protein and nutrients for muscle growth. Don't make the mistake of thinking you can cram more and more food into each meal and get good results. That would lead to an overload on your digestive system causing the excess to be converted to fat. Don't ever underestimate the power of meal frequency in your bodybuilding goals. Time and time again, diabetic research has proven the benefits of a more stable blood-sugar level, optimal absorption of food stuff, and an increased metabolic rate, all a result of ingesting more balanced meals as opposed to stuffing more into each meal. For optimal performance, bodybuilders require six small, balanced meals throughout the day. For convenience, and to make this task easier, try using a meal-replacement powder, like Myoplex Plus. Try to eat at least three or more solid meals, and use the meal-replacement powders for three meals or less per day.

> "**Each** meal must, and I repeat *must*, contain a balance of protein and complex carbohydrates in order for you to really get the most out of your weight training."

Meal Balance

I may sound like a broken record, but if you think a big bowl of pasta is a meal, or if your idea of breakfast is a bowl of oatmeal with fruit, you're dead wrong! Each meal must, and I repeat *must*, contain a balance of protein and complex carbohydrates in order for you to really get the most out of your weight training. Too many people shoot for six meals a day, but they just don't understand the important role the combination of foods plays in their ability to gain mass and drop bodyfat.

Just imagine your plate divided into thirds. One third of your plate should have a low-fat source of protein. Another third should consist of a complex carbohydrate, and the final third should be some type of fibrous vegetable. This simple technique allows you to eat the correct balance of fuel, no matter where you are.

Inconsistent Sleeping Patterns

This area is an indirect dietary consideration. You see, your diet may be sufficient to allow for adequate recuperation under normal circumstances, but if there is added stress stemming from incomplete rest periods, you are much more likely to become overtrained. Without rest, over time the body cannot sufficiently recover. Couple that with an inadequate diet and you can very easily find yourself tired, losing strength, and lacking the desire to work out. I recommend that bodybuilders try to get a solid eight hours of sleep each night. Another factor that comes into play when sleep patterns become disrupted is your ability to fit all your meals into your schedule. If you stay up too late one night and consequently sleep in the next day, you'll be less likely to have time to fit in six meals.

Vitamins and Minerals and Other Ergogenic Aids

Additional vitamins and minerals, if used sensibly, may indeed help your recovery. But if you are relying too much on pills and capsules, you need to rethink your strategy. Too many bodybuilders buy all kinds of supplements without first considering their overall nutrition programs. If their diets aren't right, the supplements are useless as far as gaining muscle goes. I'm constantly amazed at how eager athletes are to try every new supplement that comes along without first getting their dietary programs in order. So get your nutritional plan in order before you add these things to your program.

Make sure you take a well-rounded multivitamin and an additional multi-mineral. The minerals are important because many bodybuilders avoid dairy products. Extra Vitamin C and E can also be good additions to your program, since they act as strong antioxidants, which can aid in recuperation. Creatine monohydrate works very well at keeping your muscles hydrated and increasing power.

SUMMARY

There's no doubt about it, most people could train harder, more often, and more effectively if they understood the role their diets play in preventing overtraining. Advocates of training less should first focus on a person's diet to make sure the individual's inability to grow isn't stemming from poor nutritional habits. I honestly believe too many people needlessly cut back on their training frequency out of fear of overtraining. The reality is, there is no magic training program or vitamin pill that will make you grow. It's the totality of what you do on a consistent, ongoing basis that will eventually get you where you want to be.

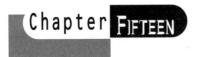

Chapter FIFTEEN

Anabolic Burst Cycling:
A Breakthrough in
Bodybuilding Nutrition

Psst... *Hey*... you wanna secret formula for some powerful "home-brew," muscle-building hormones? I don't mean the crap they sell on the streets—I mean the good stuff... <u>real</u> insulin, testosterone, insulin-like growth factor-1 (IGF-1), etc. You know... the stuff that *really* works! The juice that packs on muscle mass like nothing else in the world! Well... if you do, keep on reading because I've got some AMAZING inside info that will rock your bodybuilding world! In this chapter, I'll tell you about a "source" that will never run dry, never slip you bogus or counterfeit juice, and never rip you off. And, there's no way you could end up in any legal trouble for getting your anabolic hormones through this "connection," either. Interested? I thought so. Keep reading...

So, what is this "source"? Is it some new European pharmacy? Nope. Is it an open-minded doctor in Palm Springs? Negative. Is it a black-market 'roid dealer? Hell no! Is it a new supplement distributor? Not exactly.

This source is *your body*.

SAY WHAT?!

I'm dead serious... the <u>best</u> source of muscle-building hormones you'll ever find is your own body!

Think about it... even if you're an "average-sized" weight trainer and you've never used any synthetic physique-building drugs, it's likely that your body is made up of at least 100 lbs of skeletal muscle. (The rest is bone, blood, organs, fat, etc.) Think about where that muscle came from... It had to have been built with your body's natural anabolic hormones... right? (Where the hell else would it have come from?) So it's obvious your body has the "formula" to build muscle—*a lot of it*—with no side effects!

> **"There** is indeed a way to flood your body with a natural, powerful 'hormone cocktail' that produces substantial and rapid increases in muscle mass."

261

SPORTS SUPPLEMENT REVIEW, 3RD ISSUE•SPORTS SUPPLEMENT REVIEW, 3RD ISSUE•SPORTS SUPPLEMENT REVIEW, 3RD ISSUE•SPORTS SUPPLEMENT

•SPORTS SUPPLEMENT REVIEW, 3RD ISSUE•SPORTS SUPPLEMENT REVIEW, 3RD ISSUE•SPORTS SUPPLEMENT REVIEW, 3RD ISSUE•SPORTS SUPPLEMENT REVIEW, 3RD ISSUE•SPORTS SUPPLEMENT REVIEW, 3RD ISSUE•SPORTS SUPPLEMENT REVIEW, 3RD ISSUE•SPORTS SUPPLEMENT

ANABOLIC BURST CYCLING: A BREAKTHROUGH IN BODYBUILDING NUTRITION

ANABOLIC BURST CYCLING: A BREAKTHROUGH IN BODYBUILDING NUTRITION–ANABOLIC BURST CYCLING: A BREAKTHROUGH IN BODYBUILDING NUTRITION–ANABOLIC BURST CYCLING: A BREAKTHROUGH IN BODYBUILDING NUTRITION–ANABOLIC BURST CYCLING: A BREAKTHROUGH IN BODYBUILDING NUTRITION–ANABOLIC BURST CYCLING:

Sure, over the past 40 years, scientists have discovered how to synthetically manufacture many anabolic hormones, but could millions of years of evolution—millions of years of mutations, which developed the structure and function of your natural anabolic hormones—really be "outdone" by today's pharmaceutical science? It's *very* doubtful.

So how do we "harness" our bodies' natural muscle-building potential—how do we get these anabolic hormones that literally built our bodies to work for us in a big way? That is *the* million-dollar question! And, I recently interviewed a scientist who may very well have discovered the answer!

A REVOLUTIONARY SCIENTIFIC DISCOVERY!

There is indeed a way to flood your body with a natural, powerful "hormone cocktail" that produces substantial and rapid increases in muscle mass. In fact, researchers have shown this relatively simple muscle-building "secret" has allowed healthy test subjects, *who didn't even train with weights*, to put on 4.38 lbs of lean body mass and 2 lbs of fat in only 12 days![135] Scientists have also demonstrated, with very intricate blood analyses, that test subjects who followed this system experienced significant increases in the anabolic hormones insulin, testosterone, and IGF-1![87]

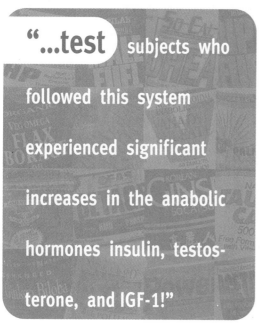

"...test subjects who followed this system experienced significant increases in the anabolic hormones insulin, testosterone, and IGF-1!"

Make no mistake, this is not a harebrained theory that was dreamed up by some bodybuilding huckster, quack, or amateur scientist. The substantiation behind this new, breakthrough bodybuilding idea is *very* compelling.

SO WHAT IS THIS BREAKTHROUGH THEORY?

Well, as I already alluded to in the introduction of this chapter, this system does not involve taking any synthetic drugs. This system is not based on any Eastern Block training secret or anything like that. It's not all that complicated; in fact, I'm amazed no one has previously discovered it, but in the 16 years I've been studying and practicing bodybuilding, I've never once seen anything written nor even discussed, in public or in private, about this muscle-building secret (that is, up until this recent interview).

Using this system, virtually every human will gain muscle mass—it doesn't matter if you're a man or a woman, and it works even if you don't train with weights[228] (but, of course, it will be much more effective when you combine it with an intense bodybuilding program).

This system produces an increase in many muscle-building hormones, which creates a powerful "anabolic cocktail"—possibly nature's perfect synergistic "stack." As *Muscle Media* writer Michael Mooney alluded to in the July 1996 issue, it is highly unlikely that taking one anabolic hormone by itself, such as insulin, growth hormone, IGF-1, or even testosterone, would create the best environment for new muscle growth. Mooney revealed how some bodybuilders are taking multiple drugs in an effort to mimic the body's natural hormonal muscle-building stack. The problems with that strategy are that it presents the potential for serious side effects as well as the legal ramifications of using these drugs (most of which are illegal). It also disrupts the natural production of these hormones, so when you stop taking them, you're basically screwed—for at least a few months, your system is thrown so out of whack that while it tries to "normalize," the muscle you gained will probably be sacrificed.

Well, with this new system, you don't have to worry about that—you're always in control. There are no side effects, and no cop will ever bust you for doing something illegal.

So, what is this breakthrough? (Drum roll, please...) It's called the ANABOLIC BURST CYCLING OF DIET AND EXERCISE (ABCDE), and it is most unique because it involves a totally revolutionary approach to bodybuilding *nutrition*. Yep... the real key to this muscle-building system is food—that stuff you get at the grocery store—the stuff that keeps you alive day in and day out and has sustained your very existence since you were weaned off your mother's milk.

Now don't worry—I'm not going to go into some long, complicated, tedious, confusing, and borderline-irrelevant discussion about things like eicosanoids, arachidonic acid, and crap like that. I don't even know what the hell that stuff is (even though I've read Dr. Barry Sears' book twice and have a pretty decent scientific background to begin with). No, the ABCDE system is damn near as simple as it sounds.

How I Discovered ABCDE

I learned about this amazing concept from a colleague named Torbjorn (pronounced Tor-b-yorn) Akerfeldt. This scientist is presently studying medicine at Uppsala University, which is located 50 miles outside of Stockholm, Sweden.

In addition to having an extensive background in sciences such as endocrinology, physiology, pharmacology, and nutrition, Torbjorn is also a pretty darn good bodybuilder himself. Thus, he understands the scientific side and the real-world applications of all aspects of this endeavor which we call bodybuilding.

Recently, Torbjorn was visiting the United States—driving from coast to coast, meeting with various research scientists and doctors at universities, exchanging data on research projects which are ongoing or are scheduled to be conducted at Uppsala University.

ANABOLIC BURST CYCLING: A BREAKTHROUGH IN BODYBUILDING NUTRITION

ANABOLIC BURST CYCLING: A BREAKTHROUGH IN BODYBUILDING NUTRITION~ANABOLIC BURST CYCLING: A BREAKTHROUGH IN BODYBUILDING NUTRITION~ANABOLIC BURST CYCLING: A BREAKTHROUGH IN BODYBUILDING NUTRITION~ANABOLIC BURST CYCLING: A BREAKTHROUGH IN BODYBUILDING NUTRITION~ANABOLIC BURST CYCLING:

Torbjorn stopped by *Muscle Media* headquarters, here in Golden, Colorado, on his way to California, and we sat down and "talked shop" for five hours. That's when I had the chance to conduct the following interview, which was definitely one of the most enlightening I've ever had the pleasure of doing.

Bill PHILLIPS What exactly is Anabolic Burst Cycling, and how does it work?

Torbjorn AKERFELDT It's primarily a new bodybuilding nutrition theory I've developed—it's quite different from anything bodybuilders are doing right now in America or Europe.

As a bodybuilder and scientist, I follow the many trends in nutrition with great interest. Sometimes people tell us to eat a high-carbohydrate diet; other times, we're told to ingest a lot of protein. Lately, we're reading that a high-fat diet is the way to go. The strange thing is, virtually all of these diets can be backed up by scientific studies.

BP How can this be—how can the positive effects of all of these diets be backed by studies?

TA Most of these studies are performed during a limited period of time, so what is actually being measured is the metabolic consequences of a *change* in the diet, and therefore, people misinterpret their results. This was one of the observations that helped me develop my theory—I noticed that scientific studies have reliably shown that when there is a drastic change in the diet, the body responds very swiftly and efficiently.

BP Isn't changing the diet often unphysiological—unnatural?

TA No, it's the opposite. Our genes have not evolved much during the last 100,000 years; thus, they are still developed for our hunter/gatherer and, more recently, pastoral ancestors, who, whenever they succeeded in killing an animal, lived on meat for a week or two. At other times, when they had bad luck hunting and a crop failed, they lived on a low-calorie diet. This selective pressure gave man adipose tissue with almost unlimited storage capacity and a very adaptive metabolism to cope with periods of different diets. So, that's what we're made for!

BP How do our bodies adapt to these changes?

TA Basically, our genes control the expression of enzymes. These enzymes control every aspect of our metabolisms, including the activation of different pathways and the rate at which chemical reactions take place in our bodies. [Outside biochemical system enzymes are often referred to as catalysts.] Evolution has given our genes the ability to control the production of these enzymes as well as their activity level. Due to this fact, the body will be able to adapt to different food intakes as well as become prepared or "primed" for a future sudden change in the diet. For example, during a calorie- [or any macronutrient] restricted period, the number and activity of enzymes which govern storage will increase, while the degrading enzymes and those which promote efficiency or utilization will decrease in activity. This is one reason you should never restrict your calorie or dietary-fat intake too much if you want to lose fat—your body will respond the opposite of how you want it to.

On the other hand, after a period of restriction, the body is now optimized for a forthcoming period of "excess" intake of calories. When this period takes place, the body will store excess calories at a tremendous rate. This applies to carbohydrates [glycogen] and is the basis for "carb loading." It also applies to fats [triglycerides] and amino acids [proteins]. Sometimes this mechanism is called "super-compensation."

However, it is important to remember that the body has a high turnover rate of enzymes; hence, the increased activity/number will disappear in a relatively short period of time—less than two weeks in most cases. Enzymes not only control the metabolism of fats, glucose, and proteins directly but also indirectly via hormones. The reason the endocrine system evolved in multicellular organisms could be to make a regulatory system that operated over a longer period of time. For example, persistent excess-calorie intake rapidly increases the release of certain anabolic hormones [to store the excess energy as muscle] with a peak after about two weeks.

According to the metabolic situation, the body has a preset program under which suitable proteins [enzymes, receptors, binding proteins, and peptide hormones] are being synthesized. This metabolic situation depends on what and how much you have been eating and the type of training during the last few days. Do you get the picture now? You have to make the body believe that an anabolic burst is necessary now and then.

The bottom line is that if your goal is to not look like an average person, you have to "trick" the body constantly in order to have different enzymatic and endocrine systems primed at different times. The timing is a very crucial factor here. That's what the ABCDE program is all about.

> "...you should never restrict your calorie or dietary-fat intake too much if you want to lose fat—your body will respond the opposite of how you want it to."

265

B P Now, let me see if I've got this straight—by eating a certain way—by changing your diet often, you can enhance muscle building? Do you follow a high-carb diet for a period of time, then switch to a high-protein diet or a high-fat diet?

T A Not exactly. The research indicates that overall energy [calorie] intake has a much greater effect on nitrogen balance [associated with muscle gain] than protein intake does.[207] I believe the same is true of carbohydrates and fats.

A good study, with test subjects having a fixed protein intake of 1.25 grams/kg/day but with different total-energy intakes, showed that an increase in calories of 15% enhanced nitrogen retention from 7.2 mg/kg/day to 23.8. When energy intake was increased to 30% above requirement, nitrogen balance rose to 33.3 mg/kg/day.[52] Basically, adding calories to the diet is anabolic, and I don't just mean it raises insulin levels—by adding just one anabolic hormone, you'll never get optimal gains in muscle. You need the whole array of anabolic hormones, and they have to be in the correct ratio to each other. This is what happens during puberty.

Few people have access or the financial wherewithal to purchase all of the necessary hormones, and certainly, no person has the knowledge of the optimal dosages in this "stack." But, your own body creates this "stack" or "hormonal milieu" when you overfeed it. Then you reach an anabolic state. While dieting, there will be a muscle anti-catabolic response that will ultimately fail with time. By combining these two states—by cycling your calorie intake over the correct period of time, your average fat mass will not increase, but your average lean body mass will go up significantly!

> "The secret to my system is acute or 'whiplash' calorie cycling. You overfeed the body for only two weeks and then diet for two weeks."

B P Okay... I think I see what you're saying... The human body has been programmed to store excess energy very efficiently when you overfeed it, so it can survive periods of famine that our ancestors regularly had to go through. Now, that sounds fine and dandy, but bodybuilders have tried high-calorie diets before, and although they do help you get big, it seems like you gain a lot more fat than muscle, and when you diet to lose the fat, you sacrifice the muscle, too. You just end up going around in circles—I've done the same thing myself. Isn't this what we're talking about?

T A No, not at all. I'm not talking about going on a "bulking diet" where you overeat for an entire season and then take 12 weeks to cut up—that doesn't work. I'm not talking about one of these ridiculous 10,000-calorie-a-day diets, either. The secret to my system is acute or "whiplash" calorie cycling. You overfeed the body for only two weeks and then diet for two weeks.

B P What's the rationale behind staying on each calorie cycle for just two weeks?

T A The two-week calorie cycles are based on scientific evidence and empirical data. In one study by Forbes, et al., entitled the "Hormonal Response to Overfeeding,"[87] it was demonstrated that when test subjects started with a maintenance-calorie-intake diet and then went on a nutrition program that provided 1,200-1,600 extra calories a day, their blood tests showed a progressive increase in IGF-1, testosterone, and insulin [which doubled in 14 days!], all in concert with an increase in lean body mass. However, the hormone levels peaked and began to decline on day 14 of the high-calorie diet! This is a *very important* observation.

By day 21, the test subjects in this study gained 3-6 lbs of lean body mass and gained a few pounds of bodyfat as well. However, these test subjects did not perform any resistance exercise, and the excess food provided only six percent of energy from protein, and the test subjects were women—we don't know yet, but the testosterone boost could be even greater in men, leading to more muscle accumulation.

B P Interesting. Are there any other studies that support your theory?

T A Yes, there are. In a 12-day study conducted by Jebb, et al., reported very recently in the *American Journal of Clinical Nutrition*,[135] entitled "Changes in Macronutrient Balance During Over- and Underfeeding Assessed by 12-Day Continuous Whole-Body Calorimetry," it was shown that when male test subjects went from a maintenance-calorie-intake diet to an overfeeding diet [approximately 3,600 total calories a day], within 12 days, they gained 4.38 lbs of lean mass and put on just 2 lbs of fat. The same study showed that when test subjects went on a pretty drastic [around 1,000 calories a day] diet for 12 days, they lost, on average, 4.6 lbs of bodyfat and only 2.4 lbs of lean mass.

As you can see, during this short overfeeding period, the amount of lean mass to fat gained was in a ratio greater than 2:1 , and in the underfeeding phase, the amount of fat versus muscle lost was 2:1.

267

REVIEW•SPORTS SUPPLEMENT REVIEW, 3RD ISSUE•SPORTS SUPPLEMENT REVIEW, 3RD ISSUE•SPORTS SUPPLEMENT

•SPORTS SUPPLEMENT REVIEW, 3RD ISSUE•SPORTS SUPPLEMENT REVIEW, 3RD ISSUE•SPORTS SUPPLEMENT REVIEW, 3RD ISSUE•SPORTS SUPPLEMENT REVIEW, 3RD ISSUE•SPORTS SUPPLEMENT REVIEW, 3RD ISSUE•SPORTS SUPPLEMENT REVIEW, 3RD ISSUE•SPORTS SUPPLEMENT REVIEW, 3RD ISSUE•SPORTS SUPPLEMENT

CHAPTER 15

ANABOLIC BURST CYCLING: A BREAKTHROUGH IN BODYBUILDING NUTRITION

ANABOLIC BURST CYCLING: A BREAKTHROUGH IN BODYBUILDING NUTRITION—ANABOLIC BURST CYCLING: A BREAKTHROUGH IN BODYBUILDING NUTRITION—ANABOLIC BURST CYCLING: A BREAKTHROUGH IN BODYBUILDING NUTRITION—ANABOLIC BURST CYCLING: A BREAKTHROUGH IN BODYBUILDING NUTRITION—ANABOLIC BURST CYCLING:

Hypothetically, if you were to follow a two-week overfeeding phase with a two-week diet, you would actually gain muscle and lose fat, even if you didn't exercise. Needless to say, if you train with weights and follow a more precise nutrition program, much less use supplements that can enhance the anabolic and anti-catabolic effects of each phase of this diet, you can continue to gain muscle, without getting fat!

Experiments I've conducted on myself and a number of my bodybuilding colleagues confirm that body composition is enhanced after each cycle.

B P **I don't understand how someone can gain muscle without working out—I mean, after you've gone through puberty, hasn't your body pretty much established how much muscle you're going to have naturally without providing some type of stimulus for new growth—without working out or taking steroids or something?**

T A When an individual who is consuming a maintenance-calorie diet [eating as much as the body's metabolism requires each day] increases calorie intake substantially, that *is* a stimulus for muscle growth—even in adults. It's somewhat of a widely accepted fallacy that when you eat too much, whether it's hamburgers, milkshakes, or even "healthy" foods like fruits, vegetables, lean meats, etc., your body's only storage compartment for these excess calories is adipose tissue [fat]. Scientific research shows that people who are overweight have more fat mass <u>and</u> more lean mass than their slender counterparts.[88]

The truth is, overfeeding your body is actually more anabolic [causes more muscle growth] than training with weights! Unfortunately, overfeeding also produces an undesirable increase in fat mass, which is contrary to what most bodybuilders seek—they work to build a lean, muscular physique, not simply one that takes up more space.

The tricky part of developing my new theory, which I've been working on for years, was to find a way to harness the body's natural "calorie-induced" anabolic potential while somehow finding a way to not increase bodyfat stores significantly. *The secret is acute calorie cycling or ABCDE.*

B P **If the body rapidly adapts to all of these different diets, won't it adapt to the ABCDE system also?**

T A I don't think it can. As long as you drastically increase calories, then reduce calories during each cycle, the body has to respond the way it's programmed to. I would recommend that someone keep doing high- and low-calorie cycles, back to back, as long as they continue to gain muscle with each cycle.

B P **Why do you suppose anabolic hormone levels peaked in Forbes' study after approximately two weeks?**

T A This has to be the body's natural response to such conditions, as it was seen in virtually all the test subjects. Exactly why this happens, no scientist can say for certain, but I have a theory: throughout the evolution of man, there have always been times of plenty followed by periods of famine. When the food supply was abundant, it became very important for the body to start up the right "metabolic program" with the right priorities, since it didn't know how long the abundance would last. In the short run, let's say over a few days, the availability of swift energy was always more important for our ancestors than muscle strength. I know some bodybuilders will not agree with me there. Anyway, the energy cost of building muscle tissue is much greater than just storing fat as triglycerides or carbohydrates as glycogen. Therefore, during the first days, the glycogen deposits will increase, and now we are coming to the interesting part: the amount of fat inside the muscle cell will increase as well, which is actually a good thing! This is why you are experiencing such a nice muscle pump the day after you have been feasting on fatty food items. Recently, research has concluded that this fat [intracellular triglycerides] has very important regulatory functions. The result will be muscle synthesis, followed by storage of the excess calories in adipose tissue.

"...we have a small time window of about 14 days—long enough for muscle hypertrophy to occur, while short enough to keep a substantial amount of fat from being stored in the adipose tissue."

Back to your question. Even though our ancestors had to be strong enough to fight and hunt, if they built too much muscle, their metabolic rates would get too high, and in the "old, old days," people with very high metabolic rates did not survive famines. Thus, the body adjusts, so after two weeks of overfeeding, the body becomes more efficient at storing excess calories in adipose cells.

Basically what I'm saying here is that we have a small time window of about 14 days—long enough for muscle hypertrophy to occur, while short enough to keep a substantial amount of fat from being stored in the adipose tissue.

By the way, have you noticed that more and more steroid-using bodybuilders are switching over to ultra-short cycles, for one to two weeks, with mega-doses? They claim the extra strength and mass they put on after this period is due only

REVIEW•SPORTS SUPPLEMENT REVIEW, 3RD ISSUE•SPORTS SUPPLEMENT REVIEW, 3RD ISSUE•SPORTS SUPPLEMENT REVIEW, 3RD ISSUE•SPORTS SUPPLEMENT

•SPORTS SUPPLEMENT REVIEW, 3RD ISSUE•SPORTS SUPPLEMENT REVIEW, 3RD ISSUE•SPORTS SUPPLEMENT REVIEW, 3RD ISSUE•SPORTS SUPPLEMENT REVIEW, 3RD ISSUE•SPORTS SUPPLEMENT REVIEW, 3RD ISSUE•SPORTS SUPPLEMENT REVIEW, 3RD ISSUE•SPORTS SUPPLEMENT REVIEW, 3RD ISSUE•SPORTS SUPPLEMENT

ANABOLIC BURST CYCLING: A BREAKTHROUGH IN BODYBUILDING NUTRITION

ANABOLIC BURST CYCLING: A BREAKTHROUGH IN BODYBUILDING NUTRITION~ANABOLIC BURST CYCLING: A BREAKTHROUGH IN BODYBUILDING NUTRITION~ANABOLIC BURST CYCLING: A BREAKTHROUGH IN BODYBUILDING NUTRITION~ANABOLIC BURST CYCLING: A BREAKTHROUGH IN BODYBUILDING NUTRITION~ANABOLIC BURST CYCLING:

CHAPTER 15

270

to water retention and will subsequently be lost. Maybe the perfect duration of an anabolic boost is around two weeks.

It's really quite fascinating when you think about it, and it's a logical theory. Can I substantiate this with rock-hard scientific data? No, not yet, but the available scientific literature offers evidence that this *is* the way the human body works.

B P **Wow... that's powerful stuff! You mentioned that you've already tried calorie cycling—how did it work? [*Torbjorn is not a small guy—he's 6'1", 225 lbs, 8% bodyfat, and he's definitely not on steroids; I guarantee it!*]**

T A It flat out works. During the two-week bulking phase, you can eat just about anything you want, which is actually fun—guilt-free ice cream and Swedish meatballs! If you begin an overfeeding program after a diet, within a matter of days, you'll notice an increase in muscle fullness and strength. It's absolutely "drug like" the way your body changes so rapidly.

During my last 2 bulking phases, I gained 7 and 6 lbs, respectively, and during both cycles, the amount of lean mass to fat was 3:1.

Of course, some of the lean mass is increased cell volume from the extra glycogen. Remember, when you start overfeeding, your body stores macronutrients in every available compartment—you store protein as muscle, fat as triglyceride in muscle and adipose tissue, and carbohydrate as glycogen, which enhances strength and muscle size.

> **"On** each cycle, you'll gain between two and five pounds of muscle, which... is a phenomenal thing to experience."

The dieting phase is fairly difficult, but restricting calorie intake for just two weeks is nothing compared to what many bodybuilders do—starving themselves for two, three, or even four months to get ready for a photo shoot or contest. Every time I get hungry, I always know it will be only a matter of days before I can eat just about anything I want again. This helps compliance a great deal.

During my dieting phases, I have been able to lose virtually all of the fat I gained on my bulking cycles while dropping only a couple pounds of lean mass. You might think of the ABCDE as a two-steps-forward, one-step-back program.

I have a number of "gym buddies" who I've had experimenting with the system, and their results have been very similar to mine. On each cycle, you'll gain between two and five pounds of muscle, which, for someone who has been training for over a decade, like I have, is a phenomenal thing to experience.

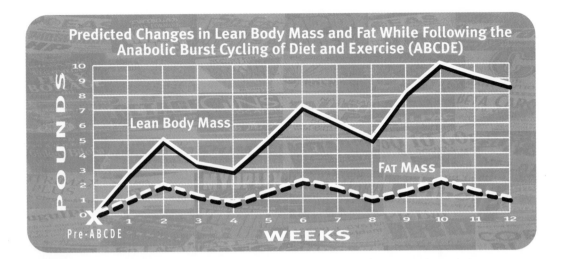

Predicted Changes in Lean Body Mass and Fat While Following the Anabolic Burst Cycling of Diet and Exercise (ABCDE)

BP **I've heard that the type of muscle you gain from consuming a high-calorie diet is structurally not the same as the muscle you gain from weight training—that it's not quality muscle. Is this true?**

TA I can't agree with that. Let me explain... During the bulking phase of the ABCDE program, several things happen. First of all, fluid, glycogen, and amino acids are loaded into the myocyte [muscle cell]. According to Häussinger's theory of cellular hydration[116, 117] and Millward's "full-bag" theory,[184] the cell will actually stretch. This stretching, or as Millward calls it, "bag filling," occurs rapidly during the bulking phase of this system. Bag enlargement is remodeling of the connective tissue. Remodeling is stimulated during the stretching or eccentric components of exercise and is further enhanced by the incredible pump you'll get while training during this phase of the diet. [*Remember how Arnold used to always say the pump meant you were growing? Maybe he was right!*]

After the cell has loaded up with glycogen, amino acids, creatine, and fluid—when it cannot store any more energy—2 things will happen as long as the endocrine environment is optimal, which it is after 10-14 days of overfeeding, according to Forbes' study.[87] The cell will start to build up the ultimate storage form of energy: namely, **actin** and **myosin**, and under the influence of IGF-1, satellite cells will start to split to create new nuclei. Try to follow me closely here—toward the end of the anabolic/bulking phase, when all of the energy stores within the myocyte are completely full, when the cell is hydrated to its maximum, when the myocyte is not inhibited by a lack of space, when the blood has a high concentration of IGF-1, when there is a high mitochondrial activity of the cell, when exercise has induced an acute local [autocrine and/or paracrine] release of growth factors, THEN the potential for satellite cells to fuse with the myocyte is increased, thus adding nuclei to the muscle cell. [*Go ahead and take a minute to read that very long, complicated sentence again... I'll wait... Okay, ready to continue? Good.*]

271

ANABOLIC BURST CYCLING: A BREAKTHROUGH IN BODYBUILDING NUTRITION

ANABOLIC BURST CYCLING: A BREAKTHROUGH IN BODYBUILDING NUTRITION~ANABOLIC BURST CYCLING: A BREAKTHROUGH IN BODYBUILDING NUTRITION~ANABOLIC BURST CYCLING: A BREAKTHROUGH IN BODYBUILDING NUTRITION~ANABOLIC BURST CYCLING: A BREAKTHROUGH IN BODYBUILDING NUTRITION~ANABOLIC BURST CYCLING:

This represents the <u>ultimate</u> quality growth of muscle, since the amount of available DNA [which makes proteins] increases. I have coined this phenomenon *neomyobolism*. It seems that the cell wants to keep a constant relationship between cell volume and number of myonuclei.[190] The myonuclear number also seems to be correlated with mitochondrial content of the cell.[279] Therefore, if you increase the number of mitochondria through exercise and elevate hormone levels, as well as increase the volume of the cell through overfeeding and using cell-volumizing supplements, like creatine and glutamine, it is logical that fusion will take place and deliver more nuclei. *Voilà*—steroid-like gains in quality muscle mass!

B P *Alrighty then...* **So what you're telling me is that the muscle you gain during the bulking phase of the ABCDE System is good muscle, and I assume you're saying it's the type of muscle that is functional and lasts—it won't disappear overnight?**

T A Exactly, and boy was I happy when, after my early experiments, I discovered that my theory on lasting muscle was confirmed.

B P **What type of macronutrient profile do you think is optimal during each phase of the diet? Do you recommend a high-protein intake, a high-carb intake, or...?**

T A The macronutrient profile of the diet is not nearly as important as the total-energy intake, but one could logically surmise that consuming a higher protein diet during the bulking phase may stimulate anabolic drive and produce even greater nitrogen retention. In the studies by Forbes and Jebb that I've already mentioned, I believe the results would have been more substantial if the subjects had been consuming more protein.[184]

The ratio of macronutrients during the anabolic phase is actually not far from the ordinary, habitual diet most people eat and is actually in concert with Dr. Erasmus' recommendations of 20% protein, 50% carbohydrates, and 30% fat. However, an even higher protein, lower carbohydrate bulking diet may also be effective, but the health aspects concern me a bit here.

I have numerous theories, which I'm developing, on how to set up "microcycles," where you consume different macronutrient profiles on different days of the two-week high-calorie and low-calorie phases. But rather than get into all those intricacies at this point, I will simply emphasize that it is very likely a substantial effect will be realized by consuming high quantities of food rich with quality protein [at least one gram per pound of bodyweight per day], carbohydrates, and unsaturated fats.

B P **What about the low-calorie phase? What type of nutrient profile do you recommend?**

T A First of all, let's backtrack a bit and go over why it's so important to have a low-calorie/dieting phase in this program. This dieting phase actually serves two very important purposes. First, we want to strip off what fat will be gained during the two-week bulking phase. This is very important, as bodybuilders want to gain muscle, not fat.

A second very important aspect of the dieting phase of this program is to "reprime" your body's enzymes and anabolic hormones. As I've already discussed, testosterone, insulin, and IGF-1 levels start to decline after about two weeks of overfeeding. In order to boost these levels again, you've got to trick the body into thinking it's necessary to store more calories as muscle tissue.

> "**In** order to boost these levels again, you've got to trick the body into thinking it's necessary to store more calories as muscle tissue."

The great thing about these short, low-calorie, two-week dieting phases is that fat loss is very efficient during this time. As Dan Duchaine has cited often in *Muscle Media*, after a few weeks of dieting, the body starts to adjust—to adapt. I'm sure you and your readers have experienced this—after a few weeks of dieting, your progress comes to a standstill, and to experience further weight loss, you have to increase calorie expenditure through exercise or further decrease energy intake, both of which may lead to an increased loss of fat <u>and</u> muscle.

As you know, fat loss is all but impossible in the presence of elevated insulin levels—a high-carbohydrate diet will severely inhibit fat oxidation. Also, if you followed a high-carbohydrate diet during the low-calorie phase, the accompanying increase in fat oxidation would make you put on a lot of fat during the next bulking phase.

Nevertheless, carbohydrates also have some very important properties during a hypocaloric diet, such as keeping GH and IGF-1 primed. Therefore, it's almost necessary to perform "microcycles" for optimal results.

B P **How many calories should somebody eat on the bulking phase and cutting program?**

T A A rough guideline—a place to start—would be to take your bodyweight times 12 [to approximate maintenance-calorie intake for an individual who's not

273
REVIEW•SPORTS SUPPLEMENT REVIEW, 3RD ISSUE•SPORTS SUPPLEMENT REVIEW, 3RD ISSUE•SPORTS SUPPLEMENT

•SPORTS SUPPLEMENT REVIEW, 3RD ISSUE•SPORTS SUPPLEMENT REVIEW, 3RD ISSUE•SPORTS SUPPLEMENT REVIEW, 3RD ISSUE•SPORTS SUPPLEMENT REVIEW, 3RD ISSUE•SPORTS SUPPLEMENT REVIEW, 3RD ISSUE•SPORTS SUPPLEMENT REVIEW, 3RD ISSUE•SPORTS SUPPLEMENT REVIEW, 3RD ISSUE•SPORTS SUPPLEMENT

CHAPTER 15

ANABOLIC BURST CYCLING: A BREAKTHROUGH IN BODYBUILDING NUTRITION

ANABOLIC BURST CYCLING: A BREAKTHROUGH IN BODYBUILDING NUTRITION~ANABOLIC BURST CYCLING: A BREAKTHROUGH IN BODYBUILDING NUTRITION~ANABOLIC BURST CYCLING: A BREAKTHROUGH IN BODYBUILDING NUTRITION~ANABOLIC BURST CYCLING: A BREAKTHROUGH IN BODYBUILDING NUTRITION~ANABOLIC BURST CYCLING:

extremely active] and add 1,500 calories to this number. For example, a person who weighs 200 lbs, like yourself, would consume about 4,000 calories a day during the bulking phase [200 x 12 = 2,400 + 1,500]. On the low-calorie phase, I would recommend consuming a number of calories equal to your bodyweight times eight. That would be about 1,600 calories for you [200 x 8 = 1,600].

This is just a rough place to start—a person's activity level [whether someone has a desk job or is a construction worker could make a BIG difference] and a person's muscle mass and metabolism also come into play. If a bodybuilder is following this recommendation and not gaining weight during a bulking phase, I would recommend increasing calorie intake by 500 calories a day, for a week, and if a substantial weight gain is not realized, I would take it up 500 more calories the next week.

Likewise, if someone is not losing bodyweight on the low-calorie phase, I would recommend decreasing calorie intake by 300 calories a day, per week.

Remember that each time you start an anabolic phase, you may need to increase your calorie intake, provided you're gaining lean body mass. For example, if you go from 190 to 195 lbs during your first anabolic and fat-burning cycle, you should add about 100 more calories to your diet per day for the next cycle.

> **"...during** the bulking phase, you should avoid aerobic exercise and conduct heavy, intense weight-training sessions."

BP What happens if you don't gain a significant amount of weight on the bulking phase or lose weight during each dieting phase?

TA I would highly recommend that all those who try this system keep track of their calories as best they can, simply by writing down what they eat each day, the time they eat it, and do their best to calculate how many calories they're consuming—this data could be recorded in a notebook or journal. Having a record of what you've done will allow you to troubleshoot your program very effectively. If you're not gaining a significant amount of weight [at least three pounds a week during the bulking phase], then you need to <u>increase</u> your calorie intake. During the cutting phase, if you don't lose weight, you need to consume less calories. It's very simple to make adjustments on this program.

In addition to keeping a journal, it would also be very beneficial to keep track of your body composition and actually maintain an updated line graph [*like the one shown on page 271*] to gauge your progress.

B P **What if you fail to gain muscle and lose fat even after making adjustments?**

T A Well, I would be amazed if that were the case. But if that happens to you, then your body's got bigger problems than the Anabolic Burst Cycling of Diet and Exercise System can solve.

B P **What about exercise? Should you perform a different type of training during the bulking phase versus the dieting cycle?**

T A This is an area that can also get quite complex, but for the time being, I think it would be sufficient to say that during the bulking phase, you should avoid aerobic exercise and conduct heavy, intense weight-training sessions. As energy, strength, and recovery levels will be heightened during this period, you might be able to train with weights five days a week. When I'm on my high-calorie/bulking phase, my strength literally goes up every workout. During intense weight training, your body further stimulates the release of testosterone and growth hormone.

During the dieting phase, it is very important to include aerobic exercise, and the best time to do this is in a fasted state; i.e., in the morning, before breakfast. Recent studies at my lab strongly support this. I have experienced excellent results doing 40 minutes of moderate-intensity aerobic exercise 4 days a week—I keep my pulse around 120 beats per minute. During aerobic exercise, your body is more likely to stimulate the production of fat-burning chemicals like epinephrine.

During this low-calorie phase, I would expect one to see good results training with weights 3 days a week, doing a more moderate-intensity program—for example, conducting 3 sets of 8-12 reps on standard exercises like dumbbell bench presses, lateral side raises, incline curls, triceps pushdowns, etc. Remember, your training goals during the low-calorie phase are to lose fat while maintaining as much muscle tissue as possible.

B P **I see—you should go all-out during the bulking phase, training heavy and hard, eating a bunch of food, then after two weeks, drop the calorie and carbohydrate intake substantially, perform regular aerobic exercise, and back off a bit on the weight training. That makes sense. What about meal frequency and supplements?**

T A I'm a proponent of frequent feeding—I think you should eat every three hours or so during the day for optimal results. This would mean you'd consume five or six meals a day.

ANABOLIC BURST CYCLING: A BREAKTHROUGH IN BODYBUILDING NUTRITION

ANABOLIC BURST CYCLING: A BREAKTHROUGH IN BODYBUILDING NUTRITION-ANABOLIC BURST CYCLING: A BREAKTHROUGH IN BODYBUILDING NUTRITION-ANABOLIC BURST CYCLING: A BREAKTHROUGH IN BODYBUILDING NUTRITION-ANABOLIC BURST CYCLING: A BREAKTHROUGH IN BODYBUILDING NUTRITION-ANABOLIC BURST CYCLING:

CHAPTER 15

ANABOLIC BURST CYCLING: A BREAKTHROUGH IN BODYBUILDING NUTRITION-ANABOLIC BURST CYCLING: A BREAKTHROUGH IN BODYBUILDING NUTRITION

In terms of supplements, this is an area where I think you can substantially increase the effects of the ABCDE Program. I'm presently writing a whole book about this system, which will spell out every aspect of this program—all my theories on nutrition, training, and supplementation will be revealed. I think I can have this book completed within the next six to eight months—I would be able to finish it sooner, but my research obligations and time in the ER make it difficult to allocate a significant number of hours to this project, even though it is one I'm quite passionate about.

As far as supplements go, creatine, HMB, glutamine, Vitamin C, and chromium would all be extremely useful as long as they are used properly.[102, 180, 193, 204, 205, 283]

B P **So whom would you recommend the ABCDE Program to?**

T A This is the type of bodybuilding program I would highly recommend to drug-free weight trainers who are trying to increase muscle mass without gaining fat. On this program, it's even possible to lose bodyfat while you gain muscle mass, but I would not recommend it for the obese.

B P **Would this program work for someone who's using steroids or who has just completed a steroid cycle?**

T A I'm not sure. I'm concerned that if someone is coming off a steroid cycle, the body's endocrine system may not function properly and will not respond to the anabolic stimulus of a hypercaloric diet.

I would have the same concern about someone who is presently using steroids—the body may not respond optimally because of all the interrupted feedback loops.

B P **What if someone tried to create his own "super-enhanced" bulking and fat-burning cycles by taking insulin, growth hormone, and fast-acting oral steroids for two weeks while consuming a lot of calories and then went on fat-burning drugs, like Cytomel and clenbuterol, and consumed a low-calorie diet for two weeks. Is it likely he would get phenomenal results?**

T A That's an interesting question. Whether we take a number of hormones or we overfeed, we create constantly elevated levels of anabolic hormones in the

> "My acute, two-week calorie cycles will produce even better results than competitive bodybuilders get from cutting up and bulking up."

bloodstream. These two states [exogenous vs. endogenous hormones] may look the same, but they are *totally different*. You see, in the former case, you add hormones to a body in homeostasis, meaning it will do a number of things to counteract the increased level, including blunt its own production of the hormones, increase the breakdown and excretion, decrease receptor sensitivity and number, increase the amount of binding proteins, and so on. While in the latter case, the body has created a hormonal environment aimed for anabolism and will not counteract itself. This way, the cycle will work very well every time you try it. I actually can't see any advantages to using drugs during the ABCDE Program.

B P **What if people are already on a high-calorie diet, or what if they're presently on a low-calorie diet and they want to try your ABCDE Program?**

T A If some of your readers are already consuming an excess number of calories, they should start the ABCDE Program with the low-calorie phase to "reprime" their anabolic systems, so to speak.

If they are already on a low-calorie diet, let's say they're getting ready for a bodybuilding contest or a photo shoot, following this would be an excellent time to start the Anabolic Burst Cycling Program with a high-calorie phase. In fact, many bodybuilders will probably recognize that they have "unintentionally" done an anabolic-burst high-calorie dieting phase already—anyone who's cut up for a contest and then "pigged out" for a few weeks afterwards will confirm he/she gained size and strength at a phenomenal rate, and not all of the weight gained was fat. Ask them—they'll confirm this!

One of the things that's often discussed in bodybuilding is that those who compete make better gains, year in and year out, than those who don't because they're forced to go on calorie cycles, albeit rather traditional, longer ones. My acute, two-week calorie cycles will produce even better results than competitive bodybuilders get from cutting up and bulking up. On this system, you're literally bulking and cutting every month.

B P **So basically, when you pig out for two weeks, your body releases testosterone, insulin, and IGF-1 to help deposit or "store" those calories as muscle tissue. Are any other hormones in the body affected by calorie cycling?**

T A Yes, most definitely. One your readers might recognize is called *leptin*. This hormone is by far the most interesting one for fat loss. Unfortunately, we develop resistance to this hormone very easily when it is present at chronically [long term] elevated levels.[46] However, this will not happen with my system. The high-calorie

CHAPTER 15

ANABOLIC BURST CYCLING: A BREAKTHROUGH IN BODYBUILDING NUTRITION

ANABOLIC BURST CYCLING: A BREAKTHROUGH IN BODYBUILDING NUTRITION~ANABOLIC BURST CYCLING: A BREAKTHROUGH IN BODYBUILDING NUTRITION~ANABOLIC BURST CYCLING: A BREAKTHROUGH IN BODYBUILDING NUTRITION~ANABOLIC BURST CYCLING: A BREAKTHROUGH IN BODYBUILDING NUTRITION~ANABOLIC BURST CYCLING:

phase "primes" the effects of leptin, so it's very effective during the fat-loss/dieting phase. There is also an increase in T_3 [the "active" form of thyroid hormone], adrenaline, and noradrenaline—all help with fat loss.

Going back and forth between low- and high-calorie diets is a fantastic way to keep your anabolic hormones and your lipolytic [fat-burning] hormones and enzymes, as well as receptors, primed at all times.

BP **You mentioned something about the importance of intramuscular/ intracellular triglyceride levels. How could having fat inside your muscle cells help you gain size and strength?**

TA This is a technically difficult question to answer. But, it's a very important subject—one you American bodybuilding experts have overlooked.

First of all, intracellular triglycerides are an important source of energy for athletes. A normal, 70-kg [154-lb] man with 15% bodyfat has close to 2 lbs of fat in his muscle cells; half of this is readily available as stored triglycerides. Athletes have an even larger amount of intracellular triglycerides and much more efficient utilization.[124] If we extrapolate this for a 220-lb bodybuilder, we'll come up with 2 lbs of triglycerides. This represents an energy reserve equal to approximately 8,000 calories—that's more than twice the energy your body stores in glycogen, which virtually everyone believes is the major "muscle fuel" for athletes.

Next, an increase in intracellular triglycerides is a trigger of protein synthesis: i.e., muscle anabolism. In other words, it's a signal that says, *"Hey, we have a steady supply of calories—it's time to build muscle!"* Not to mention high levels of triglycerides within muscle cells increase your pump <u>more</u> than when the cells are full of glycogen alone!

In a nutshell, intracellular triglycerides play a very important role in weight-training-induced muscle growth. They help trigger anabolism, they supply energy for your workouts, they help construct muscle cell membranes, and they have a cell-hydrating/cell-volumizing effect by sparing glycogen. The downside is, high levels of intracellular triglycerides will eventually lead to insulin resistance.

BP **You also mentioned something to do with stretching the connective tissue around muscle fibers in order to enhance growth. How did you come up with this theory?**

TA The "bag theory" is not mine—it was developed by a scientist named D.J. Millward, a well-known researcher who has extensively studied the muscle-building process. His immense knowledge and research could help a lot of bodybuilders.

Basically, Millward has observed three things: 1) the almost unlimited extent to which increased food intake can promote protein deposition during "catch-up growth" in malnourished patients, 2) both active and passive *stretch* will mediate anabolic and anti-catabolic influences, and 3) the cessation of normal muscle growth coincides with the cessation of bone growth.

There are "connective sheets" surrounding the individual muscle fiber [endomysium], bundles of muscle cells [perimysium], and the entire muscle [epimysium]. These sheets can be thought of as a series of "bags" acting to conduct the contractile force generated by actin and myosin in muscle fibers to the bone by the tendon.

Millward postulates that bag filling and enlargement may increase muscle development. You see, these bags have a minimum elasticity, at least compared to the cell membranes they enclose, so they'll actually inhibit muscle growth—you might think of them as very tight "girdles" that prevent the expansion of tissue.

"...intracellular triglycerides play a very important role in weight-training-induced muscle growth."

B P Doesn't "cell volumizing" help stretch these bags?

T A Not really. The anabolic state of the muscle fiber *does* depend on its state of hydration, which is secondary to the amount of osmotic [the ability to attract water] substances in the cells, such as sodium, potassium, creatine, proteins, glycogen, and free amino acids like glutamine.[115] The anabolic phase of my program is designed to maximize this cell-volumizing effect. Within a few days of starting a properly supplemented, high-calorie anabolic phase, your cells will be jam-packed with the aforementioned nutrients <u>and</u> *intracellular triglycerides*. They'll be "volumized" to the <u>max</u>. A cell will literally swell to fill the entire space of its connective-tissue compartment or, as Millward calls it, "bag." You'll feel "pumped" even when you're not training.

Interestingly, Millward believes that when this occurs, it will elicit a signal to reduce the appetite—this is just one of many regulatory feedback mechanisms that limit the rate of growth in mammals. This means that a few days into the anabolic/bulking phase of my program, you will probably not have a ferocious appetite, but you *must* keep eating if you want to grow!

Now, to build *extraordinary* muscle mass, you need to somehow stretch this "girdle" that confines your muscle tissue. The osmotic gradient over the cell membrane is not strong enough to stretch this tissue all that much; however, the blood rushing into the muscle during resistance training [i.e., the pump] *is* strong enough

ANABOLIC BURST CYCLING: A BREAKTHROUGH IN BODYBUILDING NUTRITION

ANABOLIC BURST CYCLING: A BREAKTHROUGH IN BODYBUILDING NUTRITION-ANABOLIC BURST CYCLING: A BREAKTHROUGH IN BODYBUILDING NUTRITION-ANABOLIC BURST CYCLING: A BREAKTHROUGH IN BODYBUILDING NUTRITION-ANABOLIC BURST CYCLING: A BREAKTHROUGH IN BODYBUILDING NUTRITION-ANABOLIC BURST CYCLING:

CHAPTER 15

ANABOLIC BURST CYCLING: A BREAKTHROUGH IN BODYBUILDING NUTRITION-ANABOLIC BURST CYCLING: A BREAKTHROUGH IN BODYBUILDING NUTRITION

to stretch these bags to some extent. This is how "the pump" contributes to muscle growth. It seems, as Arnold and many other famous bodybuilders have reported, the pump *is* associated with muscle growth. This is very likely due to the compartmental stretching or expansion that is induced by this swelling of muscles while they're trained and full of blood.

Millward confirms "...a key feature of skeletal muscle growth appears to be that it is limited by connective-tissue growth, which controls myofiber diameter and length." Somehow you must stretch this connective tissue—this tight girdle around muscle tissue—to experience dramatic muscle growth. This is very important. All bodybuilders must do this.

Show me a "natural" bodybuilder who is big, muscular, and cut, and you will show me a bodybuilder who has either used steroids in the past and/or has been overeating in the past; thus, he increased his potential for muscle growth by stretching the space for myofibers at one time. Once you have already expanded the connective tissue around muscles, you can be natural with a more normal calorie intake while still being relatively big.

This is what "muscle memory" is really all about. People have talked about this for decades in bodybuilding circles. They make the observation that a bodybuilder who was big in the past is able to gain a significant amount of muscle size—let's say he builds up some muscular 19-inch arms, then he stops training for a few months and loses a lot of mass, and his arms atrophy to 16½ inches. Whereas the first time it took him years to gain 2½ inches of muscular mass on his arms, this time he'll be able to add that bulk back in only a couple of months with proper training, nutrition, and supplementation. The explanation for this "muscle-memory phenomenon" is that the connective tissue around the muscle fibers has been previously stretched; thus, rapid growth is possible.

> **"...a key feature of skeletal muscle growth appears to be that it is limited by connective-tissue growth..."**

B P **This makes sense. But, if you've never had 19-inch arms, how do you get this tissue to stretch?**

T A You have to bulk up at some point. In the past, as we've discussed, this usually meant going on prolonged periods of overfeeding, basically turning yourself into a blimp, and then cutting up—going on a brutal diet for months and months. Usually, these long, painful diets caused the loss of almost all the muscle mass you gained during the bulking phase, but they did serve one purpose—they *stretched* the connective tissue around the muscles.

We know that to maximize muscle growth, we need to make sure the cell is properly hydrated and volumized. This is accomplished during the overfeeding phase of my Anabolic Burst Cycling Program. Next, you need to get a good, solid pump during the workout and, beyond that, if you're looking for greater growth, you can now apply extreme stretching *while being pumped*.

The American bodybuilding coach John Parillo has made the same observation I have—that extreme stretching when the muscle is pumped, which he refers to as "fascia stretching," results in increased muscular growth. Research at Ohio State University also demonstrates that the amount of myosin heavy chains— a very important contractile protein in skeletal muscle—is increased by stretching.[29] The result is obvious within a short period of time. Parillo's theory is that you stretch the fascia around the muscle which, according to him, is limiting muscle growth. However, research supports the idea that the endomysium and perimysium are involved in this limitation of growth—not necessarily the fascia.

What we are basically trying to do is further remodel that encumbering girdle around muscle tissue by stretching. This theory beautifully explains the perfect coordination between the lengthening of the skeleton—and thus a passive stretch of the connective tissue in muscle—and the increased muscle bulk in fast-growing teenagers. This is something few people think about, but when a teenager goes through rapid bone growth and experiences a dramatic increase in muscle mass during puberty, the muscle hypertrophy usually ends when the bones stop growing. Millward has documented that lean body mass increases in direct proportion to height in normal human beings.

Some "old-time" bodybuilders performed exercises with extreme stretching while they were pumped. I'm not sure how they figured out this was important, but some did. One of them was Arnold. He would perform dumbbell flyes on a flat bench in a relatively slow, high-rep manner after completely pumping up his chest. He could lower the dumbbells until they almost touched the floor! That's a brutal stretch. Was it a coincidence that Arnold built what was arguably one of the most well-developed pairs of pecs ever, in a day and age when steroid use was "minuscule" compared to what today's champs are using? I think not. Arnold used to really stretch out his lats while doing low rowing and high-cable pulldowns, too. And, he did pullovers which are an amazingly effective stretching exercise that you American lifters seem to have forgotten about.

You can stretch *during* your lifts *and* between them. But, I recommend extreme stretching only during the second week of the bulking phase of my system. This is when the muscles will get incredibly pumped, and recuperation will be maximal. The stretch-induced fusion and increased nuclei number peak within a week.[297] This is one of the reasons to limit the use of extreme stretching to one week.

ANABOLIC BURST CYCLING: A BREAKTHROUGH IN BODYBUILDING NUTRITION

ANABOLIC BURST CYCLING: A BREAKTHROUGH IN BODYBUILDING NUTRITION–ANABOLIC BURST CYCLING: A BREAKTHROUGH IN BODYBUILDING NUTRITION–ANABOLIC BURST CYCLING: A BREAKTHROUGH IN BODYBUILDING NUTRITION–ANABOLIC BURST CYCLING: A BREAKTHROUGH IN BODYBUILDING NUTRITION–ANABOLIC BURST CYCLING:

Another stimulus for remodeling is the breakdown of connective tissue during eccentric training. I recommend your readers review Charles Poliquin's article on this subject in the January 1996 issue of *Muscle Media* and your article on this topic in the April 1996 issue. (Back issues are available by calling 1-800-297-9776. The articles can also be found <u>free</u> on the *Muscle Media* home page at www.mm2k.com.)

By the way, to support the formation of new connective tissue after you've damaged it by pumping up and stretching, I would recommend that you take at least one gram of Vitamin C before your workouts and make sure your total daily intake is at least three grams. There is evidence that Vitamin C not only supports hydroxylation in collagen synthesis but also works almost as a growth factor in the synthesis of connective tissue.[97]

Anyway, through proper eccentric training and stretching while being pumped, you will damage the connective tissue and force it to further remodel into a "larger bag." The stretching of the fiber will stimulate membrane-bound enzyme complexes which will trigger a release of growth factors such as TGF-beta, FGF, and IGF-1 from the muscle.[185] These growth factors are all important for remodeling and synthesis of connective tissue. As I mentioned, IGF-1 and FGF stimulate the development of satellite cells and their fusion with muscle fibers to deliver nuclei, thus, new muscle mass, so long as the inner environment is optimal, which it is during the end of the anabolic phase.

Millward's theory, combined with my Anabolic Burst Cycling theory, beautifully explains what happens during puberty. To start with, there is an increase in testosterone and growth hormone. This, together with intracellular triglycerides, as mentioned earlier, will increase the amount of insulin the body releases. Insulin is the main factor responsible for transporting osmotic substances, such as glucose, amino acids, and creatine, into muscle fibers, which is why people are seeing such great results while taking creatine monohydrate with an insulin-releasing carbohydrate. Hence, the muscle will swell. At the same time, growth hormone is contributing to an increase in bone length; thus, a passive *stretch* is placed on the muscle with local IGF-1 being released. Since both GH and its insulin levels are elevated, IGF-1 production in the liver is stimulated, which adds further growth to the whole body. Are you beginning to get the picture?

During the anabolic phase of my ABCDE System, we mimic the mechanisms of pubescent metabolism. You may think I'm nagging about puberty, but I cannot emphasize enough the importance of trying to replicate this natural phenomenon. During puberty, you put on muscle, even without training, and on top of that, you keep this muscle for virtually your whole life. That's the type of quality growth that's possible with my new system.

B P So when I'm on the bulking phase of your program, my muscles are being pumped full of nutrients and fluid, so when I work out, I'll get pumped up like I'm on 'roids. And, to maximize growth during this phase, I should stretch a lot during my exercises and between them, while I'm pumped. During the second week of the bulking phase, days 7-14, I should really stretch hard and do very intense eccentric reps [negatives]. And, during this time, I might benefit from taking a gram of Vitamin C before I work out and taking a total of three grams a day.

T A Yes. Very good, Bill.

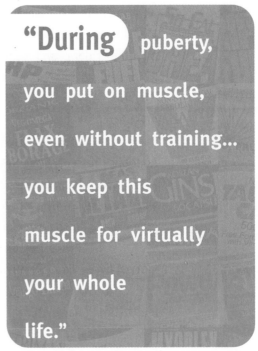

"During puberty, you put on muscle, even without training... you keep this muscle for virtually your whole life."

B P Do I need to stretch and do negatives or take Vitamin C during the cutting phase?

T A No. During the low-calorie phase, we are not trying to remodel connective tissue. The emphasis is on fat burning. Of course—for other reasons—one gram of Vitamin C daily or moderate stretching could be useful during the "non-remodeling" phase. Intense negatives, on the other hand, must be avoided.

B P Now I understand that supplements like creatine, chromium, and HMB are some of the other supplements you've experimented with. What types of supplements should someone use, and how should they use them, when following your Anabolic Burst Cycling Program?

T A Because this area has not been extensively studied, there's really no concrete data available that tells us *exactly* how various supplements such as creatine monohydrate, chromium, vanadyl sulfate, etc. work while a person is on a high- or low-calorie diet. The literature offers very little to the scientist who is interested in what type of additive effects and/or synergy might be created by using supplements in a "stacking" manner. Of course, the science of supplements which enhance performance, muscle metabolism, and fat oxidation is in its infancy. I want to make sure I preface any discussion about supplements with this information because we are largely speculating. Dan Duchaine, Dr. Mauro Di Pasquale, and you, Bill, are all familiar with the various supplements bodybuilders might benefit from, but you

ANABOLIC BURST CYCLING: A BREAKTHROUGH IN BODYBUILDING NUTRITION

ANABOLIC BURST CYCLING: A BREAKTHROUGH IN BODYBUILDING NUTRITION•ANABOLIC BURST CYCLING: A BREAKTHROUGH IN BODYBUILDING NUTRITION•ANABOLIC BURST CYCLING: A BREAKTHROUGH IN BODYBUILDING NUTRITION•ANABOLIC BURST CYCLING: A BREAKTHROUGH IN BODYBUILDING NUTRITION•ANABOLIC BURST CYCLING:

all have different theories on how those compounds should be taken. Some of these ideas come from your own personal experiences, some come from empirical [word of mouth] data, and some come from extrapolations of scientific literature. Suffice it to say, at this point we have no "proof" there is a completely right or wrong way to use supplements. What I will touch on here and discuss in more detail in my upcoming book and in future issues of your magazine, *Muscle Media,* are my <u>theories</u> of how the use of various supplements may enhance the effects of the Anabolic Burst Cycling System.

As you might have already guessed, my theory on supplement use is somewhat parallel to my theory on nutrition—*variety* is paramount. However, "random shotgunning" or taking supplements with no rhyme or reason is not the best plan either.

I believe a person can maximize the effects of supplements as well as save money by *cycling* supplements.

In Sweden, a bottle of 120 capsules of HMB costs $65! You Americans should feel lucky! I <u>have to</u> "ration" my supplement use as I am not made of money.

Nutritional supplements may act in a manner similar to drugs in that the body might adapt and eventually "override" their effects, just as it would to certain drugs. The body adapts to virtually everything, which is why, if you <u>don't</u> want to stay the same—if you want to grow—you have to constantly change things. An analogy between supplements and drugs can be made. For example, taking an antibiotic for two weeks to treat an infection is often effective. However, you cannot prevent infections by taking an antibiotic every single day for months and months. The compound would become ineffective. The same can be said of many drugs, and this may be true of supplements, too.

> **"...my theory on supplement use is somewhat parallel to my theory on nutrition—*variety* is paramount."**

Now, as far as supplements go, I would say creatine monohydrate is the most important supplement during my Anabolic Burst Cycling Program. It is virtually impossible to consume the optimal amounts of creatine through whole foods; thus, a supplement is required. My experiments lead me to theorize that creatine can be cycled. I use 20-30 grams per day during the first 6 days of a bulking phase, and then I repeat this at a lower dose of 10 grams a day for the first week of the dieting phase. By taking creatine, you fill up the myocyte, which is also known as a muscle fiber or a muscle cell, with creatine phosphate and potentiate cell volumizing. At the same time, new studies show creatine might improve insulin sensitivity and blood lipid profiles.[78]

As I mentioned, insulin sensitivity is a crucial factor for bodybuilders—both for improving body composition and maintaining proper health. Several supplements may be effective for increasing insulin sensitivity and glycogen storage. These include chromium, vanadyl sulfate, and certain fatty acids. Studies with diabetic patients involving vanadyl sulfate show that the compound continues to exert a positive effect for at least two weeks after its use has been discontinued.[57] Having this in mind, I recommend using vanadyl sulfate and chromium in a cycling pattern.

One supplement that you don't hear much about, but which I think could be valuable to bodybuilders, is sodium phosphate—the mineral form is called phosphorus. It is inexpensive but sometimes difficult to find. I suggest giving it a try, in a loading manner, for four days, consuming three or four grams a day. Several studies have shown that phosphate used this way increases both anaerobic and aerobic performance.[43, 151, 261] However, I recommend phosphate in my program because if you are deficient in intracellular phosphate during the heavy eccentric-training portion and extreme stretching—which should be conducted during the second week of the bulking phase—you may have inefficient recovery. [By the way, Phosphagen HP is fortified with phosphates.]

Furthermore, intracellular phosphate is used to make creatine phosphate and for the formation of phospholipids to meet the need for substrates of the plasma membrane of expanding muscle fibers. Another important property of phosphate is that it is the most important intracellular buffer; i.e., it will reduce the metabolic acidosis caused by intense exercise. Acidosis enhances protein breakdown and suppresses the effectiveness of growth hormone and IGF-1. In contrast, reducing the acidosis in the blood—some experts propose with bicarbonate—is probably not a good idea since there are indications that a low extracellular pH interferes with the anabolic signal for rebuilding the damaged myocyte.

Conjugated linoleic acid [CLA], a supplement which I have experimented with, may be incorporated into a cell membrane, thereby increasing the inflow of nutrients. There is also evidence that HMB has a similar ability. Both CLA and HMB may increase the amount of intracellular triglycerides, which is good so long as you can keep insulin sensitivity high. Glutamine may also play an important role in my program. Lipoic acid may have some interesting bodybuilding applications, too. HCA could also elicit a nice response in some individuals. The reason behind this is that the hypercaloric diet will eventually increase the activity of fat-storing enzymes, making the conversion of carbohydrates to fat very efficient. This could partly be blocked by using HCA during the last days of the anabolic phase. If you're over 35, you may also need to supplement with selenium since it's been shown that the age-related decrease in thyroid function is attenuated by selenium.

ANABOLIC BURST CYCLING: A BREAKTHROUGH IN BODYBUILDING NUTRITION

ANABOLIC BURST CYCLING: A BREAKTHROUGH IN BODYBUILDING NUTRITION–ANABOLIC BURST CYCLING: A BREAKTHROUGH IN BODYBUILDING NUTRITION–ANABOLIC BURST CYCLING: A BREAKTHROUGH IN BODYBUILDING NUTRITION–ANABOLIC BURST CYCLING: A BREAKTHROUGH IN BODYBUILDING NUTRITION–ANABOLIC BURST CYCLING:

B P **Are there any downsides to this program?**

T A Traditionally, high-calorie diets are associated with several undesirable effects, such as increased cholesterol levels and a greater risk of cardiovascular disease, but since the overfeeding phases are only two weeks in length and are followed by a fat-loss phase, I don't believe there will be any adverse health consequences. I think the ABCDE Program is very safe.

And, the program has numerous advantages over other diets, which make it much easier to follow, therefore more effective, such as: it offers variation, thus it won't become tedious to follow; it doesn't induce a mental state where you can't function within a social context; it's based on legitimate scientific findings; the "perfect" ratio of macronutrients in every meal is relatively unimportant; overall, the diet is relatively easy to follow; and the program allows you to make changes within the framework of the diet in regards to your personal ambitions and goals.

All of these things that I just mentioned are not true of ketogenic diets, the Zone Diet, very high-protein diets, starvation diets, very low-fat diets, high-carbohydrate diets, and high-fat diets.

SUMMARY

As you can see, you really do have access to some powerful anabolic hormones—the good stuff! You really do have a source for real insulin, IGF-1, and testosterone—a source you can use to pack on pounds of new muscle! And, now you know some things about how to tap into that source and how to use your body's natural biochemistry to build muscle size and strength faster than you might have ever imagined!

The ABCDE System just flat out makes sense. It's backed by a strong scientific theory, and before long, I predict thousands and thousands of bodybuilders will be singing the praises of this system, and we'll all be smacking ourselves in the forehead and saying, "Damn... why didn't we think of this sooner... it makes so much sense!"

CHAPTER 15

ANABOLIC BURST CYCLING: A BREAKTHROUGH IN BODYBUILDING NUTRITION–ANABOLIC BURST CYCLING: A BREAKTHROUGH IN BODYBUILDING NUTRITION–

Chapter SIXTEEN

Taking the Anabolic Burst Cycling Program for a Test Drive

After reading the last chapter, you're probably interested in giving Torbjorn Akerfeldt's exciting new program a try. This really is fascinating stuff. Akerfeldt's revolutionary theories in this area have convinced me there is more to bodybuilding nutrition than meets the eye—more to it than simply eating a high-protein diet and consuming more calories for a period of months if you want to bulk up and dieting for weeks and weeks if you want to get cut. This is exciting news for all bodybuilders—especially those of us who are training drug free and are looking for any advantage we can get—especially one that's safe and legal!

I've carefully analyzed his ideas and the science which supports them, and I've proceeded to custom design a nutrition, training, and supplementation program for my first "trial run" of the Anabolic Burst Cycling System.

In Torbjorn's forthcoming book, he'll go into great detail about micro-nutrition and supplement cycles that he is designing to maximize the effects of this program. But for now, based on my knowledge of his theories, I have put together a relatively uncomplicated program which I plan to start very soon. It's a system you may want to try as well!

Here's my plan:

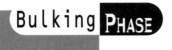

Bulking PHASE

CALORIES

I'm going to start this system by consuming 1,500 more calories per day than my maintenance energy requirements. My body burns only around 2,400-2,800 calories a day because I'm not very active. I basically sit behind a desk all day and then work out for an hour. I probably burn fewer calories each day than those of you who take part in a lot of recreational sports, have physically demanding jobs, etc. Anyway, for me, 2,400-2,800 calories a day is my maintenance intake. So, I'm going to consume around 4,000-4,200 calories per day to start with. If I don't put on at

TAKING THE ANABOLIC BURST CYCLING PROGRAM FOR A TEST DRIVE

CHAPTER 16

BURST CYCLING PROGRAM FOR A TEST DRIVE~TAKING THE ANABOLIC BURST CYCLING PROGRAM FOR A TEST DRIVE~TAKING THE ANABOLIC BURST CYCLING PROGRAM FOR A TEST DRIVE~TAKING THE ANABOLIC BURST CYCLING PROGRAM FOR A TEST DRIVE~TAKING THE ANABOLIC BURST CYCLING PROGRAM FOR A TEST DRIVE~TAKING THE ANABOLIC BURST CYCLING PROGRAM FOR A TEST DRIVE~TAKING THE

least 3 lbs the first week, I'll go up to about 4,700 calories a day the second week. My plan is to consume 6 meals every day, each with about 500 to 800 calories.

PROTEIN, CARBS, AND FAT

Torbjorn believes that on the bulking phase, a 20% protein, 50% carb, and 30% fat macronutrient profile will work well. I think I'll go with a bit more protein, but Torbjorn emphasizes that a relatively high level of carbs consumed while bulking will maximize insulin output and help promote anabolism. An example of what I'm planning for an average day on my bulking diet is indicated in the chart below.

Example of My Daily Nutrition Program
During the Bulking Phase

		Protein grams	Carb grams	Fat grams	Cal
7:30 a.m.	One bowl of oatmeal	6	25	2	144
	16 oz of skim milk	16	24	1	169
	Omelet with 2 whole eggs plus 8 egg whites with reduced-fat cheddar cheese and ½ cup mixed vegetables	55	10	20	440
	One whole grapefruit	1	19	0	80
	One gram of Vitamin C	–	–	–	–
10:00 a.m.	Myoplex Plus Deluxe mixed with 16 oz of skim milk	58	49	3	469
	One serving of Phosphagen HP	–	35	–	140
Noon	Cheeseburger with 6 oz of lean ground beef, lettuce, tomato, and mayonnaise.	58	20	39	658
	16 oz of water	–	–	–	–
3:30 p.m.	Myoplex Plus Deluxe with 16 oz of skim milk	58	49	3	469
5:00 p.m.	PR* Bar	14	19	6	190
	One gram of Vitamin C	–	–	–	–
6:00 p.m.	Workout				
7:00 p.m.	Myoplex Plus (vanilla) with 16 oz of water	42	24	2	280
	Two servings of Phosphagen HP	–	70	–	280
8:30 p.m.	Four chicken enchiladas and rice	35	93	18	668
	16 oz of water	–	–	–	–
10:30 p.m.	Two bowls of frosted Cheerios,	4	50	2	240
	12 oz of skim milk	12	18	1	128
	One gram of Vitamin C	–	–	–	–
	TOTALS	**359**	**505**	**97**	**4355**

TRAINING

As far as workouts go, I plan to do only weightlifting during the bulking phase—no aerobics. I'm going to train four times a week, lifting as much weight as possible for relatively low reps. For example, for chest, after a few warm-up sets on the flat barbell bench, I'm going to do 5 sets of between 3 and 8 repetitions with 275 to 325 lbs. Then I'm going to do dumbbell flyes—four sets of five to eight reps, using as much weight as I possibly can yet incorporating a deep stretch into the movement. And I'm going to hit the eccentric (negative) portion of each rep hard, especially during the second week of each bulking phase. I'll finish my chest work with 2 sets of pullovers, using moderate weight for 10 to 12 reps. I plan to rest a full three minutes between sets, so I'll recover my strength and be able to train heavy.

As Torbjorn explained in the last chapter, it is important to stretch the connective tissue around muscle cells as much as possible while bulking up. I'll do this by stretching between exercises and actually doing as much stretching as I can during exercises. For example, on the lat pulldown and the low-pulley row, I'll really stretch out the lats. On exercises like the dumbbell triceps extension, I'll lower the weight as far as I can behind my head and really extend those muscles, and on exercises like the dumbbell preacher curl, I'll extend the biceps muscles and stretch them out, all the way.

SUPPLEMENTS

As far as supplements go, during the anabolic phase, I'm going to have three or four servings of Phosphagen HP a day (I'll drink two right after I work out) to increase insulin output and creatine uptake by my muscle cells. I'm also going to use chromium and vanadyl sulfate in an effort to maximize insulin's anabolic actions.

Insulin is one of the main anabolic agents in this "hormone cocktail" that is elevated when you start overfeeding. I'll get the chromium and the vanadyl from the total-nutrition supplement I'll be using, which is Myoplex Plus Deluxe. I'm also going to supplement with three grams of Vitamin C a day during this bulking phase.

Cutting PHASE

CALORIES

After two weeks of overfeeding, I'm going to "shift gears" and go on a low-calorie diet. Because I'll be trying to lose fat at a very rapid pace during this two-week cutting period, I'll need to create a significant energy deficit. I think I'll have to go down to around 1,600-1,800 calories a day for 14 days in order to accomplish my objective. Basically, I'm going to starve myself. I plan to eat small meals often throughout the day.

PROTEIN, CARBS, AND FAT

During the cutting phase, I'm going to reduce my carbohydrate intake substantially. I'll be consuming a diet that will be around 40-45% protein, 40-45% carbs, and 10-20% fat.

TAKING THE ANABOLIC BURST CYCLING PROGRAM FOR A TEST DRIVE

BURST CYCLING PROGRAM FOR A TEST DRIVE•TAKING THE ANABOLIC BURST CYCLING PROGRAM FOR A TEST DRIVE•TAKING THE ANABOLIC BURST CYCLING PROGRAM FOR A TEST DRIVE•TAKING THE ANABOLIC BURST CYCLING PROGRAM FOR A TEST DRIVE•TAKING THE ANABOLIC BURST CYCLING PROGRAM FOR A TEST DRIVE•TAKING THE

An example of what an average day's food intake might be on the low-calorie phase is shown below.

Example of My Daily Nutrition Program
During the Cutting Phase

Time	Food	Protein grams	Carb grams	Fat grams	Cal
7:00 a.m.	200 mg caffeine, 25 mg ephedrine, 300 mg aspirin (on aerobic training days only)	–	–	–	–
7:30 a.m.	30 minutes aerobics on stationary bike	–	–	–	–
9:00 a.m.	Myoplex Plus with 16 oz of water mixed with	42	24	2	280
	one serving of BetaGen	–	2	–	10
11:00 a.m.	Fat-free yogurt	7	13	–	82
	Apple	–	21	–	84
	16 oz of water	–	–	–	–
12:00 p.m.	One grilled, skinless chicken breast	53	–	6	266
	One medium-sized baked potato with	5	51	–	224
	2 Tbsp ketchup	1	7	–	32
	16 oz of water	–	–	–	–
3:00 p.m.	Myoplex Plus with 16 oz of water mixed with	42	24	2	280
	one serving of BetaGen	–	2	–	10
6:30 p.m.	Weight-training workout	–	–	–	–
7:30 p.m.	One serving of BetaGen mixed with	–	2	–	10
	one serving of CytoVol	–	4	–	45
8:00 p.m.	4 oz grilled salmon	29	–	7	179
	Salad with fat-free dressing	5	3	–	32
	Steamed vegetables	3	6	–	36
	16 oz of water	–	–	–	–
10:30 p.m.	Fat-free yogurt	7	13	–	82
	One serving of BetaGen mixed with	–	2	–	10
	one serving of CytoVol	–	4	–	45
	TOTALS	**194**	**178**	**17**	**1707**

TRAINING

Four days a week I'm going to try to do a minimum of 20 minutes (but hopefully as much as 30 or 40 minutes) of aerobic exercise, on an empty stomach in the morning, to accelerate fat loss. After I work out, I'll wait about an hour before I eat (my body will continue to burn fat for fuel at an accelerated rate after exercise). By then, I'll probably *have* to eat—I'll be starving.

During this phase, I'm going to train with weights only three days a week, doing moderate weight, relatively high reps, and relatively low intensity.

My goal during this two-week period is to get rid of bodyfat while maintaining muscle mass. This phase is not about stretching the connective tissue or gaining muscle, so I'm <u>not</u> going to exaggerate the stretching components on my exercises, nor am I going to work very hard on the eccentric reps. This is not the time for beating up my muscles—protein synthesis will probably be down during this phase, and recovery will be difficult. I plan to work out Monday, Wednesday, and Friday for about 45 minutes with weights and do completely different exercises than I did during the bulking phase. And, like I said, I don't plan to really push it that hard.

SUPPLEMENTS

Because I know caffeine can stimulate the release of fatty acids for use as fuel, especially in a fasted state, as soon as I get out of bed on the mornings I'm going to be doing aerobic exercise, I plan to take 200 mg of caffeine, 25 mg of ephedrine, and one aspirin. (This is a potent fat-burning stack which works well for a lot of lifters but one which Torbjorn does not "endorse" because these are considered serious drugs in Sweden. And as a medical professional, he does not believe in the self-administration of any drugs. I have used caffeine and ephedrine before, and I tolerate them well.)

I also plan to use BetaGen (EAS' new creatine and HMB formula) and CytoVol (EAS' new Glutamine Preservation System). Because my primary goal during the dieting phase is to lose fat while attempting to minimize the loss of muscle tissue, the use of anti-catabolic supplements like glutamine and HMB is important. I'm going to use BetaGen instead of Phosphagen HP during the dieting phase because I'll be trying to keep my insulin levels relatively low and stable. (Phosphagen HP contains a good dose of carbs. BetaGen is virtually carb free.) After two straight weeks of consuming Phosphagen HP, my muscles are going to be jam-packed with creatine. I don't think they'll be able to hold any more, and consuming a maintenance dose during the fat-loss phase will ensure that my muscles don't start losing stored creatine and suffer a loss of cell volume during the dieting period.

Creatine is one supplement I would not discontinue—I'm not sure there's a good reason to stop using it. Dr. Paul Greenhaff's data from Nottingham University clearly shows that when you stop taking creatine, your muscle cells' creatine concentrations return to normal—you lose the advantage it offers. Creatine may be as important as protein, vitamins and minerals, etc. However, I think there is some justification for cycling other supplements, and I think it makes sense to use more creatine when your cells are really starting to swell, like during the bulking phase. And, I don't necessarily think it's a must to use HMB during the bulking phase— but I do think it can offer a huge benefit during the cutting cycle. Dr. Steve Nissen's research on HMB shows it has significant protein-sparing/anti-catabolic effects, and it may therefore accelerate fat loss.

I'll also have two servings of Myoplex Plus each day during this phase to make sure I'm getting enough vitamins, minerals, protein, and other important nutrients.

Throughout the program, I'm going to drink ample amounts of water—80 to 120 oz a day.

TAKING THE ANABOLIC BURST CYCLING PROGRAM FOR A TEST DRIVE

Here's a recap of my plan:

My Anabolic Burst Cycling Plan

Anabolic/Bulking Phase

DAY	1	2	3	4	5	6	7	8	9	10	11	12	13	14
						No aerobics								
	W	W	-	W	W	-	-	W	W	-	W	W	-	-
	Chest	Back		Legs	Chest			Back	Legs		Chest	Back		
	Shoulders	Bis		Calves	Shoulders			Bis	Calves		Shoulders	Bis		
	Tris	Abs			Tris						Tris			

W=Heavy Weight Training. Stretch during exercises and between. Hit eccentric hard.

Diet
around 4,000 calories each day
around 300 grams of protein
around 500 grams of carbs
(simple and complex carbs)
around 110 grams of fat

Supplements
Phosphagen HP, 3 servings a day
Myoplex Plus Deluxe, 2-3 servings a day
(contains chromium and vanadyl)
Vitamin C, 3 grams a day

Anti-Catabolic/Cutting Phase

DAY	15	16	17	18	19	20	21	22	23	24	25	26	27	28
						Day 29 (start over at day 1)								
	A	A	-	A	A	-	-	A	A	-	A	A	-	-
	W	-	W	-	W	-	-	W	-	W	-	W	-	W
	Legs		Upper		Legs			Upper		Legs		Upper		Legs
			Body					Body				Body		

A=Aerobics first thing in the morning on an empty stomach for 20-40 minutes.
Pulse 120-140 beats per minute.

Diet
around 1,800 calories each day
around 200 grams of protein
around 100-200 grams of carbs
(minimal intake of simple carbs, especially fructose)
around 20-30 grams of fat

Supplements
BetaGen, 3-4 servings a day
CytoVol, 1 right after weight-training exercise, 1 before bed each night
Myoplex Plus, 2 servings a day
Caffeine/Ephedrine/Aspirin only on aerobic training days

THE GOAL: GET BIGGER!

My goal is to put on six or seven pounds of bodyweight during the bulking phase which is a lot for me, considering I've been training for many years. According to the Anabolic Burst Cycling theory, if I do everything right, two-thirds of the weight I gain should be lean mass. During the cutting phase, I'm going to try to lose all of the fat mass I gained during the bulking phase, while hopefully retaining most of the muscle. Then, I'm going to immediately go back on another bulking phase. From what I hear, the second bulking cycle, after your body has been "primed" by a strict two-week dieting period, is when it really hits you—you notice your muscles getting drastically bigger and stronger. I'm looking forward to that!

I'll check my bodyfat and scale weight each week to gauge my body composition alterations and develop a chart like Torbjorn's on page 271.

This particular program is *my* personal version of the Anabolic Burst Cycling System. It is not Torbjorn Akerfeldt's <u>exact</u> recommendation. He has a few things he does differently—things he'll discuss in his upcoming book on this topic. But, I know many of you, like myself, are ready to take this system for a "test drive," so I thought I'd share my plan with you. I'm excited about it, and I think it's going to work great. But, who knows, I might be wrong. I'm going to give it my best shot and fill you in on all the details. It might take a little trial and error to get things fine-tuned, but I've got a logical starting point and a system I think I can live (and grow!) with.

By the time you read this, my first Anabolic Burst Cycle will be well under way. In future issues of my magazine, *Muscle Media*, I'll give you the exact details on how this program is working for me, and I'll pass along specific feedback from others who try this program, too. If you're looking for a new drug-free way to gain quality muscle mass, I highly recommend you give the program I outlined in this chapter a try!

SPORTS SUPPLEMENT REVIEW, 3RD ISSUE•SPORTS SUPPLEMENT REVIEW, 3RD ISSUE•SPORTS SUPPLEMENT REVIEW, 3RD ISSUE•SPORTS SUPPLEMENT REVIEW, 3RD ISSUE•SPORTS SUPPLEMENT REVIEW, 3RD ISSUE•SPORTS

294

Training Variety:
The Key to Bodybuilding Progress

Bodybuilders and personal trainers, athletes and coaches, and basically everyone else who has ever picked up a weight, have argued endlessly about the "best" way to train. In fact, people tend to divide themselves into opposing schools of thought on nearly every issue. For example, one camp advocates slow contraction speeds, while the other recommends ballistic, high-velocity training. Some favor high repetitions, while others espouse low reps. Other issues currently debated are machines versus free weights, compound versus isolation movements, and single versus multiple sets.

The problem is that our tendency towards "either/or" thinking leaves the majority of us in a state of perpetual confusion when it comes to designing and carrying out training programs. Many athletes find themselves constantly changing their minds on a particular aspect of training after hearing a persuasive argument by a respected expert or successful athlete. As soon as Donny Deltoid gets comfortable with one way of doing something, someone comes along and says something which totally confuses him again.

The objective of this chapter is to outline an approach for evaluating training variables. This concept was inspired by years of tackling questions from readers of my magazine and books. It's also a result of my own attempts to understand training methodology. I'm confident it will help reduce the confusion you experience when attempting to design training programs.

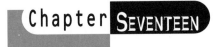

"**Many** experts recommend regular changes in programming because the body tends to rapidly adapt to a workout."

THE PRINCIPLE OF VARIATION

Change is good. Many experts recommend regular changes in programming because the body tends to rapidly adapt to a workout. I recommend variation for a different reason: all choices in training variables have specific benefits and drawbacks. For example, using one set to failure has positive features (single sets allow

TRAINING VARIETY: THE KEY TO BODYBUILDING PROGRESS

CHAPTER 17

PROGRESS•TRAINING VARIETY: THE KEY TO BODYBUILDING PROGRESS•TRAINING VARIETY: THE KEY TO BODYBUILDING PROGRESS•TRAINING VARIETY: THE KEY TO BODYBUILDING PROGRESS•TRAINING VARIETY: THE KEY TO BODYBUILDING PROGRESS•TRAINING VARIETY: THE KEY TO BODYBUILDING PROGRESS•TRAINING VARIETY: THE KEY

for higher intensities compared to multiple sets) as well as less favorable effects (the targeted motor units, although recruited, are not exhausted due to the low number of sets and small amount of time under tension). However, using a large number of sets is a trade-off as well: on the one hand, this method results in complete exhaustion of muscle fibers, yet the high volume requires lower intensity. The only way around this paradox is to regularly change your choice of training variables. In this way, you avoid the problem of adaptation and plateaus in training progress.

Let's take a look at some of the most vehemently debated issues concerning training variables. By seeing a different perspective, you'll find that there's really nothing to debate.

EXERCISE SELECTION

Free Weights Versus Machines: Pianists don't debate the relative merits of white keys versus black keys, yet many exercise articles have been written about the superiority of free weights versus machines (or vice versa). Those favoring machines cite the many resistance technologies available (such as "target loading" used by Strive equipment) offered by machines as well as the superior ability of machines to isolate the targeted muscle. Machines may also be safer when implementing techniques such as eccentrics, strip sets, and partials.

From another perspective, free weights have a greater ability than machines to involve stabilizer muscles. Consider the following training scenario, which was relayed to me by Paul Chek, an exercise and rehabilitation specialist in La Jolla, California:

> **"...regularly** change your choice of training variables. In this way, you avoid the problem of adaptation and plateaus in training progress."

Pick a moderately heavy set of dumbbells, and perform one set to failure. Immediately go to a bench, and perform a set of barbell bench presses, using the same weight, until failure. You may be surprised to find that you can continue, despite failing with the dumbbells. Finally, go to a smith machine loaded with exactly the same weight, and you'll be able to continue even further.

The explanation for the above scenario is *stabilizer muscle failure*. The dumbbell bench presses required the most stabilizer involvement, and the smith machine required the least. Hence, you'd be able to continue past the first exercise because the second and third exercises required progressively less stabilizer activity. Put plainly, when your prime movers are too strong in relation to your stabilizers, your strength output is limited, and you'll never make the progress you can and should be making.

So, there are advantages to both free weights and machines. It would make a lot more sense to spend less time wondering which method is better and more time incorporating both into your training program.

Isolation Versus Compound Movements: Isolation exercises are those which involve only one joint (such as cable curls), while compound exercises involve two or more joints (such as dumbbell bench presses or lunges). Compound exercises allow you to train more muscles with fewer exercises, which improves the efficiency of the workout from a time-management standpoint. They also tend to improve "intermuscular coordination"; i.e., the ability of different muscle groups to cooperate efficiently during a movement. On the other hand, isolation movements allow you to put the bulk of the training stress on one particular muscle or muscle group. This is very useful for therapeutic purposes and for bodybuilders who need to improve a particular muscle group. It's also useful for athletes whose sport skills are limited by weakness in a particular muscle. (For example, jumping ability is often limited by the dynamic strength of the gastrocnemius [calf] muscle.)

Clearly, all trainees need the advantages offered by both isolation and compound movements. However, athletes who emphasize one and neglect the other are likely to make limited progress, compared to what could happen with a more varied approach.

Training Load

Few Versus Many Exercises: There is an inverse relationship between the number of exercises you perform and the number of sets you can complete. In other words, as the number of exercises goes up, the number of sets of each exercise you can perform goes down. Using a large number of exercises allows you to hit additional muscle fibers within the selected muscle, theoretically leading to more complete development. But when you use many exercises, you can't do a lot of sets. Performing a small number of exercises may not recruit as many different muscle fibers, but on the positive side, it enables you to perform many more sets, allowing you to thoroughly exhaust the fibers you do use.

It's important to understand that simply recruiting a motor-unit pool (a group of muscle fibers) doesn't mean you're exhausting those motor units, which is necessary to achieve a training effect. Many "one-set-to-failure" proponents disagree with me on this point, but in my experience, motivated athletes who properly supplement their diets with creatine monohydrate can perform one set to failure and then, after five or six minutes of rest, perform another identical set. This clearly shows that the first set did not sufficiently fatigue the targeted muscle fibers.

TRAINING VARIETY: THE KEY TO BODYBUILDING PROGRESS

PROGRESS•TRAINING VARIETY: THE KEY TO BODYBUILDING PROGRESS•TRAINING VARIETY: THE KEY TO BODYBUILDING PROGRESS•TRAINING VARIETY: THE KEY TO BODYBUILDING PROGRESS•TRAINING VARIETY: THE KEY TO BODYBUILDING PROGRESS•TRAINING VARIETY: THE KEY TO BODYBUILDING PROGRESS•TRAINING VARIETY: THE KEY TO BODYBUILDING PROGRESS•TRAINING VARIETY: THE

High Versus Low Reps: Recently, a famous pro bodybuilder told me that as long as he was training as hard as he possibly could, it made no difference how many reps he performed. I waited for the punch line... I'm still waiting. Apparently, there was none. Let's examine the good and the bad when it comes to addressing the issue of time under tension.

The number of repetitions per set is perhaps the most important short-term training variable—the number of reps you do determines the intensity of work, which in turn determines the type of adaptation you'll get. Performing between one and five repetitions tends to enhance strength more than mass. When you perform between 6 and 12 repetitions, however, the most significant adaptation is increased muscular growth. Almost everyone should incorporate both repetition ranges into his or her training since muscular growth is partly a function of strength. Athletes who depend on relative strength should emphasize the 1- to 5-rep range (for example, 3 weeks of 1-5 followed by 1 week of 6-12), while bodybuilders and fitness enthusiasts should emphasize the 6- to 12-rep range (for example, 3 weeks of 6-12 followed by 1 week of 1-5).

Although high (over 15 and perhaps up to 100) repetitions do little or nothing to directly develop strength or mass, they can contribute to various metabolic processes which indirectly support strength and mass development. These processes include an enhanced ability to clear lactic acid from working muscles, which improves short-term endurance. Incidentally, a popular bodybuilding magazine recently featured a story about doing one rep per set per session! The creator of this method claims to get fantastic gains, but I suspect that you may need identical genetics to his in order to achieve the same results.

Single Versus Multiple Sets: Recently, the concept of one set to failure has received renewed interest in the bodybuilding world. Advocates of this approach argue that multiple sets decrease training intensity and increase the recovery time needed between workouts. To a large degree, they're correct. But while one set per exercise per workout does increase intensity, it also has its drawbacks. The most significant problem is that high intensity (by definition) means low volume. When training volume is insufficient, two problems arise:

1) Target muscle fibers aren't exposed to enough reps to exhaust them.

2) Since only a small amount of mechanical work occurs, damage to the sarcomeres (the microscopic working unit of the muscle cell) is limited. Micro-damage (or degradation) to muscle tissue is an important stimulus for growth.

Recent studies also suggest that multiple sets result in greater growth hormone and testosterone production than single-set protocols.

When trying to decide how many sets to perform, it helps to understand the relationship between volume and intensity in training. In a nutshell, both are needed. The problem is, you can't have high volume and high intensity in the same training session. The only way to solve the problem is to regularly *alternate* between periods of relatively high volume and periods which emphasize higher intensity.

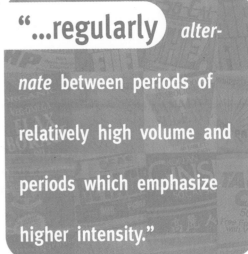

"...regularly *alternate* between periods of relatively high volume and periods which emphasize higher intensity."

Long Versus Short Training Sessions: Sometimes the letters I get shock me. Recently, I received a letter from a gentleman who claimed he had the perfect workout: he spent 20 minutes once a week in the gym! He hammered away at 8 exercises that covered every body part for between 10-20 reps per exercise. Let me say here that this will not work. Now, the amount of time you should spend in the gym is debatable—but 20 minutes a week?

I think this poor guy's "mind-muscle link" is broken! Nevertheless, although it's widely accepted that resistance-training sessions should be limited to one hour, a case can be made for doing both longer and shorter sessions. Long (up to 90-minute) workouts are useful in cases where training frequency is very limited, due to outside obligations or other reasons. For example, if you can train only once every 4 or 5 days, a 90-minute session may prove more productive than an hour or less. On the other hand, very short sessions allow you to really "bust your ass" with very high intensity and can help you fit your training program into a busy schedule. I know a lot of people who wouldn't even consider trying to work out unless they had at least 45 minutes available, but even a half hour can go a long way when time's tight. When planning your training program, start with what's ideal, and then make whatever compromises are necessary based on your unique situation.

Short Versus Long Rests Between Sets: The most commonly used rest periods range between 30 seconds and 6 minutes. Generally, when you're doing fewer repetitions, you need more rest and vice versa. However, most people rarely or never change the time between sets. Big mistake, and here's why: long rest periods allow a more complete recovery, which enables you to use the heaviest possible loads for each set, and that's necessary for strength gains. The drawback is that long rests are not time efficient. Also, if you rest too long between sets, you may begin to "cool off," which can negatively impact your workout.

Short rest periods limit the amount of weight you can use, but they also force the body to fortify its recovery mechanisms—particularly its ability to clear lactic acid from the muscles. What's in it for you? Improved body composition, better short-term endurance, and more vascularity. Short rests between sets also trim time off your workouts.

Slow Versus Fast Tempos (Contraction Speed): Exercise tempo refers to the amount of time it takes to perform a repetition. Each rep has three phases—the negative portion, where the muscle lengthens as it yields to the weight (such as lowering the dumbbells during a seated dumbbell curl); followed by a pause; and finally the positive portion, where the muscle shortens and overcomes the weight being lifted (such as lifting the dumbbells during a seated dumbbell curl). Normally, the negative portion should last longer than the positive for the best training results. You can use any tempo you like, as long as the set doesn't extend past one minute in duration. Interestingly, the *Super Slow Exercise Guild* (*SSEG*) suggests 15 seconds per rep, which would allow for only 4 reps before the set becomes an aerobic activity. Nevertheless, the *SSEG* recommends eight or more reps per set. This type of protocol would benefit an 800-meter runner or synchronized swimmer much more than it would anyone trying to gain muscular bodyweight. But it may have some sporadic value, provided it's either different or more intense than what you are used to doing.

Muscle Media Strength Guru Charles Poliquin illustrated the inherent trade-offs in contraction speeds in a 1988 article for the *National Strength and Conditioning Association Journal*:

> In North America, there are conflicting schools of thought on the optimal speed at which strength work should be performed. One school advocates high-velocity training, while another contends that strength can optimally be gained only though slowly performed repetitions. However, both schools are correct.

> Poliquin further notes that slow velocities are associated with the production of high forces which are ideal for mass gains, and fast contraction speeds favor strength development through neural improvements. (Remember, strength is important for growth since your strength level determines the percentage of muscle fibers you'll be able to recruit during a set.) Using only fast tempos or only slow tempos is akin to eating only protein for the reason that carbs aren't used for growth and repair! While that isolated fact may be true, it's only part of the total story.

"Using only fast tempos or only slow tempos is akin to eating only protein for the reason that carbs aren't used for growth and repair!"

Full Versus Partial Range of Motion: About three years ago, the book *Power Factor Training* (and the training system it describes) received quite a bit of publicity in the bodybuilding world. The authors of the book argued that movements should always be performed in one's "strongest range" of motion. This allowed for the use of heavier loads, and the authors insisted it created greater results. The Power Factor system worked for many people, and I'll tell you exactly which ones— those who always use the full range of motion when performing resistance exercises. But while a partial range of motion allows for greater loads, it also has its drawbacks. Perhaps the most significant problem is the likelihood of developing muscle imbalances, which can lead to injuries. In the squat, for example, the hamstrings and gluteals don't begin to contribute until the lifter reaches a fairly deep position—certainly below parallel. And while some coaches recommend that athletes squat only as deep as the positions they normally encounter in their sport (called "accentuation training"), overreliance on lifting only in "shallow" positions where mechanical leverages are best is a mistake. Thus, "partials" should be used as a part-time tool; they serve a purpose only when used intelligently.

SUMMARY

If I told you that in the sport of golf, there is a raging controversy over one group that uses only woods versus another that uses only irons, you'd laugh and write me off as a nut case. Yet every day I talk to people who have been at a plateau in their training for months or even years, usually due to long-term overreliance on one limited method of training. Does this sound like you? If so, your ticket to success is <u>change</u>. Remember, a mistake is only a mistake if you don't learn from it.

SPORTS SUPPLEMENT REVIEW, 3RD ISSUE~SPORTS SUPPLEMENT REVIEW, 3RD ISSUE~SPORTS SUPPLEMENT REVIEW, 3RD ISSUE~SPORTS SUPPLEMENT REVIEW, 3RD ISSUE~SPORTS

302

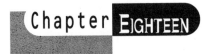

Chapter EIGHTEEN

German Volume Training:
A New Look at an Old Way
to Get Big and Strong

As we discussed in the last chapter, variety is an important component of training success—you can't use one program forever—it just doesn't work. If you're looking for a great training routine to jump start new muscle growth, you'll definitely want to read this chapter thoroughly. I'm going to tell you about an awesome training system that's hard, but it's a very effective way to pack on muscle fast!

In strength-coaching circles, this method is often called the "ten-sets method." Because it has its roots in German-speaking countries, I like to call it German Volume Training. To the best of my knowledge, this training system originated in Germany in the mid-'70's and was popularized by Rolf Feser, who was then the National Coach of Weightlifting. A similar protocol was promoted by Vince Gironda in the U.S., but regardless of who actually invented it, *it works*.

In Germany, the ten-sets method was used in the off-season to help weightlifters gain muscle mass. It was so efficient that lifters routinely moved up a full weight class within 12 weeks. It was the base program of Canadian weightlifter Jacques Demers, silver medalist in the Los Angeles Olympic Games. Jacques was known in weightlifting circles for his massive thighs, and he gives credit to the German method for achieving such a spectacular level of development.

The program works because it targets a group of motor units, exposing them to an extensive volume of repeated efforts, specifically, ten sets of a single exercise. The body adapts to the extraordinary stress by hypertrophying the targeted fibers. To say this program adds muscle fast is probably an understatement—gains of five to ten pounds or more in a few months are not uncommon—even for experienced lifters!

GOALS AND GUIDELINES

The goal of the German Volume Training method is to complete ten sets of ten reps with the same weight for certain exercises. You want to begin with a weight you could lift for 20 reps to failure if you had to. For most people, on most exercises, that would represent 60% of their 1RM load. Therefore, if you can bench press 300 lbs for 1 rep, you would use 180 lbs for this exercise.

For lifters new to this method, I recommend using the following body-part splits: Day 1: chest and back, Day 2: legs and abs, Day 3: off, Day 4: arms and shoulders, Day 5: off.

When using this program—or any other, for that matter—you should keep a detailed journal of the exact sets, reps, and rest intervals performed, and only count the repetitions completed in strict form. Here are a few more guidelines to ensure optimal progress:

Rest Intervals: When bodybuilders start with this method, they often question its value for the first several sets because the weight doesn't feel heavy enough. However, there is minimal rest between sets (about 60 seconds when performed in sequence and 90-120 seconds when performed as a superset), which causes cumulative fatigue. (Interestingly enough, you might find you get stronger again during the eighth and ninth sets—this is because of a short-term neural adaptation.) Because of the importance of the rest intervals, you should use a stopwatch to keep the rest intervals constant. This is very important, as it becomes tempting to lengthen the rest time as you fatigue.

Tempo: For exercises such as squats, dips, and chins, use a 4-0-2 tempo; this means you would lower the weight in four seconds and immediately change direction and lift for two seconds. For movements such as curls and triceps extensions, use a 3-0-2 tempo.

Number of Exercises: Only one main exercise per body part should be performed for ten sets. Therefore, select exercises that recruit a lot of muscle mass. Triceps kickbacks and leg extensions are definitely out—squats and bench presses are definitely in. For supplementary work for individual body parts (like triceps and biceps), you can do 3 sets of 10-20 reps.

Training Frequency: Because this is such an intense program, it'll take you longer to recover. In fact, if you're familiar with the writings of Peter Sisco and John Little, you'll find that the average "Power Factor Rating" of the ten-sets method is about eight billion. Consequently, *one* training session every four to five days per body part is plenty.

Overload Mechanism: Once you're able to do ten sets of ten with constant rest intervals, increase the weight on the bar by four percent to five percent, and repeat the process. Refrain from using forced reps, negatives, or partials. The volume of the work will take care of the hypertrophy. Expect to have some deep muscle soreness without having to resort to set prolongation techniques. In fact, after doing a quad and hams session with this method, it takes the average bodybuilder about five days to stop limping.

Beginner INTERMEDIATE

Phase 1 Program

This is a sample routine based on a five-day cycle. Once you've used this method for six workouts per body part, it's time to move on to a different program for a three-week period.

Day One: CHEST AND BACK

Exercise	Sets	Reps	Tempo	Rest Interval
A-1 Decline Dumbbell Presses, Semi-Supinated Grip (palms facing each other)	10	10	4-0-2	90 seconds
A-2 Chin-Ups (palms facing you)	10	10	4-0-2	90 seconds
B-1 Incline Dumbbell Flyes	3	10-12	3-0-2	60 seconds
B-2 One-Arm Dumbbell Rows	3	10-12	3-0-2	60 seconds

(A-1 and A-2 are a Superset; B-1 and B-2 are a Superset)

Note: Rest 90 seconds between each "A" set. For example, perform a set of dumbbell presses, rest 90 seconds, do a set of chin-ups, then wait 90 seconds before repeating this sequence. Rest 60 seconds between each "B" set. Incidentally, I recommend only three sets of ten in this program for the "B" exercises. The "B" exercises constitute supplementary work, and doing ten sets of them would result in overtraining.

Day Two: LEGS AND ABS

Exercise	Sets	Reps	Tempo	Rest Interval
A-1 Back Squats	10	10	4-0-2	90 seconds
A-2 Lying Leg Curls	10	10	4-0-2	90 seconds
B-1 Incline Sit-Ups	3	15-20	2-0-2	60 seconds
B-2 Seated Calf Raises	3	15-20	2-0-2	60 seconds

(A-1 and A-2 are a Superset; B-1 and B-2 are a Superset)

Note: Rest 90 seconds between each "A" set; rest 60 seconds between each "B" set.

GERMAN VOLUME TRAINING: A NEW LOOK AT AN OLD WAY TO GET BIG AND STRONG

CHAPTER 18

TO GET BIG AND STRONG-GERMAN VOLUME TRAINING: A NEW LOOK AT AN OLD WAY TO GET BIG AND STRONG-GERMAN VOLUME TRAINING: A NEW LOOK AT AN OLD WAY TO GET BIG AND STRONG-GERMAN VOLUME TRAINING: A NEW LOOK AT AN OLD WAY TO GET BIG AND STRONG-GERMAN VOLUME TRAINING: A NEW LOOK AT AN OLD

Day Three: Off

Day Four: Arms and Shoulders

	Exercise	Sets	Reps	Tempo	Rest Interval
Superset	A-1 Parallel Bar Dips	10	10	4-0-2	90 seconds
	A-2 Incline Curls	10	10	4-0-2	90 seconds
Superset	B-1 Bent-Over Dumbbell Lateral Raises*	3	10-12	2-0-X	60 seconds
	B-2 Seated Dumbbell Lateral Raises	3	10-12	2-0-X	60 seconds

(*While seated on the edge of a bench with your torso bent over, raise the dumbbells out to the side, making sure the top two knuckles—the ones closest to your thumb—are in line with your ears at the top of the movement.)

Note: Rest 90 seconds between each "A" set; rest 60 seconds between each "B" set. "X" in the tempo means to move as fast as possible, keeping the weight under control. For example, on lateral raises you would lift the weight up in two seconds then lower it quickly, but under control, then repeat.

Day Five: Off

Day Six: Start Over With Day One

Beginner Intermediate

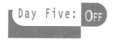

Phase 2 Program

After six of those five-day cycles, I recommend you do a three-week phase where the average set is six to eight reps, and do only four to six sets per body part over a five-day cycle, or you can do any other split that suits your recovery pattern. After this three-week block, you can return to the German Volume Training method by doing the following ten sets of six reps routine. In the exercises that are prescribed for 10 sets, use a weight you'd normally be able to do 12 repetitions with. The goal in this phase is to do ten sets of six with that weight.

Here's a sample ten sets of six reps routine:

Day One: CHEST AND BACK

	Exercise	Sets	Reps	Tempo	Rest Interval
Superset {	A-1 Incline Dumbbell Presses	10	6	5-0-1	90 seconds
	A-2 Wide-Grip Pull-Ups (palms facing away from you)	10	6	5-0-1	90 seconds
Superset {	B-1 Flat Dumbbell Flyes	3	6	3-0-1	60 seconds
	B-2 Bent-Over Rows with EZ Bar	3	6	3-0-1	60 seconds

Note: Rest 90 seconds between each "A" set; rest 60 seconds between each "B" set.

Day Two: LEGS AND ABS

	Exercise	Sets	Reps	Tempo	Rest Interval
Superset {	A-1 Bent-Knee Deadlifts	10	6	5-0-1	90 seconds
	A-2 Seated Leg Curls	10	6	5-0-1	90 seconds
Superset {	B-1 Twisting Crunches	3	12-15	3-0-3	60 seconds
	B-2 Standing Calf Raises	3	12-15	3-0-3	60 seconds

Note: Rest 90 seconds between each "A" set; rest 60 seconds between each "B" set.

Day Three: OFF

Day Four: ARMS AND SHOULDERS

	Exercise	Sets	Reps	Tempo	Rest Interval
Superset {	A-1 Parallel Bar Dips	10	6	5-0-1	90 seconds
	A-2 Incline Curls	10	6	5-0-1	90 seconds
Superset {	B-1 Bent-Over Dumbbell Lateral Raises	3	10-12	2-0-X	60 seconds
	B-2 Seated Dumbbell Lateral Raises	3	10-12	2-0-X	60 seconds

Note: Rest 90 seconds between each "A" set; rest 60 seconds between each "B" set.

GERMAN VOLUME TRAINING: A NEW LOOK AT AN OLD WAY TO GET BIG AND STRONG

TO GET BIG AND STRONG•GERMAN VOLUME TRAINING: A NEW LOOK AT AN OLD WAY TO GET BIG AND STRONG•GERMAN VOLUME TRAINING: A NEW LOOK AT AN OLD WAY TO GET BIG AND STRONG•GERMAN VOLUME TRAINING: A NEW LOOK AT AN OLD WAY TO GET BIG AND STRONG•GERMAN VOLUME TRAINING: A NEW LOOK AT AN OLD

Advanced TRAINEE

For the advanced trainee, variety is even more important; thus, I use a system called the four-percent method. That is, I increase the load four percent every workout for three workouts in a row, and I reduce the target rep by one rep for every weight increase. Then I reduce the weight four percent and increase the rep bracket to its original starting point. Since this is very mathematical, let's look at an example that will clearly illustrate this point.

Let's say you can barbell curl 100 lbs for 12 strict reps, and you haven't been able to increase the amount of reps or weight on this exercise. Here's a sample routine that would increase your curling strength:

Workout 1: 10 sets of 6 @ 110 lbs
Workout 2: 10 sets of 5 @ 115 lbs
Workout 3: 10 sets of 4 @ 120 lbs
Workout 4: 10 sets of 6 @ 115 lbs
Workout 5: 10 sets of 5 @ 120 lbs
Workout 6: 10 sets of 4 @ 125 lbs
Workout 7: Test day. At this point, you would curl 120 for 12 reps, a 9% gain over 6 workouts!

Here's an example of the German Volume Training method with the 4% method for someone who can bench press 300 lbs 10 times in strict form:

Workout 1: 10 sets of 5 @ 300 lbs
Workout 2: 10 sets of 4 @ 315 lbs
Workout 3: 10 sets of 3 @ 330 lbs
Workout 4: 10 sets of 5 @ 315 lbs
Workout 5: 10 sets of 4 @ 330 lbs
Workout 6: 10 sets of 3 @ 345 lbs
Workout 7: Test day. At this point, you would bench press 330 lbs for 10 reps.

SUMMARY

To recap, perform the Beginner/Intermediate Phase 1 Program for six weeks (six 5-day cycles). Then, progress to the Beginner/Intermediate Phase 2 Program for three weeks. After that, you'll be ready to graduate to the Advanced Program.

This program is elegant in its simplicity, but that's what the Germans do best. Just ask any Mercedes Benz or BMW owner.

For more great tips on training to gain new muscle size and strength, read *Muscle Media*. Each issue offers insights and instruction from some of the world's greatest weight-training experts!

Chapter NINETEEN

How to Set Goals
and Achieve Them!

One of the "secrets to success" in any endeavor, especially one as challenging as bodybuilding, is to use "goal-setting techniques" to help get where you want to go. These techniques really do work, and using them is not that complicated.

Make no mistake, even if you choose the best supplements and make the right decisions in terms of what type of exercise program you should follow, without setting goals and putting "positive pressure" on yourself, you'll probably never get where you want to go. How does that old saying go? *Those who fail to plan are inadvertently planning to fail.* It's really true—if you don't know where you're going, you'll never get there.

The thing is, we all have goals, whether we know it or not. No matter what they are, they have a profound effect on our lives, so you might as well acknowledge these "subconscious" objectives and bring them to the conscious level and make an effort to control them, instead of letting them control you.

Like I said, using goal-setting techniques is really not that complicated—in this short chapter, I'll tell you some simple, easy methods which I use and which you can start using *today* to help you set new goals and achieve them—to help you build muscle, lose fat, and look and feel better than ever before!

The first step (which you should start now!) is to commit to spending ten minutes a day (that's not a lot of time) writing your goals in a notebook or journal.

Start by asking yourself, "What do I want to achieve? What would I do if I knew I could not fail?" Have fun—imagine you're a kid again and your birthday is coming up and you're making out your wish list. In this state of excited anticipation, nothing is too big to ask for, nothing costs too much, and everything is within reach! Get excited!

If one of your goals is to build an awesome, muscular body, write down six things you'll have to start doing <u>this</u> <u>week</u> to reach your goal. Be specific—state

> "**Writing** down your goals and your 'Master Plan' on paper is a well-known, widely accepted method for achieving success..."

HOW TO SET GOALS AND ACHIEVE THEM!

CHAPTER 19

AND ACHIEVE THEM!•HOW TO SET GOALS AND ACHIEVE THEM!•HOW TO SET GOALS AND ACHIEVE THEM!•HOW TO SET GOALS AND ACHIEVE THEM!•HOW TO SET GOALS AND ACHIEVE THEM!•HOW TO SET GOALS AND ACHIEVE THEM!•HOW TO SET GOALS AND ACHIEVE THEM!•HOW TO SET GOALS AND ACHIEVE THEM!•HOW TO SET GOALS

HOW TO SET GOALS AND ACHIEVE THEM!•HOW TO SET GOALS AND ACHIEVE THEM!•HOW TO SET GOALS AND ACHIEVE THEM!•HOW TO SET GOALS

310

exactly how much fat you want to lose or how much muscle you want to gain and how you are going to do it.

Then, taking just two minutes, write a brief paragraph stating why you are absolutely committed to achieving this goal. Remember, this is your opportunity to accomplish something extraordinary! Seize the opportunity!

Each evening, open your journal and read what you've written on previous days. Read about your goals and, for at least five minutes, sit down someplace quiet, and visualize yourself doing the things you know will be necessary to make this dream a reality. Visualize your success with very specific and graphic details. Picture yourself completing a super-intense workout—smashing personal records by lifting more weight, in perfectly strict form, than you've ever lifted before in your life! Envision yourself following the perfect diet—feeding your body with quality nutrition and the supplements it needs to recover from your brutal workouts. Picture yourself turning down desserts and pushing away junk food that "average people" eat—things like cheesecake, French fries, and donuts. Feel the sense of confidence, control, and pride you'll have and how excited you'll be to know that you're actually doing it—you're actually following through with your plan. Imagine your physique in perfect condition—rock-hard abs, striated pecs, vascular arms, and thighs with amazing separation and cuts.

To help you visualize and focus on your goal, cut out pictures of physiques that inspire you (I collect photos of Arnold) and put them someplace you'll see them often—on your refrigerator, in your bedroom, in your office, or on a wall in your home gym (if you have one). Visualize yourself with your new body, training, walking on the beach, or whatever, and sense the excitement.

After you've "visualized" for at least five minutes, write down four things you did that day which brought you closer to achieving your goals and two things you could have done better. Promise yourself you'll improve on these weak links in the coming days and weeks.

Decide what you want—be precise—clarity is power! Take action... **desire is not enough!** Remember that even the longest journey starts with a single, small step, and never forget that procrastination kills! And, be quick to notice what's working and what's not, so you don't expend energy going in the wrong direction. Remember that short-term "failures" often provide the insight you'll need to reach your long-term goals! And, remember to "adapt" or change your approach until you achieve the results you want—flexibility gives you the power to create a new, possibly better approach.

I cannot emphasize enough how important this goal-setting exercise is. Writing down your goals and your "Master Plan" on paper is a well-known, widely accepted method for achieving success in any endeavor.

Have fun, set your goals, get motivated, and get ready to make the most incredible progress over the coming weeks that you've ever made! You *really* can do it!!

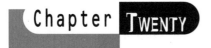

Chapter TWENTY

Frequently Asked Questions and Answers About Supplements

Q I've been seeing a lot of liquid forms of the supplement vanadyl sulfate popping up on the market. The manufacturers of these supplements claim they're more powerful and effective than the tableted versions of this product—are they?

A When vanadyl sulfate is put in a liquid suspension for more than a few hours, it may become very unstable and has the potential to convert into a toxic form of the mineral vanadium. According to EAS research consultant Anthony Almada, if you're going to use vanadyl sulfate, you should stick with the tableted, encapsulated, or a powdered version and never consume more than 45-50 mg in a 24-hour period.

"**It** wouldn't be a bad idea to use this product if you're using a low amount of DHEA..."

Q My health-food store sells DHEA chewing gum made by Genetic Evolutionary Nutrition. Is this real DHEA?

A I believe it is. Last fall I had a sample (Lot #MG0677) of this product tested by high-performance liquid chromatography (HPLC), and it showed that it contained 23 mg of DHEA per piece (label claim is 25, which is pretty darn close).

The product also contains chromium, which was tested by capillary electrophoresis (CE), and it showed that it contained over 200 mcg of chromium per piece of gum.

It wouldn't be a bad idea to use this product if you're using a low amount of DHEA, but most bodybuilders I know are using, on average, 200-600 mg/day, which would be 8-24 pieces of this gum. So, if you're using a higher dose of DHEA, it might be easier to just take capsules or tablets. But at least the product's real.

FREQUENTLY ASKED QUESTIONS AND ANSWERS ABOUT SUPPLEMENTS

ESTIONS AND ANSWERS•QUESTIONS AND ANSWERS•QUESTIONS AND ANSWERS•QUESTIONS AND ANSWERS•QUESTIONS AND ANSWERS•QUESTIONS AND ANSWERS•QUESTIONS AND ANSWERS•QUESTIONS AND ANSWERS•QUESTIONS AND ANSWERS•QUESTIONS AND ANSWERS•QUESTIONS AND ANSWERS•QUESTIONS AND ANSWERS•QUESTIONS AND ANSWERS

CHAPTER 20

Q **Do I really need whey protein over other protein sources? If I eat enough extra protein, wouldn't I be getting enough amino acids? Powdered milk is way cheaper than whey protein. Even if I need more grams of powdered milk protein to get the same nitrogen, it's cheaper than most other proteins, even with the extra amount needed.**

A In one way, you're right. All amino acids are the same (assuming they're not heat damaged, which reduces digestibility). The branched-chain amino acids (BCAA) in powdered milk are just as good as the BCAA's in whey protein. There are more BCAA's in whey than powdered milk, but if you consume enough powdered milk protein (or another protein), you can achieve the same nitrogen level in the body. Of course, you may have to consume an extra 25% (or more) of powdered milk protein to achieve the same nitrogen level. But it might be more economical to buy 125 grams of powdered milk protein than buying 100 grams of whey protein.

However, these excess aminos, because of the various limiting nondispensable aminos, will be eliminated from the body. Remember, you can't really store excess amino acids as you do fat. Extra aminos will be dealt with in three ways: the liver will cleave part of the structure into urea, which is fine, as urea is excreted in the urine. And some of the aminos can be converted into other amino acids: notably, glutamine. The rest of the partial aminos are converted into triglycerides (fat), specifically *saturated* fats. And we now know that saturated fat lowers insulin sensitivity. The really interesting question is this: does excessive protein consumption lower insulin sensitivity from the increased saturated fats in the body? This is an avenue that needs to be explored in the future, charting the various pathways of each of the dietary amino acids. I've wondered about the threshold amount of saturated fat needed to lower insulin sensitivity. Once I find this out, I could give a definitive answer about powdered milk protein. Well-made powdered milk protein can adequately supply your amino acid needs. However, it's not an efficient protein, nor does it have all of the health benefits of whey.

Q **If I'm using the low-calorie lean-mass stimulator Phosphagain (which contains creatine monohydrate), do I need to take Phosphagen or Phosphagen HP (which also contain creatine monohydrate)?**

A The three supplements you mentioned, or any supplement that contains an effective dose of creatine monohydrate, will probably help your bodybuilding efforts; however, you certainly don't have to use all three of the products you mentioned.

Each serving of Phosphagain contains about seven grams of creatine monohydrate, and a heaping teaspoon of Phosphagen contains about five grams of creatine monohydrate, and a serving of Phosphagen HP also contains about five grams of creatine monohydrate.

As long as you start with a "loading phase" of 20-30 grams of creatine monohydrate for 5-7 days, and then go to a "maintenance dose" of 5-10 grams of creatine monohydrate a day, I don't really think it makes much difference where it comes from.

Q **I read that the supplement HMB is a metabolite of the branched-chain amino acid leucine and ketoisocaproic acid (KIC). Can I get the effects of HMB by just taking leucine or KIC?**

A Probably not. Researchers currently believe only five percent of dietary leucine is converted to HMB in the body. To make 3 grams of HMB (which is believed to be the effective dose), you would have to take 60 grams of leucine or over 20 grams of KIC per day, which is not only expensive and impractical but could cause severe stomachaches.

Q **I recently saw an ad for a high-calorie "weight-gain" product that caught my attention. This ad showed some study results and claimed this was scientific proof this supplement works. Do you know if this is true?**

A I'm aware of the ad and the study you're asking about. First of all, "proof" is a very strong word—one scientific study isn't *proof* of anything. I'm very careful when using the word "proof"—in my opinion, studies offer *evidence* that something does or doesn't work. I think you would need a number of pretty solid studies before you could convince me they represent "proof" of anything.

In this study, weight trainers who used a high-calorie supplement made better gains than lifters who used no supplements.

Now, from a "scientific" standpoint, these results are not as valid as they could be because the two groups were not "blinded." That is, the non-supplement users knew they weren't getting anything, and the supplement users knew they were taking something. This leaves room for a "placebo" effect.

An inside source told me there was a third group involved in this study that just received a plain carbohydrate powder. I'm told this "control group" experienced

> "...any supplement that contains an effective dose of creatine monohydrate, will probably help your bodybuilding efforts..."

FREQUENTLY ASKED QUESTIONS AND ANSWERS ABOUT SUPPLEMENTS

ESTIONS AND ANSWERS•QUESTIONS AND ANSWERS•QUESTIONS AND ANSWERS•QUESTIONS AND ANSWERS•QUESTIONS AND ANSWERS•QUESTIONS AND ANSWERS•QUESTIONS AND ANSWERS•QUESTIONS AND ANSWERS•QUESTIONS AND ANSWERS•QUESTIONS AND ANSWERS•QUESTIONS AND ANSWERS•QUESTIONS AND ANSWERS

CHAPTER 20

314

the same results as the weight-gainer group. If that's true, I guess it means using a supplement that contains calories may help you get better results from your weight-training program *if* calories are the "limiting factor" in your program. The results also offer *evidence* that the high-calorie "gainer" supplement didn't work better than a plain carbohydrate powder.

Q I've heard a lot about the thermogenic potential of stacking caffeine and ephedrine. I've read the best way to use this stuff is in a 10:1 ratio, caffeine to ephedrine (200 mg of caffeine and 20 mg of ephedrine, 3 times a day). My problem is, I can't find a source that sells 20-mg tablets of ephedrine. They all sell 25-mg tablets. How do I get around this problem?

A Good question—but it's really not a problem at all. I'm sure you'll get the same effect from using an 8:1 ratio (which would be 200 mg of caffeine for every 25-mg ephedrine tablet). It's just not that exact of a science. If you're off by a little bit, it isn't going to matter that much. I've heard from literally hundreds of bodybuilders who use 25 mg of ephedrine for every 200 mg of caffeine they take, and they've seen great results.

However, if you want to be exact, simply take a small knife and chip off what you would estimate to be a fifth of a 25-mg tablet of ephedrine and consume the other four-fifths along with 200 mg of caffeine.

Q I have a natural show coming up, and I'm using vanadyl sulfate, creatine, glutamine, and ephedrine. Should I stop using any of these compounds before the show, and if so, when?

A Keep using the vanadyl sulfate and glutamine. I'm assuming you've already loaded with creatine, and you're probably using a smaller amount (the average is five to ten grams a day). To ensure you have the maximum fullness effect with the creatine, I suggest that you reload for five days before the show. The research has shown that large amounts of creatine are not needed once creatine is loaded into the muscle, but it may turn out that reloading could add another pound of lean body mass. I can't guarantee it, but it wouldn't hurt to try.

> "...I have never heard any bodybuilders say they received any positive effects from taking Super Blue-Green Algae."

Using ephedrine up to the show is an "iffy" proposition. I've read research pointing out that clenbuterol, a beta$_2$ agonist more potent than ephedrine, lowers insulin sensitivity. So use of clenbuterol would interfere with the carbing-up process. I don't know if the same rationale applies to ephedrine. Ephedrine is a poor beta$_2$ agonist and has a poor fit at the receptor. Most of the thermogenic action of ephedrine is not from direct stimulus at the receptor; rather, its action is caused by the generation of noradrenaline at the nerve endings. I haven't read any research linking ephedrine to insulin sensitivity. But on a wholly practical level, "cold turkey-ing" ephedrine may make you tired and depressed. You have to be at your mental best for your contest. So even though there is a logical possibility that ephedrine use will interfere with your carb-up, I suggest you stay on ephedrine, so you can remain "stable."

Q **I read about a new steroid alternative called "Cobaforte." I was excited to hear that this potent alternative to steroids has no side effects and builds muscle almost as fast as testosterone. Do you know the best dosage for this product and exactly how it should be taken?**

A I've received a number of inquiries about Cobaforte lately. Apparently, some fitness writer on the East Coast recently wrote about it in a newsletter and claimed it was a powerful steroid alternative. Unfortunately, that is not the case. Cobaforte is simply a European product that contains a deriv-ative of Vitamin B$_{12}$. It is similar to the Mexican versions of dibencozide, which go under the brand names Maxibol and Neurofor. Cobaforte works absolutely nothing like an anabolic steroid and doesn't do anything to increase muscle growth.

Q **A friend of mine recently told me about a new miracle supplement called Super Blue-Green Algae. He said it would help me gain muscle and strength and improve my health. Have you heard anything good about this product?**

A Without being hypercritical, let me just answer your question—no, I have never heard any bodybuilders say they received any positive effects from tak-ing Super Blue-Green Algae. I haven't the slightest idea why this product (I am familiar with it) would have an effect on your ability to gain muscle size and strength. I would <u>not</u> recommend this supplement.

FREQUENTLY ASKED QUESTIONS AND ANSWERS ABOUT SUPPLEMENTS

ESTIONS AND ANSWERS•QUESTIONS AND ANSWERS•QUESTIONS AND ANSWERS•QUESTIONS AND ANSWERS•QUESTIONS AND ANSWERS•QUESTIONS AND ANSWERS•QUESTIONS AND ANSWERS•QUESTIONS AND ANSWERS•QUESTIONS AND ANSWERS•QUESTIONS AND ANSWERS•QUESTIONS AND ANSWERS•QUESTIONS AND ANSWERS

Q I've heard that taurine is an important amino acid for bodybuilders. I'm taking a product called GT Fuel made by PROgenix. This supplement contains the "L" form of taurine. Is that the best kind?

A There is no "L" form of the amino acid taurine. Obviously, PROgenix doesn't know this, or they wouldn't put it on their label and in their advertisements. They advertise this "GT Fuel" with the claim "Scientifically Proven #1." Proven by whom? Where's the research? Number one at what? Whose science?

I called these people to ask them about their product, and the person I talked to didn't have a clue. They should advertise this product as "Science Free." That would be more accurate.

Q Coach Poliquin and others (including Dan Duchaine) have recommended higher doses of creatine monohydrate than are recommended on the label. For example, Coach Poliquin recommends about 40 grams a day for 7 days for a loading phase and then 20 grams a day for a maintenance dose. Do you think I'll get better results if I take this much?

A That is a good question. I know a lot of people are experimenting with different dosages of creatine monohydrate, and some contend they are getting better results, but it's hard to tell if their feedback is conclusive.

In an effort to try to provide a "scientifically valid" answer to this question, EAS is putting up a considerable amount of money to fund more research involving creatine use. Several studies will attempt to shed light on the "best" dosage of creatine monohydrate. Hopefully, the results of these studies will be available soon—I'll be sure to pass them along in future issues of *Muscle Media*.

Q I was wondering if the recommended dosage of supplements like creatine monohydrate, HMB, CLA, and vanadyl sulfate should be adjusted according to bodyweight. Do you have any information on this?

A It seems to make sense that a 125-lb woman would not need to take the same amount of HMB or creatine as a 220-lb guy. Unfortunately, no studies have been done to answer this particular question.

Logic would *seem* to dictate that if a 220-lb guy gets good results using 3 grams of HMB a day, a 125-lb woman should get good results by using 2 grams a day.

It also *seems* to make sense that if a 220-lb bodybuilder gets good results using a maintenance dose of 10 grams a day of creatine monohydrate, then a woman who weighs 125 lbs might only need 5 grams per day. I would think the same would be true for other supplements.

By the same token, guys who weigh over 220 lbs might need to take more of these supplements to get optimal results. For example, I know some big body-builders (275 pounders) use a maintenance dose of 30 grams of creatine monohydrate a day.

You can assume that the dosages we talk about most often are basically for guys who weigh between 170 and 200 lbs. If you're in that range, you probably don't need to make any adjustments. If you're not in that weight range, you might think about slightly decreasing or increasing your supplement intake in an attempt to "tailor" the dosage to fit your particular physiological needs. Hopefully, future research will provide us with more "exact" info.

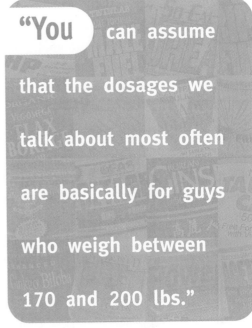

"You can assume that the dosages we talk about most often are basically for guys who weigh between 170 and 200 lbs."

Q **I've read about how the supplement creatine works even better if you can "spike" insulin levels when you take it. After reading this, I came up with the theory that injecting insulin plus taking creatine might produce remarkable results. What do you think of this theory?**

A Taking injectable insulin and loading up on creatine monohydrate may be an extremely potent muscle-size-and-strength-building stack. I've heard that some lifters use ten IU of the long-acting form of insulin first thing in the morning along with ten IU of the short-acting form, then, eight hours later, they inject one more ten IU dose of short-acting insulin. And, on top of this, they load with creatine monohydrate.

Studies have shown that insulin drives creatine into muscle cells, and it promotes additional glycogen uptake. This dramatically increases cell volume, which causes greater strength and promotes huge increases in performance.

A European performance expert I talked with said some athletes are using a new form of insulin called Humalog. This is a new insulin analog of recombinant DNA origin. This insulin analog was discovered by Lilly scientists who found that the time action of insulin could be accelerated by changing the order of two amino acids in the human insulin molecule. Humalog is designed to mimic the body's natural rapid insulin output in response to eating a meal. Current forms of injectable insulin are not absorbed as quickly as naturally occurring insulin.

FREQUENTLY ASKED QUESTIONS AND ANSWERS ABOUT SUPPLEMENTS

CHAPTER 20

ESTIONS AND ANSWERS·QUESTIONS AND ANSWERS·QUESTIONS AND ANSWERS·QUESTIONS AND ANSWERS·QUESTIONS AND ANSWERS·QUESTIONS AND ANSWERS·QUESTIONS AND ANSWERS·QUESTIONS AND ANSWERS·QUESTIONS AND ANSWERS·QUESTIONS AND ANSWERS·QUESTIONS AND ANSWERS·QUESTIONS AND ANSWERS

Unfortunately, using insulin can be extremely dangerous, and I don't recommend it to anyone—especially if you're just a "recreational" weight trainer.

Even without insulin injections, you may still be able to get a hefty boost in size and muscle strength by taking creatine monohydrate along with a simple carbohydrate source, such as grape juice or dextrose. I think 35-50 grams of a simple carbohydrate will produce a significant insulin release and will help shuttle more creatine into muscle cells.

Q What do you think of this new supplement called HGF-1?

A I don't understand what this stuff is supposed to do—I know there are no studies that show it does anything to directly improve muscle size and strength, and when I'm reviewing a supplement that has not yet been studied, I like to look for a theory—a possible mechanism of how it *might* work. I don't have any idea how this stuff could possibly aid in muscle building.

Q Why are the diets of bodybuilders typically devoid of fruits or vegetables? Are meal replacements that complete, or is it possible that there are some nutrients available in fruits or vegetables that most bodybuilders simply aren't getting?

> **"Are** *artificial* vitamins?" Chemically and structurally, there's no difference."

A There are probably a couple of reasons why bodybuilders seem to avoid fruits and vegetables. For one thing, fruits are often seen as being glycemically "incorrect." The fructose they contain is often not what is desired by bodybuilders. As far as vegetables, they often cause gas, are inconvenient, or just don't taste good unless you saturate them with butter.

I guess, ultimately, the question comes down to whether or not it's important to eat fruits and vegetables, especially if you're eating a high-tech meal-replacement product. Well, as far as the vitamin content, you're probably better off drinking the meal replacement. Unfortunately, Mother Nature doesn't regulate the nutrient content of fruits and vegetables, so, for example, the Vitamin C content of two particular oranges could vary enormously. That isn't the case with a meal-replacement drink. If the label says 50% of the RDA for Vitamin C, you can bet that it contains 50% of the RDA (provided it's a reputable brand).

The second question that probably comes to mind is, "Are *artificial* vitamins as good as *natural* vitamins?" Chemically and structurally, there's no difference. If you had a microscope powerful enough to see down to the molecular level, you'd see that "artificial" Vitamin C (or D or E or whatever) is identical to "natural" Vitamin C.

That brings us to the final question: "Is there anything found in fruits and/or vegetables that you can't get in meal-replacement drinks that might be important for overall health?" The answer is, most likely, yes. Fruits and vegetables contain *phytochemicals,* which simply means chemicals found in plants. Many of these chemicals are alleged to have certain disease-fighting properties. For instance, cruciferous vegetables (broccoli, Brussels sprouts, cabbage, cauliflower, collards, kale, kohlrabi, rutabaga, turnip greens, and turnips) contain phytochemicals called "indoles," and indoles stimulate enzymes that make the hormone estrogen less effective. *Voilà,* natural (there's that word again) Nolvadex. By the way, cooking these vegetables either frees up or creates more indoles.

So where does that bring us? There are a couple of answers. On one hand, meal-replacement drinks are better than fruits and vegetables. On the other hand, these drinks contain few, if any, phytochemicals. One thing you can do is buy bags of frozen fruits from the grocery store. Then, when you mix up your meal-replacement drinks, toss in some frozen fruit instead of ice cubes. Keep buying different types of frozen fruit or use those fruit-potpourri bags that contain just about every fruit you can find in North America. Of course, that doesn't take care of your vegetables, does it? What I do every Sunday is cook up a bunch of boneless chicken tenders and freeze them in separate plastic baggies. Then, during my grocery-store run, I buy those pre-mixed bags of garden vegetables for salads that are popular with lazy sons of bitches like myself. Whenever I feel like a snack, I thaw some chicken, pile the chicken on top of some pre-made salad, douse it with fat-free dressing, and scarf down those phytochemicals. There ya go—meal-replacement drinks and fruits and vegetables—the best of all three worlds.

Q **I mix my creatine with my workout drink in the morning, but I don't get around to drinking it until about eight hours later. Is the creatine stable enough to last this long in solution?**

A Creatine isn't totally stable in solution. So it may not be a good idea to keep it mixed with liquid for days, but there's no problem mixing it 8-12 hours before drinking it.

FREQUENTLY ASKED QUESTIONS AND ANSWERS ABOUT SUPPLEMENTS

CHAPTER 20

ESTIONS AND ANSWERS·QUESTIONS AND ANSWERS·QUESTIONS AND ANSWERS·QUESTIONS AND ANSWERS·QUESTIONS AND ANSWERS·QUESTIONS AND ANSWERS·QUESTIONS AND ANSWERS·QUESTIONS AND ANSWERS·QUESTIONS AND ANSWERS·QUESTIONS AND ANSWERS·QUESTIONS AND ANSWERS·QUESTIONS AND ANSWERS

Q **I'm interested in trying a meal-replacement drink like Myoplex Plus, but I'm lactose intolerant. Are there any drinks out there that would work for someone with my problem?**

A Myoplex Plus contains negligible amounts of lactose (it's 99% lactose free), but let's explore your problem anyhow. For some reason, lactose intolerance affects about 75% of the world population but only about 20-25% of the U.S. population. Since people with this problem lack the enzymes necessary to digest milk and milk byproducts, all the lactose hangs around the colon until mercenary bacteria find it and start to break it down. The resulting lactose fermentation and byproducts cause flatulence, diarrhea, and abdominal pain.

The development of the aforementioned symptoms depends on several factors, but most important are the dose of lactose consumed and how fast the lactose is delivered to the colon. Most people who categorize themselves as lactose intolerant avoid milk products like a vegetarian avoids "The 9th Annual Chuck Roast Lollapalooza Meat Fest" at the local Black Angus restaurant. However, recent research shows that this might not be entirely necessary. If you believe the results of a recent study reported in the *Journal of the American Dietetic Association*, small doses of lactose are tolerated well by lactose-intolerant individuals. The study showed that a small dosage of lactose, on the order of about two grams, resulted in no symptoms of intolerance. In fact, doses of up to six grams were tolerated well, even though this dosage resulted in some symptoms of intolerance (a higher rate of hydrogen detected in the breath of test subjects).

The researchers concluded that lactose-intolerant individuals could easily stomach dairy products such as hard cheeses or small servings of regular milk. If their results are correct, a serving of Myoplex Plus, with a lactose content of under one gram per serving, should pose absolutely no problem to individuals who are normally lactose intolerant.

Q **A guy at a health-food store I shop at told me the best way to supplement DHEA is by using wild yam extracts. Is this true?**

A DHEA is made commercially from a plant of the *Dioscorea* family (wild yams) found in abundance in Mexico. Extracts of this plant contain a steroidal saponin which may be converted in a laboratory, by a series of six to eight chemical reactions, into DHEA. A comparable series of reactions is not known to exist in nature and certainly ,not in the human body.

Consequently, it's very unlikely, and in my opinion, impossible, for the ingestion of extracts of the *Dioscorea* plant (or wild yams) to lead to the formation, by metabolic transformation of the relevant plant constituent, to DHEA.

Q The company I work for has a corporate "wellness center," and there's a nutritionist who works there. I was talking to her about various supplements I use. She did something called a "hair analysis" for me, where she cut a few strands of my hair, apparently took them somewhere, analyzed them, and a couple of days later, she told me she could tell from analyzing my hair that I had no nutrient deficiencies; therefore, I'm wasting my money on supplements. She said unless there's a deficiency, there's no need to use a supplement. Is it possible I could be getting all the nutrients I need just from my diet? I do try to eat right.

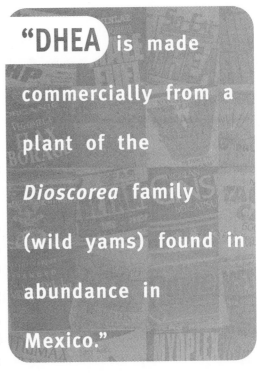

"DHEA is made commercially from a plant of the *Dioscorea* family (wild yams) found in abundance in Mexico."

A *Alrighty then...* hair analysis, huh? I didn't know anyone was still using that—what we do in our studies is have a Ugandan witch doctor come in, take pieces of your clothing and other personal property, and make a voodoo doll which captures your spirit. From there, we can study just about anything—typically we put the voodoo dolls on a Ouija Board, and if they gravitate northward, we know we're looking at Vitamin B deficiencies, and if they gravitate in a south-easterly direction, it's obvious the body has a deficiency in glucose metabolism, and so on. It's really high-tech stuff!

Seriously, the nutritionist to whom you have paid a visit probably has good intentions, but... *she's an idiot.* Hair analysis is <u>not</u>, by any stretch of the imagination, a sound, scientific way to evaluate nutrient deficiencies. Even if it were, it doesn't mean you couldn't benefit from using supplements.

The whole concept that supplementation is merely about making up for clinical vitamin/nutrient deficiencies and whatnot is so "old school" it's ridiculous. The realities of modern-day supplementation (and not just bodybuilding supplementation) are centered on a whole different philosophy—one that is based on sound, scientific theories I would liken to the study of medicine. It's an absolute, 100% valid scientific fact that supplementing the diet with extra amounts of certain nutrients produces effects which cannot be achieved with even the most "perfect" or "balanced" diet.

Now, if you ever want to try that voodoo-doll test, let me know...

321

FREQUENTLY ASKED QUESTIONS AND ANSWERS ABOUT SUPPLEMENTS

ESTIONS AND ANSWERS•QUESTIONS AND ANSWERS•QUESTIONS AND ANSWERS•QUESTIONS AND ANSWERS•QUESTIONS AND ANSWERS•QUESTIONS AND ANSWERS•QUESTIONS AND ANSWERS•QUESTIONS AND ANSWERS•QUESTIONS AND ANSWERS•QUESTIONS AND ANSWERS•QUESTIONS AND ANSWERS•QUESTIONS AND ANSWERS

Q The manager of the health-food store where I buy supplements told me there's a new "micronized" version of DHEA available. Should I be using that instead of regular DHEA?

A Micronized means the DHEA has been processed into small particles which allow it to be absorbed directly from the intestinal tract into the lymphatic system, thus bypassing the liver. Metabolism of DHEA in the liver normally converts DHEA into DHEA sulfate *and* also metabolizes it into *androgens* (such as testosterone). Thus, micronized DHEA might be better for women who want to avoid the excessive androgenic effects of DHEA, but it's *not* a better choice for bodybuilders who are using this compound in hopes of increasing testosterone levels and accelerating muscle growth.

Q A few days ago, I bought a supplement called Zebutol—my friend says it contains steroids and really works great. Do you know exactly which steroid is in Zebutol and how much I should take?

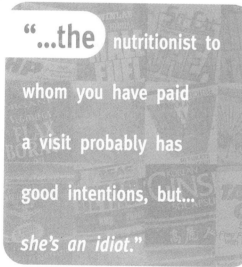

"...the nutritionist to whom you have paid a visit probably has good intentions, but... she's an idiot."

A Zebutol is promoted as a "gray-market" supplement and is distributed by ZOE Discoveries, which has been around for about five or six years. They used to sell several supplements, including a real version of clenbuterol, but I haven't seen much from them lately.

In an effort to provide you with an accurate answer to your question, on December 11, 1996, I sent a sample of this Zebutol supplement out to our lab to have it analyzed by gas chromatography (GC) and high-performance liquid chromatography (HPLC).

It's supposed to contain suma sterol extract, ten milligrams per tablet. Some people believe sterols (which are plant steroids) will produce testosterone-like effects in humans, but I don't think that's true.

Anyway, on December 27, we got the lab results back, and they couldn't find any significant traces of sterols, much less steroids, in this sample.

Bottom line—I think you've been had.

Q I picked up some prescription yohimbine when I was in Mexico. I thought it was great stuff, so when I ran out, I bought a yohimbe supplement at the health-food store. It's supposed to contain eight milligrams of yohimbine. However, when I take the yohimbe, I don't feel anything like I did with the prescription yohimbine. I've tried taking it on an empty stomach, and that doesn't help. I tried using two capsules, and that doesn't help either. Should I try three at once, or is the herbal version just a rip-off?

A Most yohimbe supplements are simply finely ground yohimbe bark. The yohimbine alkaloid (which is trapped in the bark) has very low bioavailability. Your lack of results may be because you're taking the yohimbe on an empty stomach. You would be better off taking it with some kind of animal protein, like chicken, beef, or fish along with some dietary fat. When you do this, the yohimbe supplement stays in the stomach longer, allowing the hydrochloric acid and enzymes to free the alkaloid and make it more bioavailable. An alternative approach would be to empty your yohimbe capsules in a small amount of boiling water with lemon juice. Boil it for about five minutes, and strain the goop through some coffee-filter paper. The filtered liquid should be more bioavailable than the dry powder.

Q A friend of mine is using a bodybuilding supplement called DCP. He says it's a natural product that works like Dianabol. Have you ever heard of this stuff, and do you think I should take it?

A DCP, which is an abbreviation for "dicyclopentanone," isn't a natural supplement, and I certainly wouldn't compare its effects to Dianabol's. This stuff is supposedly a non-steroidal anabolic from Russia, but the only versions I've seen on the U.S. black market are totally amateur knockoffs that have unknown ingredients.

I once took one of these "unknown pills," and within a few minutes, I became so dizzy that I damn near hit the deck.

There's no way of knowing what real DCP would do, and what's in these clandestine, underground, U.S. versions of this crap is an even greater mystery. If I were you, I wouldn't touch this stuff with a ten-foot pole.

Q Last week I bought a fat-burning supplement that contains something called "country mallow." The marketing material which came with this supplement says it is converted to ephedrine in the body. I thought ephedrine came from the herb ephedra. What's the deal?

A As you are most likely aware, ephedra and ephedrine have received a lot of bad press over the past year because some people have taken too much

FREQUENTLY ASKED QUESTIONS AND ANSWERS ABOUT SUPPLEMENTS

CHAPTER 20

ESTIONS AND ANSWERS•QUESTIONS AND ANSWERS•QUESTIONS AND ANSWERS•QUESTIONS AND ANSWERS•QUESTIONS AND ANSWERS•QUESTIONS AND ANSWERS•QUESTIONS AND ANSWERS•QUESTIONS AND ANSWERS•QUESTIONS AND ANSWERS•QUESTIONS AND ANSWERS•QUESTIONS AND ANSWERS•QUESTIONS AND ANSWERS•QUESTIONS AND ANSWERS•QUESTIONS AND ANSWERS

of the herb/drug and have suffered side effects—allegedly, some people have even died from taking too much of this central-nervous-system stimulant.

As a result, some companies have stopped using ephedra and have begun using other compounds, such as country mallow, which is also known as *Sida cordifollia*, a close cousin to ma huang, but it's found in India instead of China. Country mallow does indeed get metabolized into ephedrine and pseudoephedrine in the body.

Q **I'm on the road a lot. Any suggestions on what sports bar, if any, I should use to refuel my body before a workout? I would like something I can use as an afternoon snack before I head off to the gym.**

A It is hard to find a convenient food, but I recently came across one called the Balance Bar.

When you go to the gym to train, you want your blood sugar stable or slightly rising. If you eat foods like rice cakes (glycemic index of 133) or a banana (glycemic index of 68-82), you may feel drowsy halfway through your workout because of your body's ensuing insulin response. The Balance Bar has a glycemic index in the 30-40 range. So it's in the range of low-glycemic-index fruits like Granny Smith apples and peaches. The Balance Bar contains the combination of macronutrients endorsed by Barry "Enter the Zone" Sears and Dan Duchaine. When you are off to the gym, I recommend that you limit your food intake to foods with a glycemic index below 50. PR* Bars are pretty good, too. Both bars can be purchased at your local health-food store.

Q **It seems like all of my sins from the past have come home to roost. A recent sperm count revealed a zero count of live sperm cells. This test was taken two months after a heavy steroid cycle. Am I screwed? Will yohimbine help me?**

A Even if yohimbine helps you in the erection department (if you have such a problem), you'd still be shooting blanks. Yohimbine does nothing to raise testosterone or sperm counts. The current therapy for regenerating sperm counts (let's assume you had a normal live sperm count at one time) is a combination of HCG and Pergonal (made by Serono), which is equal parts luteinizing hormone (LH) and follicle-stimulating hormone (FSH). This is a serious medical condition, and you should see your doctor for it. <u>Don't try a do-it-yourself remedy</u>. The Sertoli cells (that make sperm, not testosterone) respond best to FSH, not LH. HCG or Clomid, which you can get easily in Mexico, won't work nearly as well as the Pergonal. I hope you have insurance because Pergonal is quite the expensive drug.

Q **Does it take longer for my body to digest a meal consisting of solid food like beef or chicken than it does to digest a protein shake?**

A Yes, usually. Whole-food proteins have to be liquefied before the stomach will release them into the small intestine. The hydrochloric acid in the stomach doesn't do the liquefying; it simply activates the various enzymes in the stomach that attack the meat. Some protein powders, such as whey protein, don't really digest in

the stomach. When dissolved in a liquid, whey will simply pass through to the intestines. However, other proteins, especially caseins, actually curdle into a solid in the stomach, similar to cottage cheese, and need further digestion to liquefy. I mention this because some protein companies state that their caseins are more soluble than whey proteins, and this is misleading because whatever superior solubility a casein has in simple water is reversed when it enters the stomach.

Q **A guy at my health-food store told me about a supplement called Goldenseal. He said it's fantastic for bodybuilders. What is it?**

A Goldenseal is an herb that contains the active ingredient *berberine*, an "isoquinolone alkaloid" which some experts believe has powerful effects, including: antibiotic activity, anti-infective activity (the ability to prevent bacteria from adhering to cells), immuno-enhancing effects, fever-lowering characteristics, and anti-cancer activity.

Goldenseal is sometimes used clinically, especially in the Orient, to treat infections and a liver disorder called cirrhosis. A lot of people in the States take it to help treat symptoms of colds and flus.

I searched the literature quite extensively, but I couldn't find any solid scientific studies that support Goldenseal's effects; however, it has a fantastic reputation as being an effective supplement for the ailments listed above.

I also searched the scientific literature extensively but was unable to come up with any direct bodybuilding applications of Goldenseal. Nonetheless, it may have

FREQUENTLY ASKED QUESTIONS AND ANSWERS ABOUT SUPPLEMENTS

ESTIONS AND ANSWERS•QUESTIONS AND ANSWERS•QUESTIONS AND ANSWERS•QUESTIONS AND ANSWERS•QUESTIONS AND ANSWERS•QUESTIONS AND ANSWERS•QUESTIONS AND ANSWERS•QUESTIONS AND ANSWERS•QUESTIONS AND ANSWERS•QUESTIONS AND ANSWERS•QUESTIONS AND ANSWERS•QUESTIONS AND ANSWERS•QUESTIONS AND ANSWERS

CHAPTER 20

indirect benefits because, obviously, if you're ill, you can't train, and the body suffers stress, which can lead to a loss of muscle tissue.

Goldenseal might be something that could help athletes maintain better health, especially during periods of intense training when the immune system can take a beating.

If you decide to try it, I would recommend that you try to find a *standardized extract* preparation. As far as dosage goes, 250-500 mg of the powdered extract, 3 times a day, is what's generally recommended, and it is advised not to exceed this dose, as it might interfere with Vitamin B metabolism. Pregnant women are also advised to avoid all *berberine*-containing plants or supplements.

Q **I've been absolutely amazed to discover how low some of these supplement companies will go to rip off consumers. I couldn't believe that lab report you talked about where the product was supposed to contain 50 grams of protein per serving and it contained only 4.6 grams. Isn't this against the law? Why doesn't the FDA or FTC shut these companies down?**

A Federal government regulatory agencies, like the FDA (Food and Drug Administration) and the FTC (Federal Trade Commission), are basically swamped. They simply don't have the manpower to go after every single company making rip-off claims. Consumer advertising is only one area in which the FTC has responsibility, and in advertising cases, it seems the FTC typically goes after the bigger companies.

Many of the top supplement companies, not just in the bodybuilding industry but also in the general-health markets, weight-loss markets, etc., have been investigated by the FTC, and in many cases, the companies investigated have entered into "consent orders." This is basically an agreement between the company and the FTC that certain "rules" will be strictly adhered to. (Many Fortune 500 companies have consent order agreements with the FTC.)

Typically, what I've seen over the years is many companies that are the greatest offenders—the ones that run the most deceptive ads—never seem to get big enough or advertise enough to be investigated by the FTC. Remember, the FTC doesn't just govern the supplement industry—it has responsibility in lots of areas from consumer advertising and consumer protection laws to antitrust and franchise regulation, just to name a few.

"**If** you found the information in this book helpful, I think you'd really enjoy *Muscle Media*."

326

The FDA is more involved with safety and effectiveness and with labeling for the products it regulates. This encompasses much more than supplements. The FDA does not "approve" supplements, so to speak. But it can take action against companies selling supplements, for labeling violations or for making drug-like claims for a supplement. (For example, if a company were selling a vitamin supplement and claiming it was a cure for cancer, that's a drug claim the FDA would crack down on.) The FDA also has the power to take supplements off the market if they've been shown to be dangerous. This is one of the things they're considering doing with ephedra (the central-nervous-system-stimulating herb which is popular in fat-loss supplements or energy products). But, the FDA has much more to do than watch over the supplement industry—they also oversee human and animal pharmaceuticals, all new medical devices and radiological health, cosmetics, toxicology, and tobacco.

I don't think the FDA nor the FTC will ever have the resources to come in and really clean house in the bodybuilding supplement industry.

Q How do I stay up to date on all the different bodybuilding supplements that come out? How do I tell which ones are real, which ones are fake, and which ones might be worth a try?

A In each issue of my magazine, *Muscle Media*, we discuss those very topics. Not only do we keep bodybuilders informed about what the best new supplements on the market are, we also expose the rip-offs, and we have regular interviews and feature stories with some of the best scientists, doctors, and other experts in the field of sports nutrition.

In each issue of *Muscle Media*, we also talk about the latest breakthroughs in training, nutrition, and virtually anything else that has to do with building muscle and losing fat. If you found the information in this book helpful, I think you'd really enjoy *Muscle Media*.

Muscle Media is distributed on newsstands everywhere, or for subscription information, please call 1-800-297-9776 (ask for Dept. #4062).

Relevant Terms AND JARGON

A number of complex words and scientific terms and jargon are used in this book. If you examine this section of the book carefully, you'll not only expand your functional vocabulary, you'll also be able to derive even more benefits from reading this book. Of course, some of you geniuses will already know all this stuff, but there's nothing wrong with a quick review; for others, some of these terms may be new, and an explanation of what they mean will help—*a lot!*

Additive Effect: This term is often used in scientific jargon when researchers are measuring the effects of two or more substances in a single study. "Additive effect" simply means the combined effect of two or more factors equals the sum of their individual effects in isolation. For example, let's say creatine monohydrate supplementation, by itself, enhances lean body mass by six pounds over a four-week period, and HMB supplementation, by itself, increases lean body mass by two pounds over a four-week period. If their effects are additive, we would expect subjects to gain eight pounds in a four-week period of time when the two products are "stacked."

ADP (Adenosine Diphosphate): This is an important chemical involved in the energy production of a cell. ADP is formed when ATP is broken down within the mitochondria (the cells' "furnaces") to provide energy for muscular contraction. In order to recreate ATP and replenish cellular energy stores, ADP must combine with creatine phosphate.

"All Natural": This is gym jargon for athletes who have not used anabolic steroids for a particular period of time. Usually, natural athletic competitions are open to athletes who have not used steroids or other banned ergogenic aids for a period of no less than 12 months.

Assimilation: This is the process by which foods are absorbed and utilized by the body.

ATP (Adenosine Triphosphate): This is a high-energy molecule stored in muscle and other cells in the body. When a muscle cell needs energy to contract, ATP is broken down to ADP to provide this energy. ATP can be thought of as the actual fuel that makes muscles move. Oxygen and glucose contribute to the formation of ATP. Many distributors of the supplements alleged to be performance-enhancing or ergogenic aids claim the supplements increase oxygen or glucose delivery to the cells. This would, in turn, increase the usable fuel in the form of ATP, hence increasing the duration of muscular endurance.

Aerobic: This means "requiring oxygen." Aerobic metabolism occurs during low-intensity, long-duration exercises, like jogging.

Amino Acids: These are a group of nitrogen-containing, carbon-based organic compounds that serve as the building blocks from which protein (and muscle) is made.

Anabolic: This term refers to promoting anabolism, which is the actual building process of tissues, mainly muscle, in the body. This might occur through the body's own natural reactions to muscular work and proper nutrition or through the introduction of drugs. Anabolism occurs by taking substances from the blood that are essential for growth and repair and using them to stimulate reactions which produce tissue synthesis.

Anabolic Steroids: These are synthetic versions of the male hormone testosterone, a hormone that controls many functions and occurs naturally in the body. Among these functions is the promotion of anabolism. Steroids mimic this naturally occurring event but have the ability to do so at an accelerated rate. Through drastic metabolic changes in the body, anabolic steroids speed up protein synthesis, reduce catabolism, and increase muscle mass and strength in athletes who train with weights. Steroids not only exert their effects on muscles but unfortunately affect many other parts of the body as well. This is why dramatic gains in muscularity are often accompanied by serious side effects.

Anaerobic: This word means "without oxygen." Anaerobic metabolism in muscle tissue occurs during explosive activities like weightlifting or sprinting.

Anti-Catabolism: This is the halting of cellular breakdown in the body. A number of effective nutritional supplements such as glutamine, AKG, and HMB, as well as anabolic steroids, may help promote anti-catabolism. Slowing down the breakdown of protein tips the scales of protein metabolism in favor of new muscle growth.

Anti-Proteolysis: This is a specific type of anti-catabolism: namely, the slowing or halting of protein (muscle) breakdown in the body.

RELEVANT TERMS AND JARGON

Antioxidants: These are little dudes that minimize tissue oxidation and help control free radicals and their nasty effects.

Attenuate: This verb means to weaken, diminish, or reduce. This term is often used to describe the diminishing effect of a drug or supplement over time. For example, if you take the herb ephedra every day, its positive effects "attenuate"— they diminish.

Bioavailability: This is the ease at which nutrients can be absorbed. (This differs from potency.)

Biochemical Reaction: This term refers to the broad range of chemical reactions which take place in all living organisms. Examples of biochemical reactions which occur within the human body are the conversion of blood sugar into energy, the effects of testosterone on muscle cell growth, and nerve impulse reaction, to name only a few of thousands.

Biological Value (BV): This is a measure of protein quality, assessed by how well a given food or food mixture supports nitrogen retention in humans.

Body Composition: This is the percentage of your body composed of fat versus fat-free mass. Very sensitive methods of body composition measurements, including DEXA, can actually subdivide body composition into more specific categories, such as percentage of bone mineral, body water, hair, etc.

Buffer: This is a substance that minimizes changes in hydrogen-ion concentration (pH). Buffers such as sodium phosphate are used by athletes to help reduce lactic-acid buildup during strenuous exercise.

Carbohydrates: These are organic compounds containing carbon, hydrogen, and oxygen. They're a very effective fuel source for the body. The different types of carbohydrates include starches, sugars, and fibers and are classified into three groups—monosaccharides, disaccharides, and polysaccharides. Carbohydrates contain four calories per gram. Glucose—blood sugar—is a carbohydrate used by every cell in the body as fuel.

Catabolic: This is the opposite of anabolic. It means the breakdown of tissue. Catabolic states occur with disease, infection, injury, intense training, strict dieting, and immobilization. Catabolic conditions are not conducive to lean muscle mass gains; in fact, they typically cause a loss of lean muscle mass.

Catabolism: This refers to the breakdown or loss of muscle and other bodily tissues.

Chelating Agents: These are soluble organic compounds that can fit certain metallic ions into their molecular structure. These are often used to increase the absorption of minerals within the body. For example, amino acids are very commonly used as chelating agents for iron and other poorly absorbed minerals.

Cholesterol: This is a type of lipid which, although most widely known as a "bad fat," implicated in promoting heart disease and stroke, is a vital component in the production of many steroid hormones in the body. It also plays a vital role in proper cell-membrane structure and functioning. It's a substrate for bile-acid synthesis, as well as sex-hormone and Vitamin D synthesis. There are different types of cholesterol: namely, HDL and LDL (HDL being the "good" form and LDL being the "bad" form).

Coenzyme: This is a substance which works with an enzyme to promote the enzyme's activity. Many coenzymes have vitamins as part of their structures.

Complete Proteins: These are proteins which contain all the essential amino acids in the right balance.

Cortisol: This is one of the primary catabolic hormones in the body. However, catabolism, or the breakdown of body tissue, is not the only function of cortisol. It is typically secreted in response to physical trauma or prolonged stress. Its functions include controlling inflammation, increasing muscular catabolism and glycolysis (the energy-yielding conversion of glucose to lactic acid), suppressing immune response, and maintaining normal vascular circulation and renal function, among others. Suppressing cortisol production at key times during the day may help bodybuilders avoid excess muscle breakdown. But, you need some cortisol to survive.

Creatine Phosphate (CP): This is an inorganic phosphate molecule which binds with ADP to form ATP. Supplementing with creatine monohydrate helps increase your muscle's CP reserves, which is good!

Cytokine: This term is used to describe a broad range of molecular protein messenger cells. The cytokine family of proteins includes interleukins (powerful anti-carcinogenic agents), interferons (which can be very effective against viral infection), IGF-1 (insulin-like growth factor-1), etc. Cytokines act directly on cells and are very potent agents which can elicit massive changes in cellular function.

RELEVANT TERMS AND JARGON

VANT TERMS AND JARGON~RELEVANT TERMS AND JARGON~RELEVANT TERMS AND JARGON~RELEVANT TERMS AND JARGON~RELEVANT TERMS AND JARGON~RELEVANT TERMS AND JARGON~RELEVANT TERMS AND JARGON~RELEVANT TERMS AND JARGON~RELEVANT TERMS AND JARGON~RELEVANT TERMS AND JARGON~RELEVANT TERMS AND JARGON~RELEVANT TERMS AND JARGON~RELEVANT TERMS

Deficiency: This is a suboptimal level of one or more nutrients that are essential for good health, most often seen with vitamins. Many natural supplements that are marketed to athletes as ergogenic aids are effective at enhancing performance if an individual is deficient in that nutrient. A deficiency can be caused by poor nutrition, increased bodily demands (especially from intense training), or both.

DEXA: This term stands for "dual-energy x-ray absorptiometry." DEXA is a form of total-body x-ray, which is used to determine body composition. This is probably the most accurate method available for measuring bodyfat, lean body mass, bone mineralization, and body water content. This is a very expensive procedure; however, it's an important part of quality clinical trials.

Dextrose: This is simply another name for glucose—the terms are interchangeable (see glucose).

Dipeptides: These are protein fragments made up of only two amino acids.

Disaccharide: This is a carbohydrate compound made up of two sugars. Examples are sucrose (table sugar), lactose (milk sugar), and maltose.

Diuretic: This term can describe any product that increases the amount of urine excreted by the body. Natural diuretics include black tea, coffee, guarana, and dandelion.

Drug: This is the generic name for any substance (except food) used for the prevention, diagnosis, and/or treatment of a disease, as well as the relief of symptoms. The word medicine is usually preferred to describe therapeutic drugs to distinguish them from the addictive drugs which are used illegally.

DSHEA: This is a term which stands for the "Dietary Supplement Health and Education Act of 1994." This law was established by Congress and states that "dietary supplements" are defined as: vitamins, minerals, herbs, or other botanicals (except tobacco), amino acids, any "dietary substance for use by man to supplement the diet by increasing the total dietary intake," and "a concentration, metabolite, constituent, extract, or combination of any of the above-listed ingredients."

Efficacious: This means producing the desired effect—that "it works."

Electrolytes: These are substances which, in solution, are capable of conducting electricity. These charged particles are present throughout the body and are involved in many activities such as regulating the distribution of water inside and outside cells in the body. Examples include the bulk minerals, potassium, sodium, and chloride.

332

Empirical Data: This is information based on observation and experience, not scientific reasoning. Empirical data is often very accurate, although it is not accepted as scientifically sound; however, no area of science is devoid of a real-world/empirical component.

Energy: This is the capacity to do work. The energy in food is chemical energy: it can be converted to mechanical, electrical, or heat energy. Energy is sometimes measured in "calories."

Endogenous: This term refers to things that occur naturally in the body. For example, the testosterone your body produces naturally is "endogenous."

Enzyme: This is a protein molecule that acts as a "helper" in thousands of chemical reactions in the body, including: digestion of food, hormone production, muscle cell repair—literally thousands and thousands of things.

Ergogenic: This word refers to something that can increase muscular work capacity. Natural supplements which can increase some aspect of athletic performance are said to be ergogenic or performance-enhancing aids.

Essential Fatty Acids (EFA's): These are fats that our bodies can't make, so we must obtain them through our diets. These fats (which include linoleic and linolenic acid) are very important to hormone production, as well as cellular synthesis and integrity. Good sources of these fats are flaxseed oil and safflower oil.

Exogenous: This term refers to things originating outside of the body. For example, if you took a DHEA pill, it would be an "exogenous" source of that hormone.

Fat: This is one of the macronutrients. Fat contains nine calories per gram; it has the most calories of all the macronutrients. Dietary fats may also be referred to as lipids or triglycerides. Fats serve a variety of functions in the body; they act as structural components for all cell membranes, as well as supply necessary chemical substrates for hormone production. There are two types of fat—saturated "bad" fat and unsaturated "good" fat.

Fat-Free Mass (FFM): This refers to all portions of body tissues not containing fat. These tissues include all skeletal bones and muscles, skin, organs, and body water, as well as hair, blood, and lymph. Fat-free mass is a term used frequently in the texts of clinical studies. Often, an increase in fat-free mass equals an increase in skeletal muscle.

333

•SPORTS SUPPLEMENT REVIEW, 3RD ISSUE•SPORTS SUPPLEMENT REVIEW, 3RD ISSUE•SPORTS SUPPLEMENT REVIEW, 3RD ISSUE•SPORTS SUPPLEMENT REVIEW, 3RD ISSUE•SPORTS SUPPLEMENT REVIEW, 3RD ISSUE•SPORTS SUPPLEMENT REVIEW, 3RD ISSUE•SPORTS SUPPLEMENT REVIEW, 3RD ISSUE•SPORTS SUPPLEMENT REVIEW, 3RD ISSUE•SPORTS SUPPLEMENT

RELEVANT TERMS AND JARGON

VANT TERMS AND JARGON~RELEVANT TERMS AND JARGON~RELEVANT TERMS AND JARGON~RELEVANT TERMS AND JARGON~RELEVANT TERMS AND JARGON~RELEVANT TERMS AND JARGON~RELEVANT TERMS AND JARGON~RELEVANT TERMS AND JARGON~RELEVANT TERMS AND JARGON~RELEVANT TERMS

Free-Form Amino Acids: These are structurally <u>un</u>linked, individual amino acids.

Free Radicals: These are troublemakers. They're highly reactive molecules possessing unpaired electrons which are produced during metabolism of food and energy production and are believed to contribute to the molecular damage and death of vital body cells. Free radicals may be a factor in aging or disease and may ultimately contribute to death. Antioxidants help neutralize free radicals.

Fructose: This is the main type of sugar found in fruit. It's sweeter than sucrose (table sugar) and has a low glycemic index (GI). In other words, eating fructose won't cause nearly as dramatic a release of insulin as glucose (dextrose). Eating a high-fructose diet may increase blood fats. Because of its low glycemic index and because it's metabolized mostly in the liver, fructose is often used as a sugar substitute for diabetics.

Full-Spectrum Amino Acids: These are supplements which contain a combination of all of the essential amino acids.

Glycemic Index (GI): This is a measure of the extent to which a food raises the blood sugar (glucose) level as compared with white bread, which has a GI of 100. Glucose (dextrose) scores a 138, brown rice an 81, and fructose (fruit sugar) is all the way down at 31.

Glycogen: This is the principal storage form of carbohydrate energy (glucose) which is reserved in muscles and in the liver. When your muscles are full of glycogen, they look and feel full/pumped.

Growth Hormone (GH): This is a hormone that is naturally released by the pituitary gland; it is an anabolic hormone. GH promotes muscle growth and the breakdown of bodyfat for energy. GH levels are high in children and in teens but diminish greatly after age 20. Some sports supplements are supposed to increase the amount of GH which is naturally released in the body and therefore create an anabolic state and increase fat burning in the athlete. Unfortunately, most have little effect.

Glucagon: This is a hormone which is responsible for helping maintain proper blood sugar levels. When blood sugar levels go too low, glucagon activates glucose production in the liver, as well as regulates the release of glycogen from muscle cells. Eventually it may cause the catabolism of muscle cell proteins for glucose. This is considered a catabolic hormone.

Glucose: This is the simplest sugar molecule. It's also the main sugar found in blood and is used as a basic fuel for the body. When you eat complex carbs, they're broken down by the body into glucose. Glucose is also found in various fruits, but not in as high concentrations as sucrose and fructose, two other sugars. However, when you eat too much glucose, it's converted to fatty acids and triglycerides by the liver and adipose (fatty) tissue. Due to its quick absorption by the body, it's often used as an invigorating and strengthening agent in many medicinal formulations. It will cause your body to release a rapid and large amount of insulin to counteract the large influx of sugar.

HDL: This stands for "high-density lipoprotein." It's one of the subcategories of cholesterol—typically thought of as the "good" cholesterol. HDL cholesterol is the form which is typically used to clear fats from the system, therefore not lending itself to the formation of crud in your arteries that can cause heart attacks. You may be able to raise your HDL cholesterol levels by ingesting quality unsaturated fats like flaxseed oil. Exercise has also been shown to increase HDL levels.

Hormones: These are substances in the body which are very important to bodybuilders. Two important hormone-producing organs are the pituitary gland and the testes. Hormones regulate various biological processes through their ability to activate or deactivate enzymes. Examples of this regulation are the effect of the testosterone hormone on the enzymatic activity relating to protein production of muscle cells. Other hormones, such as insulin and glucagon, control blood sugar levels and energy storage in the body. Hormones can be made of proteins (like insulin and growth hormone) or cholesterol (like testosterone and estrogen).

Hydrolysis: This is a chemical reaction where water reacts with a substance to change it to another substance or substances. For instance, if you add sodium acetate to water, it hydrolyses into sodium ions and acetate ions.

Hypertrophy: This means to increase in size. Muscular hypertrophy is the increase in size of the muscle cells.

Hypoglycemia: This is low blood sugar/glucose levels, resulting in anxiety, fatigue, perspiration, delirium, and in severe cases, coma. Hypoglycemia occurs most commonly in diabetics where it is due to either insulin overdose or inadequate intake of carbohydrates. Temporary hypoglycemia is common in athletes and can be overcome with the ingestion of carbohydrates.

Incomplete Proteins: These are proteins that lack or are low in one or more of the essential amino acids.

RELEVANT TERMS AND JARGON

VANT TERMS AND JARGON~RELEVANT TERMS AND JARGON~RELEVANT TERMS AND JARGON~RELEVANT TERMS AND JARGON~RELEVANT TERMS AND JARGON~RELEVANT TERMS AND JARGON~RELEVANT TERMS AND JARGON~RELEVANT TERMS AND JARGON~RELEVANT TERMS AND JARGON~RELEVANT TERMS

Insulin: This is an anabolic hormone secreted by the pancreas that aids the body in maintaining proper blood sugar levels and promoting glycogen storage. Insulin secretion speeds the movement of nutrients through the bloodstream and into muscle for growth. When chronically elevated, as with a high-carbohydrate diet, insulin can cause you to gain fat. However, short bursts of insulin, caused by consuming high-glycemic carbs, may help enhance the uptake of nutrients like creatine and glutamine by muscle cells.

Jargon: This is specialized language concerned with a particular subject. For example, surfers say "hang ten" which refers to... well... I don't know what it refers to, but that's what jargon is—words and catch phrases certain "insiders" know but others don't.

Ketones: These are organic chemical compounds resulting from the breakdown of triglycerides. They are used as an energy source in the body during very-low-carbohydrate diets.

Lactic Acid: This is a molecule produced from glucose during anaerobic metabolism. When oxygen becomes available, lactic acid can be completely broken down to carbon dioxide and water. Lactic-acid buildup is a primary cause of muscle fatigue. Supplements that limit lactic-acid buildup may enhance athletic performance.

Lean Body Mass (LBM): This is another term which describes fat-free mass (see fat-free mass).

LDL: This stands for "low-density lipoprotein" and is a subcategory of cholesterol, typically thought of as the "bad" cholesterol. LDL is the type of cholesterol that circulates throughout the bloodstream and may cause heart disease. Levels of LDL cholesterol can be elevated by ingestion of saturated fats and a lack of exercise.

Limiting Factor: This is an element that prevents a process or reaction from taking place. For example, a lack of protein in the diet can be a "limiting factor" for muscle growth.

Linolenic Acid: This is an essential fatty acid and, more precisely, an omega-3 polyunsaturated fatty acid. It is found in high concentrations in flaxseed oil.

Linoleic Acid: This is an essential fatty acid and, more specifically, an omega-6 polyunsaturated fatty acid. Good sources of this fatty acid are safflower oil and soybean oil.

Lipid: This is simply another name for dietary fats or triglycerides.

Lipogenic: This means making bodyfat (literally translated "fat producing"). This is bad.

Lipolysis: This term refers to the chemical breakdown of bodyfat by enzymes which results in stored bodyfat being used as fuel by the body. This is good.

Lipolytic: This term is usually used to describe something with fat-burning effects. It literally means "to disintegrate fat."

Luteinizing Hormone (LH): This is a powerful hormone which, in men, stimulates the testes to make testosterone. (Yeah!) In gals, LH induces ovulation.

Macronutrients: These are the nutrients that we ingest in large (macro means "big") quantities on a regular basis. These include proteins, carbohydrates, fats, and I guess, water. All of these macronutrients are necessary to sustain life.

Malabsorption: This big word means bad absorption of nutrients from the digestive tract. This can result in vitamin deficiencies, loss of weight, and poor health. Malabsorption can be caused by intestinal diseases or lack of digestive enzymes.

Meal-Replacement Powders (MRP's): These are a category of supplements which contain protein, carbohydrates, vitamins, minerals, and other key nutrients which are used to replace a regular-food meal for purposes of weight loss, weight gain, or increasing dietary nutrient intake. These supplements may also be referred to as "total-nutrition products," "engineered foods," or "superfoods." (Try finding that definition in Webster's!)

Metabolic Rate: This refers to the rate you convert energy stores into working energy in the body. In other words, it's how fast your "whole system" runs. The metabolic rate is controlled by a number of factors, including: muscle mass (the greater your muscle mass, the greater your metabolic rate), caloric intake, exercise, and use of stimulant or depressant chemicals.

Metabolism: This is a frequently used term which refers to the utilization of nutrients by the body for both anabolic and catabolic processes. It's the process by which substances come into the body and the rate at which they are utilized.

Micronutrients: These are dietary nutrients which we ingest in relatively small (micro means "small") amounts compared to macronutrients. Examples of micronutrients include vitamins and minerals. Many micronutrients are essential dietary nutrients

RELEVANT TERMS AND JARGON

VANT TERMS AND JARGON~RELEVANT TERMS AND JARGON~RELEVANT TERMS AND JARGON~RELEVANT TERMS AND JARGON~RELEVANT TERMS AND JARGON~RELEVANT TERMS AND JARGON~RELEVANT TERMS AND JARGON~RELEVANT TERMS AND JARGON~RELEVANT TERMS AND JARGON~RELEVANT TERMS AND JARGON~RELEVANT TERMS

which perform vital functions in the body. Micronutrients are typically ingested in gram quantities or less.

Minerals: These are naturally occurring, inorganic substances that are essential for human life and play a role in many vital metabolic processes.

Monosaccharide: This is a simple carbohydrate made up of one sugar molecule. Examples are glucose and fructose.

Muscle Fatigue: This is the failure of a muscle to continue to perform work, caused by muscle ATP depletion. Lactic-acid buildup also plays a role in muscle fatigue. Some natural supplements marketed to athletes have the ability to postpone muscle fatigue, thus increasing the work potential of the muscle—one of the most potent is creatine, which increases the availability of ATP, which is used for energy.

Myocyte: This means "muscle cell."

Natural: This term is often used to refer to foods or supplements that are not highly refined and which do not contain chemical fertilizers or artificial flavors and colors. The word natural has no legal definition in food supplementation though.

Net Protein Utilization (NPU): This is a method of evaluating protein quality by comparing the amount animals retained to the amount they ingested. Evaluation parameters are digestibility and essential amino acid content. (Don't worry, I don't understand it either.)

Neurotransmitter: This is a substance that is released at the end of one nerve cell when a nerve impulse arrives there. Neurotransmitters diffuse across the gap to the next nerve cell and alter the membrane of that cell in such a way that it becomes less or more likely to fire. Examples include adrenaline and serotonin. Adrenaline is responsible for the "fight-or-flight" response and is an excitatory neurotransmitter; serotonin is the opposite—it makes you sleepy.

Nitrogen: This is an element that distinguishes proteins from other substances and allows them to form various structural units in our bodies, including enzymes and muscle cells.

Nitrogen Balance: This is when a person's daily intake of nitrogen from proteins equals the daily excretion of nitrogen: a negative nitrogen balance occurs when the excretion of nitrogen exceeds the daily intake and is often seen when muscle is being lost. A positive nitrogen balance is often associated with muscle growth.

Nutrients: These are components of food that help nourish the body: that is, they provide energy or serve as "building materials." These nutrients include carbohydrates, fats, proteins, vitamins, minerals, water, etc.

Omega-3: This is the name of the first spacecraft that landed on the moon. (Nah, I'm just kidding—I was seeing if you were paying attention. This chapter is boring, huh?!) Omega-3 is actually a name for a certain fatty acid. The "3" designates where the first double-bond is located in the fatty acid carbon chain. Linolenic acid is an example of an omega-3 fatty acid.

Omega-6: This is another name for a fatty acid. "Omega-6" refers to the first double-bond on a fatty acid chain which is located at the sixth carbon acid. Linoleic acid is an example of an omega-6 fatty acid.

Optimal Nutrition: This is a term you need to know. It means the *best possible nutrition*; distinct from merely adequate nutrition which is characterized by no overt deficiency. This term describes people free from marginal deficiencies, imbalances, and toxicities, and who are not at risk for such. All athletes making an effort to increase muscle growth naturally must try to achieve optimal nutrition. In many cases, this requires supplementation of protein, vitamins and minerals, and possibly other conditionally essential nutrients such as glutamine and creatine.

Over-The-Counter (OTC): This refers to substances that do not require a prescription to be obtained legally.

Oxidation: This is the process of cellular decomposition and breakdown. Oxidation produces free radicals.

Oxygen Debt: What this means to me is "out of breath." It's a deficiency of oxygen in working muscles when performing exercise that is so demanding the cardiovascular system cannot deliver oxygen fast enough to the muscles to support aerobic metabolism. The debt must be repaid by rapid breathing after the activity slows down or stops. Oxygen debt leads to anaerobic metabolism, which leads to lactic-acid buildup and muscle fatigue.

Peptide: This is a compound made up of two or more amino acids. Protein molecules are broken down into peptides in the gut and absorbed in that form.

RELEVANT TERMS AND JARGON

VANT TERMS AND JARGON~RELEVANT TERMS AND JARGON~RELEVANT TERMS AND JARGON~RELEVANT TERMS AND JARGON~RELEVANT TERMS AND JARGON~RELEVANT TERMS AND JARGON~RELEVANT TERMS AND JARGON~RELEVANT TERMS AND JARGON~RELEVANT TERMS AND JARGON~RELEVANT TERMS AND JARGON~RELEVANT TERMS

Pineal Gland: This is an endocrine gland that functions mainly in the secretion of melatonin and a few other peptide hormones.

Phytochemical: This term means "plant chemical." It's used to refer to a broad spectrum of bio-active plant compounds which are typically used in herbal preparations and a variety of other nutrition supplements.

Placebo: This is a harmless, "inactive" substance which may be given in the place of an effective drug or substance, especially to "control groups" in clinical studies. In many cases, individuals using a placebo will react positively as though they were using an efficacious compound. Some of the positive effects performance athletes experience while using natural supplements are attributed to a "placebo effect." Basically, if you strongly believe a supplement will work, there is a chance that belief alone will produce positive results. It is even theorized that many of the positive effects athletes experience while using anabolic steroids can be attributed to a placebo effect. This is why it's important to do placebo-controlled scientific studies—to separate real effects from "placebo effects."

Polypeptides: These are proteins formed by the union of three or more (usually many) amino acids.

Polysaccharides: These are carbohydrates containing a large number of "sugar groups." Starch, glycogen, dextrin, and cellulose are examples.

Precursors: These are compounds from which another compound is formed. For example, the hormone androstenedione is a direct precursor to testosterone production in the body.

Prohormone: This term refers to a class of chemicals typically found inside various glands in the body, such as the pituitary and adrenal glands. These chemicals are the direct precursors to hormone production: e.g., proinsulin is the direct precursor to insulin. DHEA and melatonin are also prohormones.

Prostaglandins: These are "hormone-like" chemicals produced in the body. Their structure is much like that of a fatty acid, and they exhibit a wide range of actions on things like blood pressure, water balance, immune system reactions, inflammation, etc. Their synthesis, in almost all tissues in the body, is partially controlled by fatty acid intake.

Proteins: These are highly complex nitrogen-containing compounds found in all animal and vegetable tissues. They are made up of amino acids and are essential for growth and repair in the body. A gram of protein contains four calories. Those from animal sources are high in biological value since they contain the essential amino acids. Those from vegetable sources contain some but not all of the essential amino acids. Proteins are broken up by the body to produce amino acids which are used to build new proteins. Proteins are the building blocks of muscle, enzymes and some hormones.

Protein Efficiency Ratio (PER): This is a measure of protein quality assessed by determining how well a given protein supports weight gain in laboratory animals: namely, rats. The PER is probably not the best rating system because it overestimates methionine needs due to the greater need for methionine in rats for hair production, but, whatever.

Pure: This term is often used to refer to supplements that are unadulterated—that have no other ingredient in them except that which is stated on the label.

Saturated Fats: These are bad fats. They are called "saturated" because they contain no open spots on their "carbon skeletons." Saturated fats include myristic acid, palmitic acid, stearic acid, arachidic acid, and lignoceric acid. These bad fats have been shown to raise cholesterol levels in the body. Sources of these fats include animal foods and hydrogenated vegetable oils, such as margarine. These fats serve no biological function in the body, other than to supply calories.

Stacking: This term refers to taking two or more compounds at once in an attempt to maximize results.

Sublingual: This means "beneath the tongue." Several supplements available to athletes are made to be taken in this manner. This occasionally results in better absorption. Some suggest hormonal preparations be taken sublingually to avoid the harsh environment of the gut.

341

Sucrose: This is most commonly known as table sugar. Industrially, sucrose is derived from sugar cane or sugar beets. When you eat it, the body breaks sucrose into fructose and glucose. Consequently, it has some of the properties of fructose and some of the properties of glucose. Eating it will elicit a rapid insulin response but not as high as that caused by glucose.

Supplement: This is a term used to describe a preparation such as a pill, powder, or liquid which contains nutrients. A supplement is to be used as part of a person's daily food intake to either supply adequate or supraphysiological levels of a nutrient.

Supraphysiological: This big word means amounts greater than normally found in the body. For example, a person consuming ten grams of creatine monohydrate per day will create supraphysiological levels of creatine in muscle cells.

Synergistic: This term refers to an action that is created when things "cooperate" with one another: that is, one supplement could enhance or multiply the effectiveness of another supplement. Many vitamins have been found to be synergistic. Creatine plus carbs is synergistic, as is caffeine plus ephedrine, in the right amounts.

Testes: This term refers to the male reproductive organs. The testes are where many of the hormones that regulate growth, such as testosterone, are produced.

Testosterone: This is *the* anabolic hormone produced primarily by the testes in men, which makes muscles grow. It literally separates the men from the boys.

Thermogenic: This term means heat producing or fat burning. Taking a thermogenic agent will speed up the metabolism, raise core body temperature, and accelerate calorie expenditure.

Triglyceride: This is the scientific name for a common dietary fat. The backbone of the molecule is a glycerol molecule which is connected to three fatty acid molecules. Triglycerides are also called fats or lipids.

Tripeptides: These are protein fragments which are three amino acids long.

Unsaturated Fats: These are "good" fats. They are called unsaturated because they have one or more open "carbon spots." Unsaturated fats can be divided into two categories: polyunsaturated fats and monounsaturated fats. Unsaturated fats have been shown to help reduce cholesterol and triglyceride levels in the blood. This category of fats includes the essential fatty acids linoleic and linolenic. The main sources of these fats are from plant foods, such as safflower, sunflower, and flaxseed oils.

Up-regulate: This term basically means "increase." For example, creatine monohydrate appears to have the ability to up-regulate or increase the muscle's ability to replenish energy stores.

Vitamins: These are organic compounds which are vital to life, indispensable to bodily function, and needed in minute amounts. They are non-caloric essential nutrients. Many of them function as coenzymes, supporting a multitude of biological functions.

VO₂max: This is the maximum volume of oxygen an individual can consume per minute of work. It is often used to evaluate an athlete's cardiovascular efficiency and, thus, performance capacity.

The End: That means this section is over. (Thank God!)

References CITED

1   A.S. Abraham, et al., "The Effects of Chromium Supple-mentation on Serum Glucose and Lipids in Patients With and Without Non-Insulin Dependent Diabetes," *Metabolism* 41 (1992) : 768-771.

2   N. Abumrad, et al., "ß-Hydroxy ß-Methylbutyrate Increases Fatty Acid Oxidation by Muscle Cells," *FASEB J.* 11.3 (1997) : A381.

3   Z. Acs, et al., "Role of Hypothalamic Factors (Growth-Hormone-Releasing Hormone and Gamma-Aminobutyric Acid) in the Regulation of Growth Hormone Secretion in the Neonatal and Adult Rat," *Neuroendocrinology* 52.2 (1990) : 156-160.

4   M. Allard, "Treatment of Old Age Disorders with Ginkgo Biloba Extract," *La Presse Medicale* 15.31 (1986) : 1540.

5   J.F. Aloia, et al., "Calcium Supplementation With and Without Hormone Replacement Therapy to Prevent Postmenopausal Bone Loss," *Annals. Intern. Med.* 120 (1994) : 97-103.

6   J.L. Ambrus, et al., "Absorption of Exogenous and Endogenous Proteolytic Enzymes," *Clin. Pharmacol. Thera.* 8.3 (1967) : 362-368.

7   R.A. Anderson, "Chromium, Glucose Tolerance, and Diabetes," *Biol. Trace Elem. Res.* 32 (1992) : 19-24.

8   R.A. Anderson, et al., "Effects of Supplemental Chromium on Patients with Symptoms of Reactive Hypoglycemia," *Metabolism* 36 (1987) : 351-355.

9   Anonymous Author, "The Role of Growth Hormone in the Action of Vitamin B_6 on Cellular Transfer of Amino Acids: A Review," *Nutr. Rev.* 37 (1979) : 300-301.

10   S.M. Antelman, et al., "Tail Pinch Induced Eating, Gnawing and Licking Behavior in Rats: Dependence on the Nigrostriatal Dopamine System," *Brain Research* 99 (1975) : 319-337.

11   M. Araghiniknam, et al., "Antioxidant Activity of Dioscorea and Dehydroepiandrosterone (DHEA) in Older Humans," *Life Sci.* 59.11 (1996) : 147-157.

12   A. Astrup, et al., "Pharmacology of Thermogenic Drugs," *Am. J. Clin. Nutr.* 55.1 (1992) : 246S-248S.

13   A. Astrup, et al., "The Effect and Safety of an Ephed-rine/Caffeine Compound Compared to Ephedrine, Caffeine and Placebo in Obese Subjects on an Energy Restricted Diet," *Int. J. Obes.* 16.4 (1992) : 269-277.

14   A. Astrup, et al., "The Effect of Ephedrine/Caffeine Mixture on Energy Expenditure and Body Composition in Obese Women," *Metabolism: Clinical and Experimental* 41.7 (1992) : 686-688.

15   M. Auguet, et al., "Bases Pharmacologiques de l'Impact Vasculair de l'Extrait de Ginkgo Biloba," *La Presse Medicale* 15.31 (1986) : 1524.

16   M.S. Bahrke, et al., "Evaluation of the Ergogenic Properties of Ginseng," *Sports Med.* 18.4 (1994) : 229-248.

17   P.D. Balsom, et al., "Creatine Supplementation and Dynamic High-Intensity Intermittent Exercise," *Scan. J. Med. Sci. Sports* 3 (1993) : 143-149.

18   P.D. Balsom, et al., "Skeletal Muscle Metabolism During Short-Duration High-Intensity Exercise: Influence of Creatine Supplementation," *Acta. Physiol. Scand.* 154.3 (1995) : 303-310.

19   P. Balsom, et al., "Creatine in Humans with Special Reference to Creatine Supplementation," *Sports Med.* 18.4 (1994) : 268-280.

20   C.A. Barth, et al., "Endocrine Responses to Animal and Vegetable Protein," *Milk Proteins* (New York: Springer Verlag, 1989) 62-67.

21   F. Battaini and A. Peterkofsky, "Histidyl-Proline Diketop-iperazine as Endogenous Brain Peptide that Inhibits $(Na^+ + K^+)$ATPase," *Biochem. Biophys. Res. Commum.* 94 (1980) : 240-247.

22   I. Beladi, et al., "In Vitro and In Vivo Antiviral Effects of Flavonoids," In: *Flavonoids and Bioflavonoids*, L. Farkas, et al., (Eds.) (New York, NY: Elsevier, 1982) 443-450.

23   M.A. Belury and J.P. Vanden, "Protection Against Cancer and Heart Disease by the Dietary Fatty Acid, Conjugated Linoleic Acid: Potential Mechanisms of Action," *Nut. Dis. Update* 1.2 (In Press, 1997).

24   B. Benendonk, *The Gold, The Glory...and The Decay* (Horten, Norway: Hilton Publishing, 1993).

25   D. Benton, et al., "The Impact of Long-Term Vitamin Supplementation on Cognitive Functioning," *Psychophar-macol.* 117 (1995) : 298-305.

26   J.W. Berg, et al., "Epidemiology of Gastrointestinal Cancer," *Proc. Natl. Cancer Congr.* 7 (1973) : 459-463.

27   M. Berlan, et al., "Plasma Catecholamine Levels and Lipid Mobilization Induced by Yohimbine in Obese and Non-Obese Women," *Int. J. Obes.* 15.5 (1991) : 305-315.

28   F. Bloomstrand, et al., "Administration of Branched-Chain Amino Acids During Sustained Exercise. The Effects on Performance and Plasma Concentrations of Some Amino Acids," *J. Appl. Physiol.* 68 (1991) : 83-88.

29   E.R. Blough, et al., "Developmental Myosin Expression in Fast Quail Muscle After Wing Weighting and Unweighting," *Med. Sci. Sports Exerc.* 27.5 (1995) : S142.

30   A. Bonati, "How and Why Should We Standardize Phytopharmical Drugs for Clinical Validation?" *J. Ethnopharmacol.* 32 (1991) : 195-197.

31   D. Bordin, et al., "High Intensity Physical Exercise Induced Effects on Plasma Levels of Copper and Zinc," *Biol. Trace Elem. Res.* 36.2 (1993) : 129-134.

32   I.G. Borisova, et al., "Action of Antioxidants on Physical Work Capacity and Lipid Peroxidation in the Body," *Farmakol. Toksikol.* 52.4 (1989) : 89-92.

33   M. Borkman, et al., "The Relationship Between Insulin Sensitivity and the Fatty Acid Composition of Skeletal-Muscle Phospholipids," *N. Engl. J. Med.* 328 (1993) : 238-244.

34   G. Bounous, et al., "Immunoenhancing Property of Dietary Whey Protein in Mice: Role of Glutathione," *Clin. Invest. Med.* 12.3 (1989) : 154-161.

35 G. Bounous, et al., "Whey Proteins in Cancer Prevention," *Cancer Lett.* 57.2 (1991) : 91-94.

36 G. Bounous, et al., "The Influence of Dietary Whey Protein on Tissue Glutathione and the Diseases of Aging," *Clin. Invest. Med.* 12.6 (1989) : 343-349.

37 M. Braga, et al., "Pancreatic Enzyme Replacement Therapy in Post-Pancreatectomy Patients," *Int. J. Pancreatol.* 5 Suppl. (1989) : 37-44.

38 L. Breum, et al., "Comparison of an Ephedrine/Caffeine Combination and Dexfenfluramine in the Treatment of Obesity: A Double-Blind Multi-Center Trial in General Practice," *Int. J. Obes.* 18 (1994) : 99-103.

39 L.R. Brilla and T.F. Haley, "Effect of Magnesium Supplementation on Strength Training in Humans," *J. Amer. Coll. Nutr.* 11.3 (1992).

40 G.J. Brisson, *Lipids in Human Nutrition.* (Inglewood, NY: Burgess, 1981).

41 J.G. Brook, et al., "Dietary Soya Lecithin Decreases Plasma Triglyceride Levels and Inhibits Collagen- and ADP-Induced Platelet Aggregation," *Biochem. Med. Metabol. Biol.* 35 (1986) : 31-39.

42 S.P. Bydlowski, et al., "A Novel Property of an Aqueous Guarana Extract (Paullinia Cupana): Inhibition of Platlet Aggregation In Vitro and In Vivo," *Braz. J. Med. Biol. Res.* 21.3 (1988) : 535-538.

43 R. Cade, et al., "Effects of Phosphate Loading on 2,3-Diphosphoglycerate and Maximal Oxygen Uptake," *Med. Sci. Sports Exerc.* 16.3 (1984) : 263-268.

44 D.R. Campbell and M.S. Kurzer, "Flavonoid Inhibition of Aromatase Enzyme Activity in Human Preadipocytes," *J. Steroid Biochem. Mol. Biol.* 46.3 (1993) : 381-388.

45 F.P. Cappuccio, et al., "Epidemiologic Association Between Dietary Calcium Intake and Blood Pressure: A Meta-Analysis of Published Data," *Am. J. Epidemiol.* 142 (1995) : 935-945.

46 J.K. Caro, et al., "Decreased Cerebrospinal-Fluid/Serum Leptin Ratio in Obesity: A Possible Mechanism for Leptin Resistance," *Lancet* 348.9021 (1996) : 159-161.

47 A. Casey, et al., "Creatine Supplementation Favourably Affects Performance and Muscle Metabolism During Maximal Intensity Exercise in Humans," *Am. J. Physiol.* 271 (1996) : E31-37.

48 F. Cavagnini, et al., "Effect of Acute and Repeated Administration of Gamma Aminobutyric Acid (GABA) on Growth Hormone and Prolactin Secretion in Man," *Acta Endocrinol.* 93.2 (1980) : 149-154.

49 K. Chandan, et al., "Oxidative Stress After Human Exercise: Effect of N-Acetylcysteine Supplementation," *J. Appl. Physiol.* 76.6 (1994) : 2570-2577.

50 R.M. Chandler, et al., "Dietary Supplements Affect the Anabolic Hormones After Weight-Training Exercise," *J. Appl. Physiol.* 76.2 (1994) : 839-845.

51 L.P. Chepkii, et al., "The Pharmacological Correction of Disorders of the Oxygen Transport Function of the Blood in Peritonitis Patients," *Anesteziol. Reanimatol.* 1 (1990) : 47-50.

52 A.N. Chiang, et al., "Excess Energy and Nitrogen Balance at Protein Intakes Above the Requirement Level in Young Men," *Am. J. Clin. Nutr.* 48 (1988) : 1015-1022.

53 S.F. Chin, et al., "Conjugated Linoleic Acid is a Growth Factor for Rats as Shown by Enhanced Weight Gain and Improved Feed Efficiency," *J. Nutr.* 124.12 (1994) : 2344-2349.

54 B. Chua, et al., "Effect of Leucine and Metabolites of Branched-Chain Amino Acids on Protein Turnover in Heart," *J. Biol. Chem.* 254 (1979) : 8358-8362.

55 S.P. Clancy, et al., "Effects of Chromium Picolinate Supplementation on Body Composition, Strength, and Urinary Chromium Loss in Football Players," *Int. J. Sport Nutr.* 4.2 (1994) : 142-153.

56 P.M. Clarkson and E.M. Haymes, "Exercise and Mineral Status of Athletes: Calcium, Magnesium, Phosphorus, and Iron," *Med. Sci. Sports Exerc.* 27.6 (1995) : 831-843.

57 N. Cohen, et al., "Oral Vanadyl Sulfate Improves Hepatic and Peripheral Insulin Sensitivity in Patients with Non-Insulin-Dependent Diabetes Mellitus," *J. Clin. Invest.* 95.6 (1995) : 2501-2509.

58 H. Cole, "Enzyme Activity May Hold the Key to Cataract Activity," *JAMA* 254.8 (1985) : 1008.

59 A. Constantinescu, et al., "Alpha-Lipoic Acid Protects Against Hemolysis of Human Erythrocytes Induced by Peroxyl Radicals," *Biochem. Mol. Biol. Int.* 33.4 (1994) : 669-679.

60 B. Contempre, et al., "Effect of Selenium Supplementation on Thyroid Hormone Metabolism in an Iodine and Selenium Deficient Population," *Clin. Endocrinol.* 36 (1992) : 579-583.

61 J.D. Cook and E.R. Monson, "Vitamin C, the Common Cold, and Iron Absorption," *Am. J. Clin. Nutr.* 30 (1977) : 235-241.

62 J.D. Cook and S.R. Lynch, "The Liabilities of Iron Deficiency," *Blood* 68 (1986) : 803-809.

63 A. Cordova and M. Alvarez-Mon, "Behaviour of Zinc in Physical Exercise: A Special Reference to Immunity and Fatigue," *Neurosci. Biobehav. Rev.* 19.3 (1995) : 439-445.

64 D.L. Costill, et al., "Acid Base Balance During Repeated Bouts of Exercise: Influence of HCO_3," *Int. J. Sport Nutr.* 5 (1984) : 225-231.

65 R.F. Crampton, et al., "Rates of Absorption by Rat Intestine of Pancreatic Hydrolysates of Proteins and Their Corresponding Amino Acid Mixtures," *Clin. Sci.* 41 (1971) : 409-417.

66 R. Crellin, et al., "Folates and Psychiatric Disorders: Clinical Potential," *Drugs* 45 (1993) : 623-636.

67 L. Cynober, "Ornithine Alpha-Ketoglutarate in Nutritional Support," *Nutrition* 7.5 (1991) : 313-322.

68 P.A. Daly, et al., "Ephedrine, Caffeine, and Aspirin: Safety and Efficacy for Treatment of Human Obesity," *Int. J. Obes.* 17.1 (1993) : S73-S78.

69 R. DeMeersman, et al., "Sympathomimetics and Exercise Enhancement: All in the Mind?" *Pharmacol. Biochem. Behav.* 28.3 (1987) : 361-365.

70 P. Di Mascio, et al., "Lycopene as the Most Efficient Biological Carotenoid Singlet Oxygen Quencher," *Arch. Biochem. Biophysics* 274 (1989) : 532-538.

71 F. Di Silverio, et al., "Evidence that Serenoa Repens Extract Displays Antiestrogenic Activity in Prostatic Tissue of Benign Prostatic Hypertrophy," *Eur. Urol.* 21 (1992) : 309-314.

72 M. Dimitrov, et al., "The Use of Tribestan With Rams Affected With Sexual Disturbances," *Vet. Med. Nauki.* 24.5 (1987) : 102-110.

73 E. Dolev, et al., "Longitudinal Study of Magnesium Status of Israeli Military Recruits," *Magnes. Trace Elem.* 10.5-6 (1991-1992) : 420-426.

74 J.M. Dony, et al., "Effect of Chronic Aromatase Inhibition by Delta 1-Testolactone on Pituitary-Gonadal Function in Oligozoospermic Men," *Andrologia* 18.1 (1986) : 69-78.

75 F. Dray, et al., "Role of Prostaglandins on Growth Hormone Secretion: PGE2 a Physiological Stimulator," *Adv. Prostaglandin & Thromboxane Res.* 8 (1980) : 1321-1328.

REFERENCES CITED

NCES CITED▶REFERENCES CITED▶REFERENCES CITED▶REFERENCES CITED▶REFERENCES CITED▶REFERENCES CITED▶REFERENCES CITED▶REFERENCES CITED▶REFERENCES CITED▶REFERENCES CITED▶REFERENCES CITED▶REFERENCES CITED▶REFERENCES CITED▶REFERENCES CITED▶REFERENCES CITED▶REFERENCES CITED▶REFERENCES CITED▶

76   A. Drovanti, et al., "Therapeutic Activity of Oral Glucosamine Sulfate in Osteoarthritis: A Placebo-Controlled, Double-Blind Investigation," *Clin. Ther.* 3 (1980) : 260-272.

77   A.G. Dulloo and D.S. Miller, "The Thermogenic Properties of Ephedrine/Methylxanthine Mixtures: Human Studies," *Int. J. Obes.* 10 (1986) : 467-481.

78   C.P. Earnest, et al., "High-Performance Capillary Electrophoresis-Pure Creatine Monohydrate Reduces Blood Lipids in Men and Women," *Clin. Sci.* 91 (1996) : 113-118.

79   C.P. Earnest, et al., "The Effect of Creatine Monohydrate Ingestion on Anaerobic Power Indices, Muscular Strength, and Body Composition," *Acta Physiol. Scand.* 153.2 (1995) : 207-209.

80   R. Englisch, et al., "Induction of Glucose Transport into Rat Muscle by Selenate and Selenite: Comparison to Insulin," *Diabetologia* 38.1 Suppl. (1995) : A133.

81   V.F. Fairbanks and E. Beutler, *"Iron," In: Modern Nutrition in Health and Disease, 7th Edition.* M.E. Shils and V.R. Young (Eds.) (Philadelphia, PA: Lea and Febiger, 1988) 193-226.

82   E.B. Fern, et al., "Effects of Exaggerated Amino Acid and Protein Supply in Man," *Experientia* 47 (1991) : 168-172.

83   M.L. Ferrandiz and M.J. Alcaraz, "Anti-Inflammatory Activity and Inhibition of Arachidonic Acid Metabolism by Flavonoids," *Agents Action* 32 (1991) : 283-287.

84   R.J. Fessenden and J.S. Fessenden, "The Biological Properties of Silicon Compounds," *Adv. Drug Res.* 4 (1987) : 95.

85   D.A. Fisher, "Physiological Variations in Thyroid Hormones: Physiological and Pathophysiological Considerations," *Clin. Chem.* 42.1 (1996) : 135-139.

86   P.J. Flakoll, et al., "Influence of Alpha-Ketoisocaproate on Lamb Growth, Feed Conversion, and Carcass Composition," *J. Animal Sci.* 69.4 (1991) : 1461-1467.

87   G.B. Forbes, et al., "Hormonal Response to Overfeeding," *Am. J. Clin. Nutr.* 49.4 (1989) : 608-611.

88   G.B. Forbes, et al., "Lean Body Mass in Obesity," *Int. J. Obes.* 7.2 (1983) : 99-107.

89   W.A. Forsythe, "Soy Protein, Thyroid Regulation, and Cholesterol Metabolism," *J. Nutr.* 123.3 (1995) : 619S-623S.

90   J.E. Friedman and P.W.R. Lemon, "Effect of Chronic Endurance Exercise on the Retention of Dietary Protein," *Int. J. Sports Med.* 10 (1989) : 118-123.

91   G.P. Galloway, et al., "Gamma-Hydroxybutyrate: An Emerging Drug of Abuse That Causes Physical Dependence," *Addiction* 92.1 (1997) : 89-96.

92   M.L.G. Gardner, "Gastrointestinal Absorption of Intact Proteins," *Ann. Rev. Nutr.* 8 (1988) : 329-350.

93   M.L. Garg, et al., "Fish Oil Prevents Change in Arachidonic Acid and Cholesterol Content in Rat Caused by Dietary Cholesterol," *Lipids* 24.4 (1989) : 266-270.

94   R. Gatnau, et al., "Effect of Excess Dietary Leucine and Leucine Catabolites on Growth and Immune Response in Weanling Pigs," *J. Animal Sci.* 73 (1995) : 159-165.

95   B. Gebner, et al., "Study of the Long-Term Action of a Ginkgo Biloba Extract on Vigilance and Mental Performance as Determined by Means of Quantitative Pharmaco-EEG and Psychometric Measurements," *Arzneimittel-forschung* 35.9 (1985) : 1459-1465.

96   G. Gerra, et al., "Gamma Hydroxybutyric Acid (GHB) and Neuroendocrine Function in Humans," *Neuroendocrinology Letters* 16.1 (1994) : 55-63.

97   J.C. Gessin, "Regulation of Collagen Synthesis in Human Dermal Fibroblasts in Contracted Collagen Gels by Ascorbic Acid, Growth Factors, and Inhibitors of Lipid Peroxidation," *Exp. Cell Res.* 206.2 (1996) : 283-290.

98   E. Ginter, "Optimum Intake of Vitamin C for the Human Organism," *Nutr. Health* 1 (1982) : 66-77.

99   K. Gohil, et al., "Effect of Exercise Training on Tissue Vitamin E and Ubiquinone Content," *J. Appl. Physiol.* 63.4 (1987) : 1638-1641.

100 A.L. Goldberg and T.W. Chang, "Regulation and Significance of Amino Acid Metabolism in Skeletal Muscle," *Fed. Proc.* 37 (1978) : 2301-2307.

101 H. Goranzon and E. Forsum, "Effect of Reduced Energy Intake Versus Increased Physical Activity on the Outcome of Nitrogen Balance Experiments in Man," *Am. J. Clin. Nutr.* 41 (1985) : 919-928.

102 A.L. Green, et al., "Creatine Ingestion Augments Muscle Creatine Uptake and Glycogen Synthesis During Carbohydrate Feeding in Man," *J. Physiol* 491 (1996) : 63P-64P.

103 A.L. Green, et al., "Carbohydrate Ingestion Augments Skeletal Muscle Creatine Accumulation During Creatine Supplementation in Man," *Am. J. Physiol.* (In Press, 1997).

104 A.L. Green, et al., "Carbohydrate Ingestion Augments Creatine Retention During Creatine Feeding in Humans," *Acta Physiol. Scand.* 158 (1996) : 195-202.

105 B. Greenberg, *The DHEA Discovery: Wonder Hormone of the Nineties.* (Los Angeles, CA: Majesty Press, 1996).

106 P.L. Greenhaff, et al., "The Influence of Oral Creatine Supplementation on Muscle Phosphocreatine Resynthesis Following Intense Contraction in Man," *J. Physiol.* 467 (1993) : 75P.

107 P.L. Greenhaff, et al., "Influence of Oral Creatine Supplementation on Muscle Torque During Repeated Bouts of Maximal Voluntary Exercise in Man," *Clin. Sci.* 84 (1993) : 565-571.

108 G.K. Grimble, et al., "Effect of Peptide Chain Length on Absorption of Egg Protein Hydrolysates in the Normal Human Jejunum," *Gastroenterology* 92 (1987) : 136-142.

109 J.L. Groff, et al., *Advanced Nutrition and Human Metabolism.* (New York: West Publishing Co., 1995).

110 L. Guarner, et al., "Fate of Oral Enzymes in Pancreatic Insufficiency," *Gut* 34.5 (1993) : 708-712.

111 M. Halberstam, et al., "Oral Vanadyl Sulfate Improves Insulin Sensitivity in NIDDM but Not in Obese Nondiabetic Subjects," *Diabetes* 45.5 (1996) : 659-666.

112 E.K. Hamalainen, et al., "Decrease of Serum Total and Free Testosterone During a Low-Fat, High-Fiber Diet," *J. Steroid Biochem.* 18.3 (1983) : 369-370.

113 R.C. Harris, et al., "Elevation of Creatine in Resting and Exercised Muscle of Normal Subjects by Creatine Supplementation," *Clin. Sci.* 83 (1992) : 367-374.

114 A. Hartman, et al., "Vitamin E Prevents Exercise-Induced DNA Damage," *Mutations Research* 346.4 (1995) : 195-202.

115 D. Häussinger, "The Role of Cellular Hydration in the Regulation of Cell Function," *Biochem. J.* 313 (1996) : 697-710.

116 D. Häussinger, et al., "Cellular Hydration State: An Important Determinant of Protein Catabolism in Health and Disease," *Lancet* 341.8856 (1993) : 1330-1332.

117 D. Häussinger, et al., "Cell Swelling Inhibits Proteolysis in Perfused Rat Liver," *Biochem. J.* 272.1 (1990) : 239-242.

118 D. Häussinger, "Nutritional State and the Swelling-Induced Inhibition of Liver Proteolysis in Perfused Rat Liver," *Nutr. J.* 126 (1996) : 395.

119 B. Havsteen, "Flavonoids, A Class of Natural Products of High Pharmacological Potency," *Biochem. Pharmacol.* 32 (1983) : 1141-1148.

120 H. Hikiho, et al., "Antihepatotoxic Actions of Flavonolignans from Silybum Marianum Fruits," *Planta Medica* 50 (1984) : 248-250.

121 I. Hindmarch, "Activity of Ginkgo Biloba Extract on Short-Term Memory," *La Presse Medicale* 15.31 (1986) : 1562-1592.

122 L. Hobbs and E.H. Ford, *Ephedrine & Caffeine: The Ideal Diet Pill?* (Irvine, CA: Pragmatic Press, 1996).

123 G. Hocman, "Chemoprevention of Cancer: Selenium," *Int. J. Biochem.* 20 (1988) : 123-132.

124 H. Hoppeler, et al., "The Ultrastructure of the Normal Human Skeletal Muscle: A Morphometric Analysis on Untrained Men, Women and Well Trained Orienteers," *Eur. J. Appl. Physiol.* (West Germany) 344.3 (1973) : 217-232.

125 M.K. Horwit, et al. (Eds.), *Modern Nutrition in Health and Disease, 6th Edition.* (Philadelphia, PA: Lea & Febiger, 1980).

126 E. Hultman, et al., "Muscle Creatine Loading in Man," *J. Appl. Physiol.* 81 (1996) : 232-237.

127 A.R. Ibrahim and Y.J. Abul-Hajj, "Aromatase Inhibition by Flavonoids," *J. Steroid Biochem. Mol. Biol.* 37.2 (1990) : 257-260.

128 D.M. Ingram, et al., "Effect of Low-Fat Diet on Female Sex Hormone Levels," *JNCI* 79.6 (1987) : 1225-1229.

129 Institute of National Hygiene, Academy of Preventive Medicine, Beijing, China (Unpublished research).

130 J.L. Ivy, "Muscle Glycogen Synthesis Before and After Exercise," *Sports Med.* 11 (1991) : 6-19.

131 D.S. Jacobs, et al., *Laboratory Test Handbook with Disease Index.* (Hudson, OH: Lexi-Comp. Inc., 1996).

132 S. Jacob, et al., "Enhancement of Glucose Disposal in Patients With Type 2 Diabetes by Alpha-Lipoic Acid," *Arzneimittel-forschung* 45.8 (1995) : 872-874.

133 A. Jain, et al., "Effect of Ascorbate or N-Acetylcysteine Treatment in a Patient with Hereditary Glutathione Synthetase Deficiency," *J. Pediatr.* 124 (1994) : 229-233.

134 B. Jansson, "Dietary, Total Body, and Intracellular Potassium-to-Sodium Ratios, and Their Influence on Cancer," *Cancer Detect. Prevent.* 14 (1991) : 563-565.

135 S.A. Jebb, et al., "Changes in Macronutrient Balance During Over- and Underfeeding Assessed by 12-Day Continuous Whole-Body Calorimetry," *Am. J. Clin. Nutr.* 64.3 (1996) : 259-266.

136 G.N. Jenkins, "Molybdenum," In: *Trace Elements and Dental Disease,* M.E.J. Curzon and T.W. Cutress (Eds.) (Boston, MA: John Wright, 1983) 149-166.

137 C.S. Johnston and B. Luo, "Comparison of the Absorption and Excretion of Three Commercially Available Sources of Vitamin C," *J. Am. Diet. Assoc.* 94 (1994) : 779-781.

138 G.R. Katts, et al., "The Effects of Chromium Picolinate Supplementation on Body Composition in Different Age Groups," *Age* 14.40 (1991) : 138.

139 K.T. Khaw and E. Barrett-Connor, "Dietary Potassium and Stroke-Associated Mortality," *N. Engl. J. Med.* 316 (1987) : 235-240.

140 R. Kinscherf, et al., "Low Plasma Glutamine in Combination with High Glutamate Levels Indicate Risk for Loss of Body Cell Mass in Healthy Individuals: The Effect of N-Acetyl-Cysteine," *J. Mol. Med.* 74 (1996) : 393-400.

141 L. Kiremidjian-Schumacher and G. Stotsky, "Selenium and Immune Responses," *Environmental Res.* 42 (1987) : 277-303.

142 L. Kiremidjian-Schumacher, et al., "Supplementation with Selenium and Human Immune Cell Functions; II, Effect on Cytotoxic Lymphocytes and Natural Killer Cells," *Biol. Trace Elem. Res.* 41 (1994) : 115-127.

143 H.A. Kleinveld, et al., "Failure of N-Acetylcysteine to Reduce Low-Density Lipoprotein Oxidizability in Healthy Subjects," *Eur. J. Clin. Pharmacol.* 43 (1992) : 639-642.

144 R.C. Klesges, et al., "Changes in Bone Mineral Content in Male Athletes: Mechanisms of Action and Intervention Effects," *JAMA* 276.3 (1996) : 226-230.

145 L.M. Klevay, "Dietary Copper: A Powerful Determinant of Cholesterolemia," *Medical Hypothesis* 24 (1987) : 83-105.

146 A.M. Kligman, et al., "Oral Vitamin A in Acne Vulgaris," *Int. J. Derm.* 20 (1981) : 278-285.

147 H. Korpela, et al., "Effect of Selenium Supplementation After Acute Myocardial Infarction," *Res. Commun. Chem. Pathol. Pharmacol.* 65 (1989) : 249-252.

148 K. Kozak-Collins, et al., "Sodium Bicarbonate Ingestion Does Not Improve Performance in Women Cyclists," *Med. Sci. Sports Exerc.* 26.12 (1994) : 1510-1515.

149 M.V. Krause and K.L. Mahan, *Food, Nutrition and Diet Therapy, 7th Edition.* (Philadelphia, PA: W.B. Saunders, 1984).

150 R.B. Kreider, et al., "Effect of Ingesting a Lean Mass Promoting Supplement During Resistance Training on Isokinetic Performance," *Med. Sci. Sports Exerc.* 28 (1996) : S36.

151 R.B. Kreider, et al., "Effects of Phosphate Loading on Metabolic and Myocardial Responses to Maximal and Endurance Exercise," *Int. J. Sport Nutr.* 2.1 (1992) : 20-47.

152 R. Kreider, et al., "Effects of Ingesting Supplements Designed to Promote Lean Tissue Accretion on Whole & Regional Body Composition Alterations During Resistance-Training," *FASEB J.* (1995) : A1015.

153 R.B. Kreider, et al., "Effects of Ingesting Supplements Designed to Promote Lean Tissue Accretion on Body Composition During Resistance Training," *Int. J. Sport Nutr.* 6.3 (1996) : 234-246.

154 N.I. Krinsky, "Antioxidant Function of Carotenoids," *Free Rad. Biol. Med.* 7 (1989) : 627-635.

155 R. Kuijer, "Influence of Constituents of Proteoglycans on Type II Collagen Fibrillogenesis," *Coll. Relat. Res.* 5.5 (1985) : 379-391.

156 J. Lacey and D. Wilmore, "Is Glutamine a Conditionally Essential Amino Acid?" *Nut. Rev.* 48 (1990) : 297-309.

157 F.A. Lederly, "Oral Cobalamin for Pernicious Anemia: Medicine's Best Kept Secret," *JAMA* 265 (1991) : 94-95.

158 P.W.R. Lemon and F.J. Nagle, "Effects of Exercise on Protein and Amino Acid Metabolism," *Med. Sci. Sports Exer.* 13 (1981) : 141-149.

159 R. Levy, et al., "Early Results from Double Blind, Placebo Controlled Trial of High Dose Phosphatydylcholine in Alzheimer's Disease," *Lancet* 1 (1982) : 474-476.

160 M.C. Linder (Ed.), *Nutritional Biochemistry and Metabolism With Clinical Applications, 2nd Edition.* (Norwalk, CN: Appleton & Lange, 1991) 281.

161 M.I. Lindinger, "Potassium Regulation During Exercise and Recovery in Humans: Implications for Skeletal and Cardiac Muscle," *J. Mol. Cell Cardiol.* 27.4 (1995) : 1011-1022.

162 S. Low, et al., "Responses of Glutamine Transport in Cultured Rat Skeletal Muscle to Osmotically Induced Changes in Cell Volume," *J. Physiol.* 492.3 (1996) : 877-885.

163 M. Maebashi, et al., "Therapeutic Evaluation of the Effect of Biotin on Hyperglycemia in Patients with Non-Insulin Dependent Diabetes Mellitus," *J. Clin. Biochem. Nutr.* 14 (1993) : 211-218.

REFERENCES CITED

NCES CITED•REFERENCES CITED•REFERENCES CITED•REFERENCES CITED•REFERENCES CITED•REFERENCES CITED•REFERENCES CITED•REFERENCES CITED•REFERENCES CITED•REFERENCES CITED•REFERENCES CITED•REFERENCES CITED•REFERENCES CITED•REFERENCES CITED•REFERENCES CITED•REFERENCES CITED•REFERENCES CITED•REFERENCES CITED•REFERENCES CITED•

164 V.B. Mahesh and R.B. Greenblatt, "The In Vivo Conversion of Dehydroepiandrosterone and Androstenedione to Testosterone in the Human," *Acta Endocrinologica* 41 (1962) : 400-406.

165 C. Malm, et al., "Supplementation with Ubiquinone-10 Causes Cellular Damage During Intense Exercise," *Acta Physiol. Scand.* 157 (1996) : 511-512.

166 G. Marchesini, et al., "Anticatabolic Effect of Branched-Chain Amino Acid-Enriched Solutions in Patients with Liver Cirrhosis," *Hepatology* 2 (1982) : 420-425.

167 B. Martinez and E.J. Staba, "The Physiological Effects of Aralia, Panax, and Eleutherococcus on Exercised Rats," *Jpn. J. Pharmacol.* 35 (1984) : 79-85.

168 J. Masquelier, et al., "Stabilization of Collagen by Procyanidolic Oligomers," *Acta Therap.* 7 (1981) : 101-105.

169 J. Masquelier, "Procyanidolic Oligomers," *J. Parfums. Cosm. Arom.* 95 (1990) : 89-97.

170 S. Matsugo, et al., "Elucidation of Antioxidant Activity of Alpha-Lipoic Acid Toward ·Hydroxyl Radical," *Biochem. Biophys. Res. Commun.* 208.1 (1995) : 161-167.

171 T.E. McAlindon, et al., "Relation of Dietary Intake and Serum Levels of Vitamin D to Progression of Osteoarthritis of the Knee Among Participants in the Framingham Study," *Annals of Internal Medicine* 125.5 (1996) : 353-359.

172 M.J. McKenna, "Effects of Training on Potassium Homeostasis During Exercise," *J. Mol. Cell Cardiol.* 27.4 (1995) : 941-949.

173 L. McNaughton, et al., "A Comparison of Chinese and Russian Ginseng as Ergogenic Aids to Improve Various Facets of Physical Fitness," *Int. Clin. Nutr. Rev.* 9 (1989) : 32-37.

174 S.L. Meacham, et al., "Effect of Boron Supplementation on Blood and Urinary Calcium, Magnesium and Phosphorus, and Urinary Boron in Athletic and Sedentary Women," *Am. J. Clin. Nutr.* 61.2 (1995) : 341-345.

175 S.L. Meacham, et al., "Effect of Boron Supplementation on Bone Mineral Density and Dietary, Blood, and Urinary Calcium, Phosphorus, Magnesium, and Boron in Female Athletes," *Environ. Health Perspect.* 102.7 Suppl. (1994) : 79-82.

176 K.J. Meador, "Evidence for a Central Cholinergic Effect of High-Dose Thiamine," *Ann. Neurol.* 34 (1993) : 724-726.

177 K.J. Meador, "Preliminary Findings of High-Dose Thiamine in Dementia of Alzheimer's Type," *J. Geriatr. Psychiatry Neurol.* 6 (1993) : 222-229.

178 R.B. Meese, et al., "The Inconsistent Effects of Calcium Supplements Upon Blood Pressure in Primary Hypertension," *Am. J. Med. Sci.* 294 (1987) : 219-224.

179 R. Mendosa and T. Griffin, *The Glycemic Index Solution* (Australia: Hodder Headline Australia Pty Ltd., 1996).

180 W. Mertz, "Chromium in Human Nutrition: A Review," *J. Nutr.* 123 (1993) : 626-633.

181 S. Milanov, et al., "Tribestan Effect on the Concentration of Some Hormones in Serum of Healthy Subjects," Unpublished Research.

182 A. Militello, et al., *Effect of Taurine Administration on Amino Acid and 3-Methylhistidine Concentrations in Man* (Vienna, Austria: 41st International Congress on Amino Acids, 1995).

183 P. Miller, et al., "The Effect of Intensive Training and ß-Hydroxy ß-Methylbutyrate (HMB) on the Physiological Response to Exercise in Horses," *FASEB J.* 11.3 (1997) : A290.

184 D.J. Millward, "The Endocrine Response to Dietary Protein: the Anabolic Drive on Growth," *Milk Protein* (1989) : 49-61.

185 D.J. Millward, et al., "A Protein-STAT Mechanism for Regulation of Growth and Maintenance of Lean Body Mass," *Nutr. Res. Rev.* 8 (1995) : 93-120.

186 E. Mindell and C. Colman, *Earl Mindell's Herb Bible.* (New York, NY: Simon & Shuster Inc., 1992) 12.

187 P. Monteleone, et al., "Blunting by Chronic Phosphatidylserine Administration of the Stress-Induced Activation of the Hypothalamo-Pituitary-Adrenal Axis in Healthy Men," *Eur. J. Clin. Pharmacol.* 41 (1992) : 385-388.

188 M. Morrison, "Therapeutic Applications of Chondroitin-4-Sulfate, Appraisal of Biologic Properties," *Foila Angiol* 25 (1977) : 225-232.

189 J.E. Nestler, et al., "Dehydroepiandrosterone Reduces Serum Low Density Lipoprotein Levels and Body Fat But Does Not Alter Insulin Sensitivity in Normal Men," *J. Clin. Endocrinol. Metab.* 66.1 (1988) : 57-61.

190 F.P. Moss, "The Relationship Between the Dimension of the Fibers and the Number of Nuclei During Normal Growth of Skeletal Muscle in the Domestic Fowl," *Am. J. Anat.* 122 (1968) : 555-564.

191 R.T. Mossop, "Effects of Chromium (III) on Fasting Blood Glucose, Cholesterol, and Cholesterol HDL Levels in Diabetics," *Centr. Afr. J. Med.* 29 (1983) : 80-82.

192 D. Müller-Wieland, et al., "Inhibition of Fatty Acid Synthesis by Stimulation of Alpha- and Beta-Adrenergic Receptors in Human Mononuclear Leukocytes," *Horm. Metab. Res.* 26.4 (1994) : 169-172.

193 M.T. Murray, *Encyclopedia of Nutritional Supplements.* (Rocklin, CA: Prima Publishing, 1996).

194 R. Murray, et al., "Responses to Varying Rates of Carbohydrate Ingestion During Exercise," *Med. Sci. Sports Exerc.* 23.6 (1991) : 713-718.

195 N.R. Musso, et al., "Yohimbine Effects on Blood Pressure and Plasma Catecholamines in Human Hypertension," *Am. J. Hypertens.* 8.6 (1995) : 565-571.

196 National Institutes of Health Workshop, *"The Role of Dietary Supplements for Physically Active People"* (Bethesda, MD: Natcher Conference Center, 1996).

197 National Research Council, *Recommended Dietary Allowances, 10th Edition* (Washington, D.C.: National Academy Press, 1989).

198 F.H. Neilsen, "Ultratrace Elements in Nutrition," *Annu. Rev. Nutr.* 4 (1984) : 21-41.

199 F.H. Neilsen, et al., "Effect of Dietary Boron on Mineral, Estrogen, and Testosterone Metabolism in Postmenopausal Women," *FASEB J.* 1 (1987) : 394-397.

200 H.S. Nelson, et al., "Subsensitivity to Ephedrine Following the Administration of Epinephrine and Ephedrine to Normal Individuals," *J. Allergy Clin. Immunol.* 55.5 (1975) : 299-309.

201 K.M. Neuzil, et al., "Safety and Pharmocokinetics of Vitamin A Therapy for Infants with Respiratory Syncytical Infections," *Antimicrob. Agents Chemother.* 39 (1995) : 1191-1193.

202 M.G. Neuman, et al., "Protective Effect of Silymarin on the Hepatocellular Toxicity of Acetaminophen in Human Cell Lines In-Vitro," *Clin. Invest. Med.* 14.4 (1991) : A20.

203 W.Y. Ning, et al., "Effect of Ciwujia (Radix Acanthopanacis Senticosus) Preparation on the Stamina of Mice," *J. Hygiene Res.* (published in Chinese) 25 (1996) : 176.

204 S.L. Nissen, et al., "Effect of ß-Hydroxy ß-Methylbutyrate (HMB) Supplementation on Strength and Body Composition of Trained and Untrained Males Undergoing Intense Resistance Training," *FASEB J.* 10.3 (1996) : A287.

205 S.L. Nissen, et al., "The Effect of the Leucine Metabolite ß-Hydroxy ß-Methylbutyrate on Muscle Metabolism During Resistance-Exercise Training," *J. Appl. Physiol.* 81.5 (1996) : 2095-2104.

206 S.L. Nissen, et al., "Effect of Feeding ß-Hydroxy ß-Methylbutyrate (HMB) on Body Composition and Strength of Women," *FASEB J.* 11 (1997) : A150.

207 E.B. Oddoye, et al., "Nitrogen Balance Studies in Humans: Long-Term Effect of High Nitrogen Intake on Nitrogen Accretion," *J. Nutr.* 109.3 (1979) : 363-377.

208 R. Olinescu, et al., "Comparative Study of the Presence of Oxidative Stress in Sportsmen in Competition and Aged People, as Well as the Preventive Effect of Selenium Administration," *Rom. J. Intern. Med.* 33.1-2 (1995) : 47-54.

209 P. Ostaszewksi, et al., "The Effect of the Leucine Metabolite 3-Hydroxy 3-Methyl Butyrate (HMB) on Muscle Protein Synthesis and Protein Breakdown in Chick and Rat Muscle," *J. Anim. Sci.* 74.1 (1996) : 138.

210 L. Packer, et al., "Alpha-Lipoic Acid as a Biological Antioxidant," *Free Radic. Biol. Med.* 19.2 (1995) : 227-250.

211 G. Paolisso, et al., "Pharmacologic Doses of Vitamin E Improve Insulin Action in Healthy Subjects and Non-Insulin-Dependent Diabetic Patients," *Am. J. Clin. Nutr.* 57 (1993) : 848-852.

212 M. Pariza, et al., "Conjugated Linoleic Acid (CLA) Reduces Body Fat," *FASEB J.* 10.3 (1996) : A560.

213 W.S. Parkhouse and D.C. McKenzie, "Possible Contribution of Skeletal Muscle Buffers to Enhance Anaerobic Performance: A Brief Review," *Med. Sci. Sports Exerc.* 16.4 (1984) : 328-338.

214 R. Pasquali and F. Casimirri, "Clinical Aspects of Ephedrine in the Treatment of Obesity," *Int. J. Obes.* 17.1 (1993) : S65-S68.

215 R. Pasquali, et al., "Effects of Chronic Administration of Ephedrine During Very-Low-Calorie Diets on Energy Expenditure, Protein Metabolism, and Hormone Levels in Obese Subjects," *Clin. Sci.* 82.1 (1992) : 85-92.

216 R. Pasquali, et al., "Chronic Beta-Receptor Stimulation Prevents Nitrogen Loss During Semistarvation in Obese Subjects," *Int. J. Obes.* 13.1 (1989) : 151.

217 R.A. Passwater, *Lipoic Acid: The Metabolic Antioxidant.* (New Canaan, CT: Keats Publishing, Inc., 1995).

218 T. Pelikanova, et al., "Insulin Secretion and Insulin Action are Related to the Serum Phospholipid Fatty Acid Pattern in Healthy Men," *Metab. Clin. Exp.* 38 (1989) : 188-192.

219 C.L. Phillips, et al., "Effects of Ascorbic Acid on Proliferation and Collagen Synthesis in Relation to the Donor Age of Human Dermal Fibroblasts," *J. Invest. Dermatol.* 103.2 (1994) : 228-232.

220 P. Pola, et al., "Carnitine in the Therapy of Dyslipidemic Patients," *Curr. Ther. Res., Clin. Exp.* 27.2 (1980) : 208-216.

221 P. Pola, et al., "Statistical Evaluation of Long-Term L-Carnitine Therapy in Hyper-Lipo Proteinemias," *Drugs Under Exp. Clin. Res.* 9.12 (1983) : 925-934.

222 D.A. Porter, et al., "The Effect of Oral Coezyme Q10 on the Exercise Tolerance of Middle-Aged Untrained Men," *Int. J. Sports Med.* 16.7 (1995) : 421-427.

223 *Protein Quality Evaluation*, Report of the Joint FAO/WHO Expert Consultation, FAO/WHO, 1989.

224 S. Pyke, et al., "Severe Depletion in Liver Glutathione During Physical Exercise," *Biochem. Biophys. Res. Comm.* 139 (1986) : 926-931.

225 E. Racz-Kotilla, et al., "The Action of Taraxacum Officinale Extracts on the Body Weight and Diuresis of Laboratory Animals," *Planta Medica* 26 (1974) : 212-217.

226 G.K. Radda, "Control of Energy Metabolism During Muscle Contraction," *Diabetes* 45.1 (1996) : S88-S92.

227 G.K. Radda, "Phosphorus-31 Nuclear-Magnetic-Resonance Studies on Energy Metabolism in Intact Mammalian Tissue," *Biochem. Soc. Trans.* 9.3 (1981) : 213-214.

228 E. Ravussin, et al., "Short-Term, Mixed-Diet Overfeeding in Man: No Evidence for 'Luxuskonsumption,'" *Am. J. Physiol.* 249.5 (1985) : E470-E477.

229 M.J. Reed, et al., "The Role of Free Fatty Acid in Regulating the Tissue Availability and the Synthesis of Sex Steroids," *Prostaglandins Leukot. Essent. Fatty Acids* 48 (1993) : 111-116.

230 T.J. Rhim, et al., "Comparison of the Effects of Pulsatile and Constant Testosterone on the Secretion of Gonadotropins in the Ram," *Endrocrinology* 132.6 (1993) : 2399-2406.

231 R.J. Richardson and S.D. Murphy, "Effect of Glutathione Depletion on Tissue Deposition of Methylmercury in Rats," *Toxicol. Appl. Pharmacol.* 31 (1975) : 505-519.

232 E.A. Richter, et al., "Enhanced Muscle Glycogen Metabolism After Exercise: Modulation by Local Factors," *Amer. J. Physiol.* 246 (1984) : E476-E482.

233 T. Rivas, et al., "Role of Amino Acid-Induced Changes in Ion Fluxes in the Regulation of Hepatic Protein Synthesis," *J. Cell. Physiol.* 163.2 (1995) : 277-284.

234 W.B. Robertson, et al., "Augmentation of Collagen Synthesis by Ascorbic Acid In Vitro," *Biochem. & Biophys.* 49 (1961) : 404-406.

235 G.D. Rosa, et al., "Regulation of Superoxide Dismutase Activity by Dietary Manganese," *J. Nutr.* 110 (1980) : 795-804.

236 L. Rosa, et al., "Effect of a Chronic Diet Supplementation of Ornithine, Citrulline and Arginine on Exercise Performance and Metabolism," *Med. Sci. Sports Exerc.* 28.5 (1996) : S82.

237 E. Roth, et al., "Glutamine: An Anabolic Effector," *J. Parent. Ent. Nutr.* 14 (1990) : 1305-1365.

238 S.J. Rudzki, et al., "Gastrointestinal Blood Loss in Triathletes: Its Etiology and Relationship to Sports Anaemia," *Aust. J. Sci. Med. Sport* 27.1 (1995) : 3-8.

239 F.M. Ruggiero, et al., "Effect of Aging and Acetyl-L-Carnitine on the Lipid Composition of Rat Plasma and Erythrocytes," *Biochem. Biophys. Res. Comm.* 170.2 (1990) : 621-626.

240 J.C. Rupp, et al., "Effect of Sodium Bicarbonate Ingestion on Blood and Muscle pH and Exercise Performance," *Med. Sci. Sports Exerc.* 15 (1983) : 115.

241 R. Sahelian and D. Tuttle, *Creatine: Nature's Muscle Builder* (Garden City Park, NY: Avery Publishing Group, 1997).

242 P.D. Saltman and L.G. Strause, "The Role of Trace Minerals in Osteoporosis," *J. Am. Coll. Nutr.* 12.4 (1993) : 384-389.

243 T. Sandor and A. Lanthier, "The In Vitro Transformation of 4-Androstene-3,7-dione to Testosterone by Surviving Human Ovarian Slices," *Can. J. Biochem. Physiol.* (1960) : 445-447.

244 H.E. Scaglia, et al., "Altered Testicular Hormone Production in Infertile Patients with Idiopathic Oligoasthenospermia," *J. Andro.* 12.5 (1991) : 273-280.

245 B. Schwitters and J. Masquelier, *OPC in Practice: Biflavanols and Their Application.* (Rome, Italy: Alfa Omega, 1993).

246 J. Serkedjieva, "Inhibition of Influenza Virus Protein Synthesis by a Plant Preparation from Geranium Sanguineum L.," *Acta Virol.* 39.1 (1995) : 5-10.

REFERENCES CITED

NCES CITED•REFERENCES CITED•REFERENCES CITED•REFERENCES CITED•REFERENCES CITED•REFERENCES CITED•REFERENCES CITED•REFERENCES CITED•REFERENCES CITED•REFERENCES CITED•REFERENCES CITED•REFERENCES CITED•REFERENCES CITED•REFERENCES CITED•REFERENCES CITED•REFERENCES CITED•REFERENCES CITED•REFERENCES CITED•

247 I. Setnikar, et al., "Pharmacokinetics of Glucosamine in Man," *Arzeim Forsch* 43.10 (1993) : 1109-1113.

248 G.B. Shah and R.K. Goyal, "Effect of Yohimbine in Congestive Cardiac Failure," *Indian J. Pharmacol.* 26.1 (1994) : 41-43.

249 S. Shutler, "The Cholesteral-lowering Effects of Legumes II: Effects of Fiber, Sterols, Saponins, and Isofavones," *Human Nutr. Food Sci. Nutr.* 41F (1987) : 87-102.

250 K.H. Sidney and N.M. Lefcoe, "The Effects of Ephedrine on the Physiological and Psychological Responses to Submaximal and Maximal Exercise in Man," *Med. Sci. Sports* 9.2 (1977) : 95-99.

251 T. Silverstone and E. Goodall, "The Clinical Pharmacology of Appetite Suppressant Drugs," *Int. J. Obes.* 8.1 (1984) : 23-33.

252 I. Sipila, et al., "Supplementary Creatine as a Treatment for Gyrate Atrophy of the Choroid and Retina," *N. Engl. J. Med.* 304 (1981) : 867-870.

253 B. Sjodin, et al., "Biochemical Mechanisms for Oxygen Free Radical Formation During Exercise," *Sports Med.* 10.4 (1990) : 236-254.

254 D.J. Smith and D. Roberts, "Effects of High Volume and/or Intense Exercise on Selected Blood Chemistry Parameters," *Clin. Biochem.* 27.6 (1994) : 435-440.

255 J.A. Smith, "Exercise, Training and Red Blood Cell Turnover," *Sports Med.* 19.1 (1995) : 9-31.

256 I.P. Snider, et al., "Effects of Coenzyme Athletic Performance System as an Ergogenic Aid on Endurance Performance to Exhaustion," *Int. J. Sport Nutr.* 2.3 (1992) : 272-286.

257 O. Spigset, "Coenzyme Q10 (Ubiquinone) in the Treatment of Heart Failure. Are Any Positive Effects Documented?" *Tidsskr Nor Laegeforen* 114.8 (1994) : 939-942.

258 R.T. Stanko and S.A. Adibi, "Inhibition of Lipid Accumulation and Enhancement of Energy Expenditure by the Addition of Pyruvate and Dihydroxyacetone to a Rat Diet," *Metabolism* 35 (1986) : 182-186.

259 R.T. Stanko, et al., "Body Composition, Energy Utilization, and Nitrogen Metabolism with a 4.25-MJ/d Low-Energy Diet Supplemented with Pyruvate[1-3]," *Am. J. Clin. Nutr.* 56 (1992) : 630-635.

260 R.D. Starling, et al., "Effect of Inosine Supplementation on Aerobic and Anaerobic Cycling Performance," *Med. Sci. Sports Exerc.* 28 (1996) : 1193-1198.

261 L. Stewart, et al., "Phosphate Loading and Effects on VO_2max in Trained Cyclists," *Research Quarterly* 61 (1990) : 80-84.

262 K.X. Stopozyk, *Preseglad Lekasski* 25 (1969) : 723.

263 J. Stout, et al., "The Effects of Endurox Supplementation on Critical Power" (in review, 1997).

264 J.R. Stout, et al., "The Effects of a Supplement Designed to Augment Creatine Uptake on Anaerobic Reserve Capacity" (*NSCA National Conference Abstract,* 1997).

265 J.R. Stout, et al., "The Effects of a Supplement Designed to Augment Creatine Uptake on Exercise Performance and Fat-Free Mass in Football Players" (*ACSM Conference Abstract,* 1997).

266 V. Stroescul, et al., *Metabolic and Hormonal Responses in Elite Female Gymnasts Undergoing Strenuous Training and Supplementation with Supro® Brand Isolated Soy Protein* (Brussels, Belgium: Second International Symposium on the Role of Soy in Preventing and Treating Chronic Disease, 1996).

267 G.T. Sunderland, et al., "A Double-Blind, Randomized Placebo-Controlled Trial of Hexopal in Primary Raynaud's Disease," *Clin. Rheumatol.* 7 (1988) : 46-49.

268 F. Susnik, "Present State of Knowledge of the Medicinal Plant Taraxacum Officinale," *Med. Razgledi* 21 (1982) : 323-328.

269 J.W. Suttie, "Vitamin K and Human Nutrition," *J. Am. Diet. Assoc.* 92 (1992) : 585-590.

270 S. Takahashi, et al., "Effect of L-5-Hydroxytryptophan on Brain Monoamine Metabolism and Evaluation of its Clinical Effect in Depressed Patients," *J. Psychiat. Res.* 12 (1975) : 177-187.

271 M.J. Tapadinhas, et al., "Oral Glucosamine Sulfate in the Management of Arthrosis: Report on a Multi-Centre Open Investigation in Portugal," *Pharmatherapeutica* 3 (1982) : 157-168.

272 U. Tarp, et al., "Selenium Treatment in Rheumatoid Arthritis," *Scand. J. Rheumatol.* 14 (1985) : 364-368.

273 G.T. Taylor, et al., "Testosterone in a Cyclodextrin-Containing Formulation: Behavioral and Physiological Effects of Episode-Like Pulses in Rats," *Pharmaceutical Research* 6.7 (1989) : 641-646.

274 Tin-May-Than, et al., "The Effect of Vitamin B_{12} on Physical Performance Capacity," *Br. J. Nutr.* 40 (1978) : 269-273.

275 S. Toubro, et al., "Safety and Efficacy of Long-Term Treatment with Ephedrine, Caffeine and an Ephedrine/Caffeine Mixture," *Int. J. Obes.* 17.1 (1993) : S69-72.

276 D.E. Trentham, et al., "Effects of Oral Administration of Type II Collagen on Rheumatoid Arthritis," *Science* 261 (1993) : 1727-1730.

277 H. Tritschler (Munich, Germany: *Diabetic Neuropathy Conference,* 1995).

278 M.F. Tsan, "Modulation of Endothelial GSH Concentration: Effect of Exogenous GSH and GSH Monoethyl Ester," *J. Appl. Physiol.* 66 (1989) : 1029-1034.

279 B.S. Tseng, et al., "Cytoplasm-to-Myonucleus Ratios and Succinate Dehydrogenase Activities in Adult Rat Slow and Fast Muscle Fiber," *Cell Tissue Res.* 275 (1994) : 39-49.

280 R.G. Tucker, et al., "The Influence of Sleep, Work, Diuresis, Heat, Acute Starvation, Thiamine Intake and Bed Rest on Human Riboflavin Excretion," *J. Nutr.* 72 (1960) : 251-261.

281 T.E. Tuormaa, "Adverse Effect of Zinc Deficiency: A Review from the Literature," *J. Orthomol. Med.* 10 (1995) : 149-162.

282 M.R. Valetto, et al., "Reproducibility of the Growth Hormone Response to Stimulation with Growth Hormone-Releasing Hormone Plus Arginine During Lifespan," *Eur. J. Endocrin.* 135.5 (1996) : 568-572.

283 M. Varnier, et al., "Stimulatory Effect of Glutamine on Glycogen Accumulation in Human Skeletal Muscle," *Amer. J. Physiol.* 269.2 (1995) : E309-E315.

284 R.A. Vigersky and A.R. Glass, "Effects of Delta-1 Testo Lactone on the Pituitary Testicular Axis in Oligo Spermic Men," *J. Clin. Endocrinol. Metab.* 52.5 (1981) : 897-902.

285 J.S. Volek and W.J. Kraemer, "Creatine Supplementation: Its Effect on Human Muscular Performance and Body Composition," *J. Strength and Condit. Res.* 10.3 (1996) : 200-210.

286 S. Vom Dahl and D. Häussinger, "Nutritional State and the Swelling-Induced Inhibition of Proteolysis in Perfused Rat Liver," *J. Nutr.* 126.2 (1996) : 395-402.

287 M.D. Vukovich and G.D. Adams, "Effect of ß-Hydroxy ß-Methyl Butyrate (HMB) on VO_2 Peak and Maximal Lactate in Endurance Trained Cyclists" (*ACSM Conference Abstract,* 1997).

288 M.D. Vukovich, et al., "The Effect of Dietary ß-Hydroxy ß-Methyl Butyrate (HMB) on Strength Gains and Body Composition Changes in Older Adults," *FASEB J.* 11.3 (1997) : A376.

289 J.L. Walberg, et al., "Macronutrient Content of a Hypoenergy Diet Affects Nitrogen Retention and Muscle Function in Weight Lifters," *Int. J. Sports Med.* 9 (1988) : 261-266.

290 J.B. Walker, "Creatine: Biosynthesis, Regulation and Function," *Adv. Enzymol. Relat. Areas Mol. Med.* 50 (1979) : 177-242.

291 J.G. Warner, et al., "Combined Effects of Aerobic Exercise and Omega-3 Fatty-Acids on Plasma Lipids in Hyperlipidemic Subjects," *Clin. Res.* 34.2 (1986) : 806A.

292 C. Weber, et al., "Effect of Dietary Coenzyme Q10 as an Antioxidant in Human Plasma," *Mol. Aspects Med.* 15 Suppl. (1994) : 97-102.

293 M.A. Weiner and J. Weiner, *Herbs That Heal: Prescription for Herbal Healing* (Mill Valley, CA: Quantum Books, 1994).

294 T.C. Welbourne, "Increased Plasma Bicarbonate and Growth Hormone After an Oral Glutamine Load," *Am. J. Clin. Nutr.* 61.5 (1995) : 1058-1061.

295 D. Wilkes, et al., "Effect of Induced Metabolic Alkalosis on 800m Racing Time," *Med. Sci. Sports Exerc.* 15.4 (1983) : 277-280.

296 J.R. Wilson, et al., "Contribution of Potassium to Exercise-Induced Vasodilation in Humans," *J. Appl. Physiol.* 77.6 (1994) : 2552-2557.

297 P.K. Winchester, et al., "Satellite Cell Activation in the Stretch-Enlarged Anterior Latissimus Dorsi Muscle of the Adult Quail," *Am. J. Physiol.* 260.2 (1991) : 206-212.

298 A. Witschi, et al., "The Systemic Availability of Oral Glutathione," *Eur. J. Clin. Pharmacol.* 43 (1992) : 667-669.

299 J. Wojcicki, et al., "Clinical Evaluation of Lecithin as a Lipid-Lowering Agent," *Phytotherapy Res.* 9 (1995) : 597-599.

300 C. Wolfman, et al., "Possible Anxiolytic Effects of Chrysin, a Central Benzodiazepine Receptor Ligand Isolated from Passiflora Coerulea," *Pharmacol. Biochem. Behav.* 47.1 (1994) : 1-4.

301 R. Wurtman, et al., *Choline and Lecithin in Brain Disorders, Nutrition and the Brain, Vol. 5.* (New York, NY: Raven Press, 1979).

302 S.S.C. Yen, et al., "Replacement of DHEA in Aging Men and Women: Potential Remedial Effects," *N.Y. Acad. Sci.* 774 (1995) : 128-142.

303 S. Zarkova, *Tribestan: Experimental and Clinical Investigations* (Sofia, Bulgaria: Sopharma Chemical Pharmaceutical Research Institute, 1981).

304 K.M. Zawadzki, et al., "Carbohydrate-Protein Complex Increases the Rate of Muscle Glycogen Storage After Exercise," *J. Appl. Physiol.* 72.5 (1992) : 1854-1859.

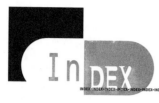

INDEX-

353

Tripeptides, 165, 342
Triphosphate, 49, 328
Troponin, 192
Tryptophan, 62, 128, 164-166, 168-169, 174-175, 178-180, 185-186
Turmeric, 86, 152
TwinLab, 94, 100, 148, 200, 204-205, 211-214, 218, 246, 250
Tylenol, 156
Tyrosine, 62, 135, 166, 174-175, 178

U

Ultimate Nutrition, 100, 205-206, 351
Ultimate Orange, 203, 219, 351
Unipro, 206
University of Florida, 212
University of Memphis, 7, 73, 104, 254
University of Nebraska, 7, 57, 104, 254
University of Nottingham, 51, 59, 104
University of Pittsburgh, 39-40
University of Texas, 80
University of Wisconsin, 104
University of Wisconsin-Madison, 181
Unsaturated fat, 95, 272, 333, 335, 342
Urea, 166, 256, 312

V

V2G, 94, 141, 215, 240-241
Valine, 81, 164, 169-170
Vanadium, 142-143, 311
Vanadyl sulfate, 10, 14, 33, 35, 94, 111, 141-143, 218-220, 227, 240, 283, 285, 289, 292, 311, 314, 316, 345-346, 351
Vasodilation, 129, 140, 214, 351
Vegetarian, 50, 128, 130, 136, 185, 320
Victory Super Mega Mass 2000, 220, 351
Vitamin A, 122-125, 152, 221, 347-348
Vitamin B, 154, 321, 326
Vitamin B$_1$, 127
Vitamin B$_2$, 128
Vitamin B$_3$, 128
Vitamin B$_5$, 129
Vitamin B$_6$, 128-130, 172, 344
Vitamin B$_{12}$, 118, 130, 185, 315, 350
Vitamin C, 18, 74, 86-88, 90, 118, 122, 124-126, 136, 144, 189-190, 259, 276, 282-283, 288-289, 292, 318-319, 345-347
Vitamin D, 122, 126-127, 331, 348
Vitamin E, 86, 88, 125-127, 182, 214, 346, 349
Vitamin K, 127, 350
VO$_2$max, 69, 343, 350

Volumize, 52-53, 71, 80, 83, 172, 279, 281, 284
Vukovich, Dr. Mathew, 69, 170, 350

W

Walls, Mike, 204
Water soluble, 37, 63, 72, 86, 122, 128, 130, 192, 246
Weider, 39, 94, 100, 148, 196-197, 200, 203-204, 206-208, 214, 220, 246, 250, 351
Weight gain, 108, 119, 197, 203, 212, 313, 314
Weight Gainer 900, 351
Weight loss, 76-77, 326
Weightlifting, 138, 194, 225, 262, 288, 303, 329, 344
Whey peptide, 103
Whey protein, 10, 61-65, 80, 94, 110, 189, 214-215, 222, 225, 227, 242, 246, 249, 312, 325, 344-345
White willow bark, 154-155
Worldwide Sport Nutrition, 217, 351

X

X-Plode, 100, 220, 351

Y

Yogurt, 74, 167, 211, 290
Yohimbe, 100, 151, 214, 221, 235-237, 322-323
Yohimbine, 30, 100, 151, 214, 235, 237, 322-324, 344, 348-349

Z

Zebutol, 322
Zinc, 122, 125, 143-144, 208, 214, 344-345, 350
Zumpano, Michael, 197

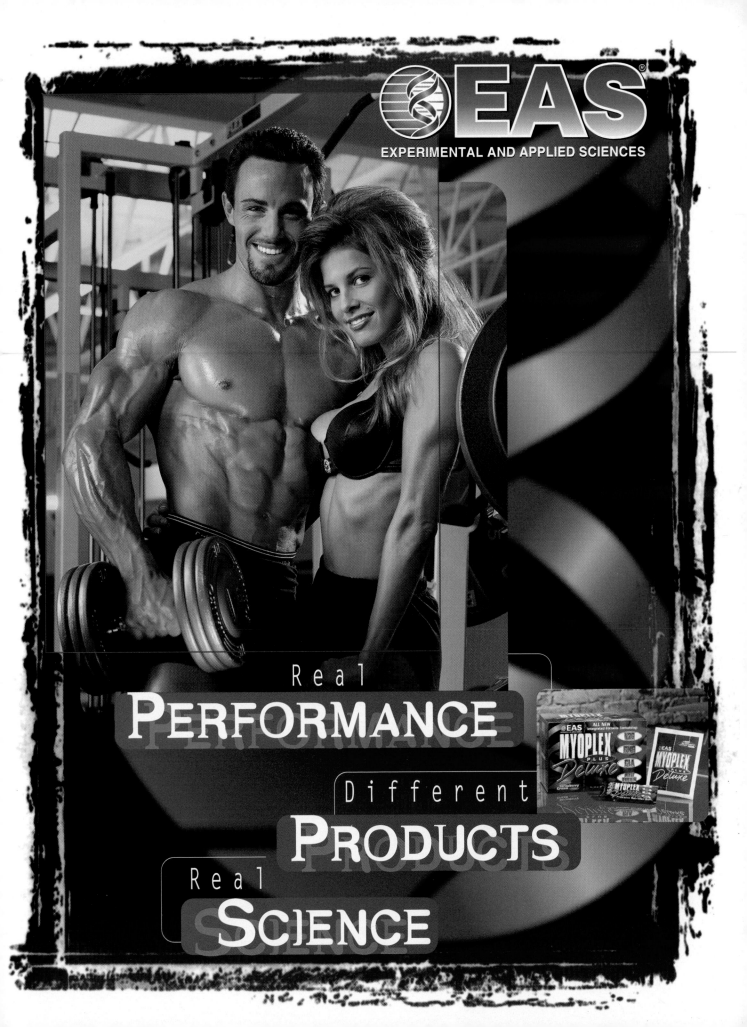

SCIENCE

makes the difference

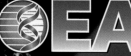 **is committed to providing the** marketplace with credible information and reliable products that enhance muscle metabolism and sports performance. We aim to foster understanding and responsible use of nutritional supplements that have been scientifically designed to enhance the positive effects of exercise and a healthy lifestyle.

Our mission is to be unparalleled in the knowledge of scientific nutritional research, in the design and formulation of effective and safe nutritional supplements, in the collaborative support of university-level clinical research on our products, and in the application of this research to the marketplace. Aiming to further expand and refine our nutritional and metabolic performance product line, EAS assigns high priority to supporting original research collaborations.

A portion of every dollar consumers spend on EAS supplements goes to fund additional university research that will hopefully identify new and perhaps even better drug-free ways to build muscle size and strength and enhance performance.

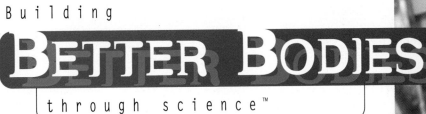

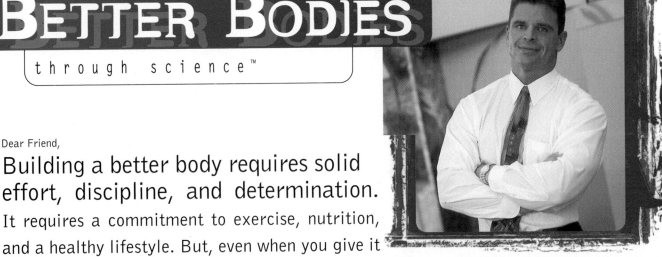

Dear Friend,

Building a better body requires solid effort, discipline, and determination.

It requires a commitment to exercise, nutrition, and a healthy lifestyle. But, even when you give it your best, progress isn't guaranteed. I'm sure from time to time you've experienced a plateau or slow progress. I know I have—it's frustrating.

I guess that's why we're all looking for that extra edge—something that will help us get better results faster. And, today more than ever before, bodybuilders and athletes like us are turning to supplements (instead of drugs) for that extra advantage.

The good news is, over the past few years, legitimate scientific research has shown that supplements can make a difference—a big difference! The right ones can boost athletic performance as well as increase gains in size and strength. The science of supplements really is moving forward at an encouraging pace.

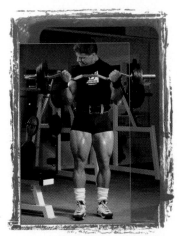

The bad news is, not all supplements work—there are some companies which sell products that are, well... to put it bluntly... *garbage*. They're not based on anything that has to do with science, and some of these supplements don't even contain what their labels claim, much less do what their advertisements suggest. Make no mistake, it can be a real chore trying to sort it all out.

I'm often asked what makes EAS different from the others—why has EAS so rapidly become the hottest brand in the sports nutrition business?

The answer can be found in our commitment to *science*. From the very beginning, EAS set out to build the most effective, scientifically designed, university-tested supplements on the market. And, we have made an extraordinary effort to make this happen. I firmly believe the reason EAS products are so popular among athletes and fitness buffs of all kinds—from bodybuilders (novice and advanced) to professional football players to gold-medal-winning, world-champion athletes—is because EAS products work in the real world as well as they do in the university laboratories where they are subjected to rigorous trials.

I share your passion for building a better body, and I understand you *demand* products that work as hard as you do. That's why I feel very confident in highly recommending these powerful supplements to anyone who wants to build a better body. I believe EAS products are the best available, and I'm confident that if you use them along with an effective exercise and nutrition program, you'll see and feel the difference these supplements can make! In fact, I guarantee it!

Very sincerely,

Bill Phillips

Bill Phillips
CEO, EAS

continued →

There is no
questioning whether or not Phosphagen produces dramatic
results in the laboratory and in the real world;
it does, and
it works *fast*.

Shawn Phillips

EAS Executive, drug-free athlete, and Phosphagen fanatic.

PHOSPHAGEN™

the original creatine supplement

The research scientists at EAS started

a whole new era in sports nutrition when, in 1993, they introduced the first creatine monohydrate supplement to the sports nutrition market under the brand name Phosphagen.

Phosphagen was the first creatine product shown in university studies to increase lean mass and strength in weight-training athletes.[4]

Over the past four years, numerous university studies have confirmed creatine helps athletes increase size and muscle strength, even in the most rigorous trials.[1,7,8]

Phosphagen is a nutrient formed from three specific amino acids and is also found in various whole foods, such as red meat. (Phosphagen is derived from sources free of animal products.) Phosphagen saturates muscle tissue with creatine, an essential precursor component of muscle energy production. By increasing muscle creatine concentrations, athletes can recover more quickly between bouts of intense physical activity, such as weight training.[7]

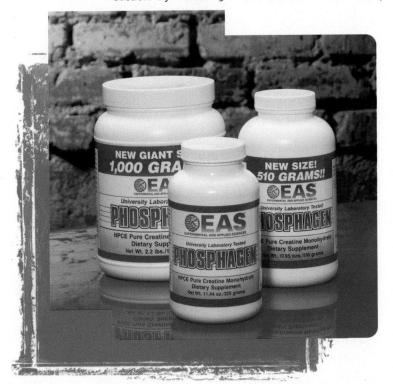

Over 95% of the body's creatine pool is stored inside muscle cells. And, leading scientists believe most athletes can store more creatine than is normally obtained from the diet. Phosphagen supplementation helps "saturate" your muscles with creatine. When the muscle holds extra creatine, it has more reserve fuel for intense exercise which can result in substantial increases in power. (Many Phosphagen users report significant increases in strength after using Phosphagen for only a week.)

It's also believed that when a muscle cell takes in more creatine, it also brings water along with it. This promotes a phenomenon called cell volumizing or cellular hydration. When a muscle cell is hydrated, it gets bigger, and this may create improved conditions for new muscle growth.[10,11]

Cell volumizing does not involve water retention outside of cells—the type that can produce a puffy look. It promotes *intra*cellular hydration. Think of your muscle cells as individual water balloons (muscles are made up of 70% water). If you can get more water *inside* of them, they get bigger and firmer—if you let water out, they get smaller and softer. When muscles start to swell with creatine and water, and then you train with weights, it can cause an extraordinary "pump."

There is no questioning whether or not Phosphagen produces dramatic results in the laboratory and in the real world; it does, and it works *fast*. That is undoubtedly why Phosphagen has been such an amazingly popular product—it remains the number one creatine supplement on the market and is used by tens of thousands of serious bodybuilders and other athletes to gain that "extra edge."

continued →

A recent
university study showed
Phosphagen HP may
significantly enhance
athletic performance.

Shannon
Sharpe

All-pro tight end/receiver, Denver Broncos—
bench presses 470 lbs—uses Phosphagen HP daily.

PHOSPHAGEN HP™

In 1995, the EAS research and development team took creatine supplementation

a step further with the introduction of Phosphagen HP—High Performance Creatine Transport System.™ This product was developed based on the latest research conducted by scientists in Europe, which showed high-glycemic carbohydrates (which cause a natural release of the anabolic hormone insulin) significantly enhance muscle creatine uptake.[5,6]

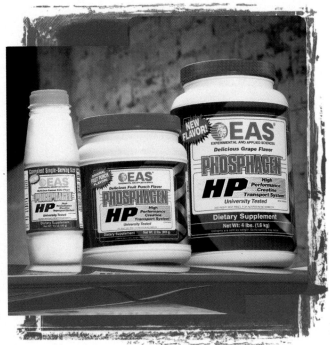

Further scientific evidence has shown that even athletes who don't respond to regular creatine monohydrate supplementation are likely to become "responders" when they consume creatine along with a carbohydrate source that increases insulin.

In a recent EAS-funded university study, scientists compared the effects of Phosphagen HP to those of regular creatine monohydrate and discovered both supplements enhance lean mass and strength compared with a placebo, but Phosphagen HP produces up to 160% greater gains in lean mass.[19] In this study, Phosphagen HP also significantly improved sprint time (in a 100-meter dash) and maximum vertical jump, while supporting a reduction in bodyfat greater than that seen with the placebo or creatine by itself.

Phosphagen HP contains pure creatine monohydrate; the high glycemic, insulin-releasing carbohydrate dextrose; and sodium from sodium phosphate (a critical nutrient for proper creatine transport) and is available in three refreshing flavors: lemon-lime, grape, and fruit punch.

PHOSPHAGEMS™ NEW!

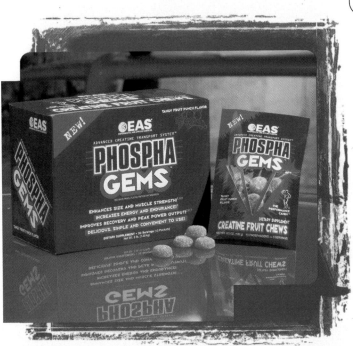

Another new EAS product, designed along the same scientific theory as

Phosphagen HP, is the new "performance candy," PhosphaGems. These creatine "fruit chews" are not your ordinary candy—this supplement contains a special high-glycemic carbohydrate blend and over five grams of creatine per serving. When you eat PhosphaGems, the special blend of carbs causes a rapid increase of insulin (very similar to how Phosphagen HP works), which promotes the uptake of creatine and glucose by muscle tissue. This, in turn, may cause an increase in lean mass and strength above and beyond using creatine by itself.

One of the great things about PhosphaGems is that you can take them with you anywhere—in your gym bag, briefcase, your car when you travel, etc. They're great for post-workout energy and a creatine boost or for snacking throughout the day. PhosphaGems really are delicious—they're sweet, tart, and chewy. (They taste like regular candy, but they're definitely not!)

continued →

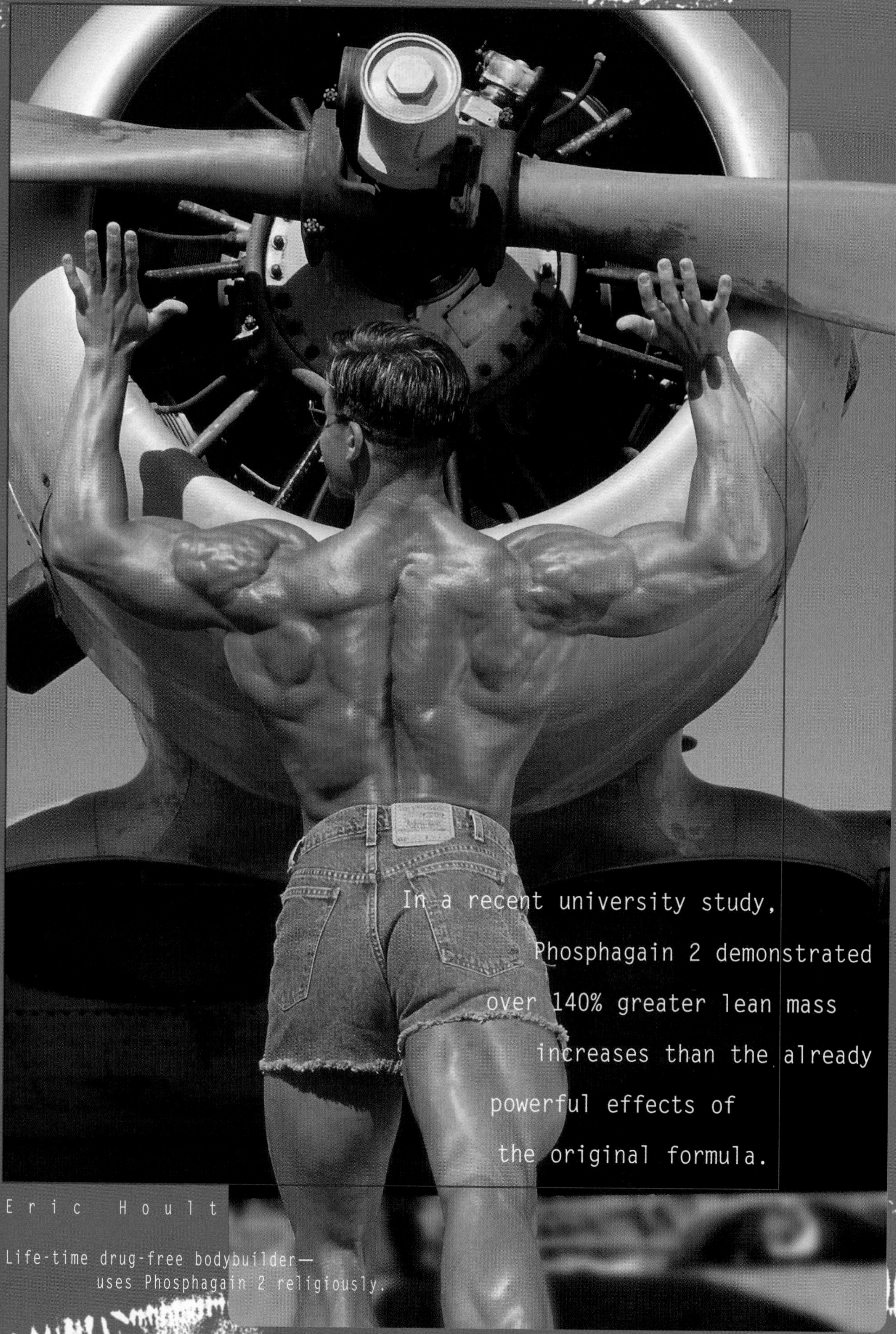

In a recent university study,
Phosphagain 2 demonstrated
over 140% greater lean mass
increases than the already
powerful effects of
the original formula.

Eric Hoult

Life-time drug-free bodybuilder—
uses Phosphagain 2 religiously.

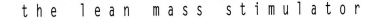

PHOSPHAGAIN®

the lean mass stimulator

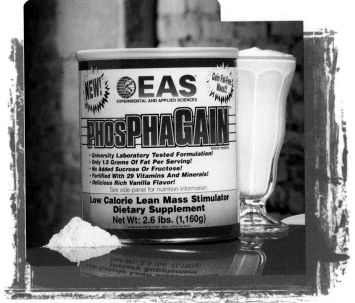

In 1994, the world of

weight-gain powders was forced to

go on a crash diet: mega-calories; unsubstantiated

hype; and bloated, ever-growing waistlines

fell prey to the original *hypo*caloric (*low* calorie) university-tested[12] lean-mass-stimulator Phosphagain® This supplement was designed to help weight trainers gain lean mass *without* putting on fat.

Since its introduction, Phosphagain has become an extremely popular bodybuilding supplement, and numerous attempts to duplicate this revolutionary formulation have been made, but Phosphagain is still the ONLY one shown in published university studies to increase lean body mass without increasing fat, the latter being the unsightly downside of even the most popular mega-calorie weight gainers.

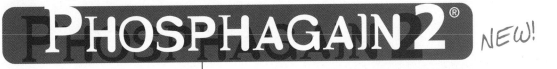

PHOSPHAGAIN2® NEW!

a new and improved formula

Following the revolution of

weight gainers came the *evolution* of lean mass

stimulators: Phosphagain 2.® Phosphagain 2 is at the leading edge

of lean-mass-building supplements, delivering 25% more protein in

the form of Nitrogenin 2,™ a modified carbohydrate profile for even better tolerability and a comprehensive array of micronutrients, including 29 vitamins and minerals. At the heart of the Phosphagain 2 formula is an improved and expanded version of Phosphagain's unique, patent-pending biochemical matrix which includes: Phosphagen™ (HPCE pure creatine monohydrate), yeast RNA, L-glutamine, alpha-ketoglutarate (AKG), and taurine. These biomolecules support cell volumizing, glutamine preservation, and lean-mass augmentation.

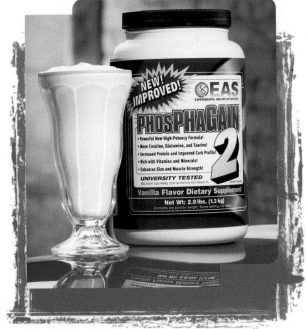

At EAS we believe the best way to compare one product to another is to allow the objective hands of university scientists to test their effects "head to head" on muscle size and strength in weight-training athletes. (Advertisements with tally sheets comparing quantities do not automatically equal greater results.) In a recent university study, Phosphagain 2 demonstrated over 140% greater lean-mass increases than the already powerful effects of the original formula.[13] University data, combined with impressive results in the real world, indicate Phosphagain 2 will be a powerful supplement for athletes looking to gain size and strength *without* putting on fat.

Phosphagain 2 is available in new, convenient 20-serving containers in rich vanilla, strawberry cream, and deluxe chocolate flavors, which all make a delicious, high-nutrient shake.

continued →

University studies
show HMB may promote
gains in muscle
size and strength and
accelerate fat loss.

Joe
Lazzaro

Bodybuilding champion—
devoted HMB user.

HMB™

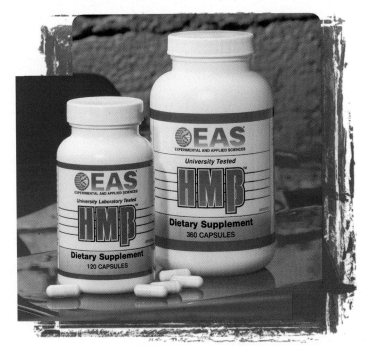

This supplement is

definitely the state of the art in drug-free bodybuilding. HMB (beta-hydroxy beta-methylbutyrate) is a patented amino acid metabolite that was discovered by research scientists at Iowa State University. University studies have shown that when intensely trained athletes supplement their diets with HMB, they gain significantly more lean mass and strength than athletes using a placebo.[14,15] These two studies also showed that HMB may help accelerate fat loss that occurs secondary to strenuous exercise.

Scientists theorize that HMB may suppress protein breakdown that follows intensive exercise, producing an anti-catabolic effect. By reducing muscle tissue breakdown, HMB may tip the scales of protein turnover in favor of new muscle growth.

EAS was the first company to bring HMB to the market. Since then, it has been written up in numerous health and fitness magazines, hundreds of newspapers, and it's been featured on dozens of TV news programs as an exciting, breakthrough supplement which might allow bodybuilders and fitness buffs to get better results faster from the time they spend exercising.

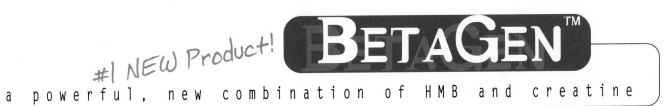

BetaGen™

#1 NEW Product!

a powerful, new combination of HMB and creatine

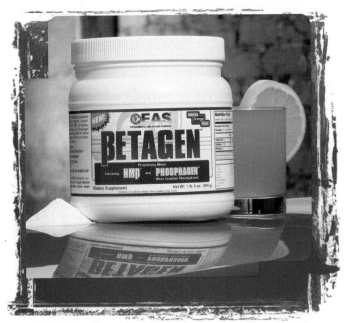

The concept behind this new

EAS supplement is rather simple—it didn't take any Nobel Prize winners to come up with this one. But, sometimes the simplest ideas are the best ones.

Virtually any bodybuilder who's been following the "supplement news" over the past year knows creatine monohydrate and HMB are probably the two most effective supplements on the market right now. Creatine has been shown to work in study after study, and HMB is developing an impressive track record of its own. Both of these products have been shown to produce dramatic results in the laboratory and in the real world.

BetaGen is an exclusive formula, available only from EAS, that contains pure creatine monohydrate and HMB, as well as the cell-volumizing amino acids glutamine and taurine—the two most abundant free amino acids in muscle tissue.

BetaGen is a powdered drink mix that is very convenient to use and has a delicious orange flavor. Simply pour a serving of it into a small glass of water, stir it up, and drink it down. Or, you can add it to a protein drink, a milk shake, or a meal-replacement powder. It not only offers tremendous convenience but also great value.

(BetaGen was designed for use as a creatine maintenance-dose supplement. Phosphagen HP is probably the best product for creatine loading, which you should do the first week you take creatine.)

continued →

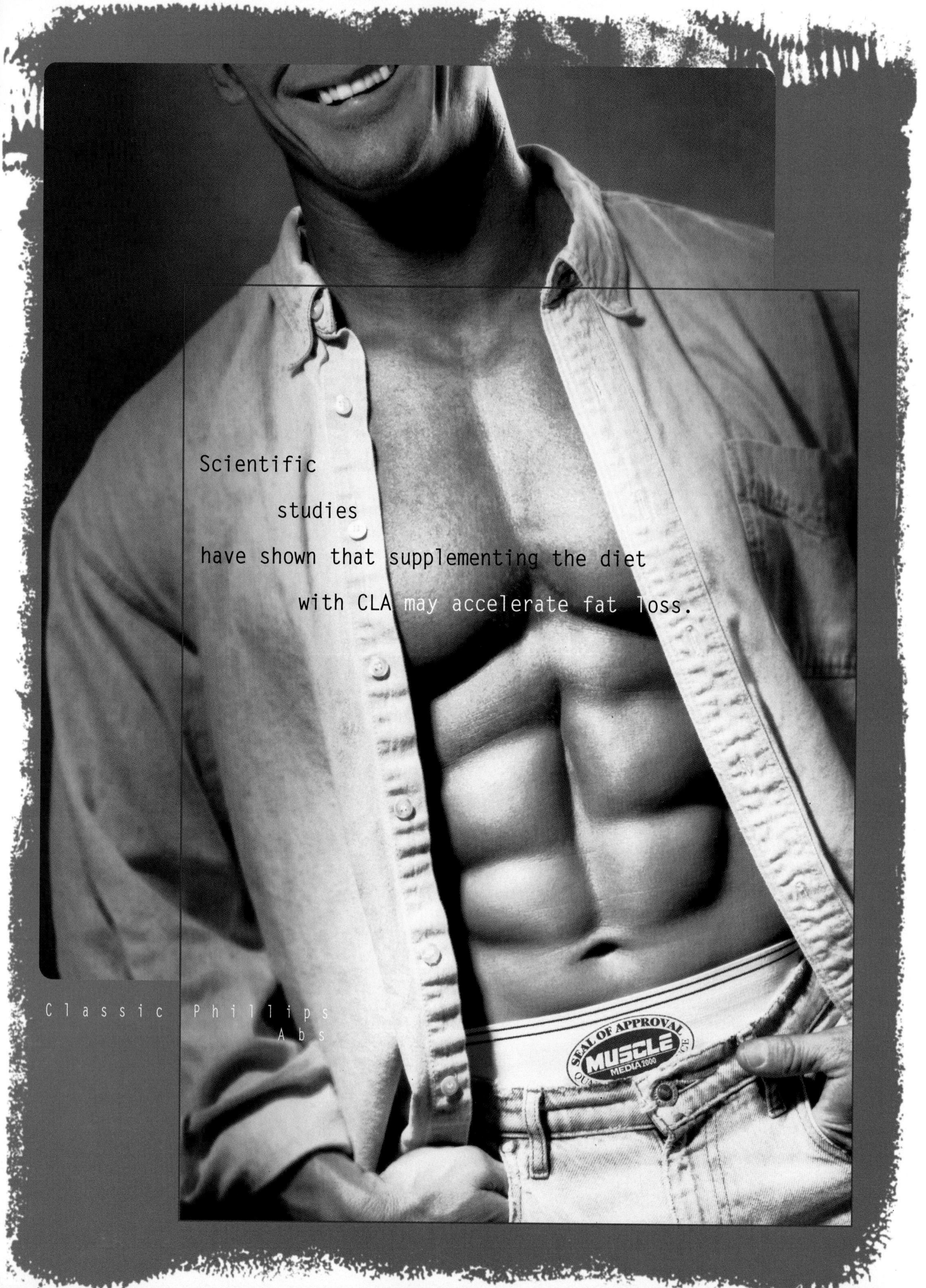

Scientific
studies
have shown that supplementing the diet
with CLA may accelerate fat loss.
Classic Phillips Abs
SEAL OF APPROVAL
MUSCLE
MEDIA 2000

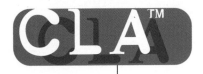

CLA™

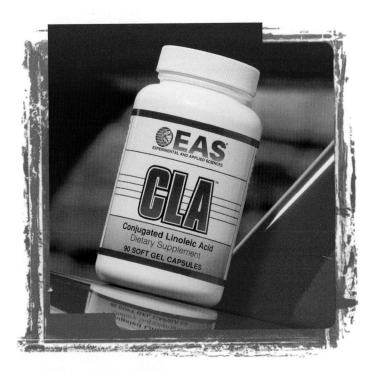

CLA (conjugated linoleic acid) is a naturally

occurring nutrient which scientists have discovered exerts a positive effect on protein and fat metabolism.[9,16] Controlled scientific studies have shown that supplementing the diet with CLA may accelerate fat loss,[17] increase lean body mass, and have potent antioxidant properties.

Based on these results, scientists hypothesize that CLA, possibly acting to enhance metabolic activity at the cellular membrane level, may allow those who exercise and follow a healthy lifestyle to lose fat and gain muscle definition faster. EAS introduced CLA to the supplement market in 1996 and was the first company to fund human clinical studies (which are ongoing at two major universities) involving this patented dietary supplement.

V2G™

The researchers behind EAS introduced vanadyl sulfate to the nutritional

supplement industry in 1989. V2G catapulted vanadyl sulfate into the next generation, creating a new frontier in vanadyl action and synergism. This was achieved through the addition of the selenate form of the essential trace mineral selenium (which has been shown to mimic several of the actions of vanadyl while being twice as potent as other forms of selenium) and taurine, a non-protein amino acid, which also supports the actions of vanadyl through distinct and specific mechanisms.

V2G was designed to support carbohydrate metabolism by potentiating the effects of insulin, a potent anabolic hormone which helps shuttle glucose and amino acids into muscle tissue and stimulate glycogen and protein synthesis.

V2G users frequently report that within a week or two of regular use of this supplement, their muscles feel fuller and more "pumped," which anecdotally confirms the scientific hypothesis behind this supplement—that V2G increases the amount of glycogen (your body's stored form of glucose energy) that's being pushed into muscle cells, making them bigger and stronger.

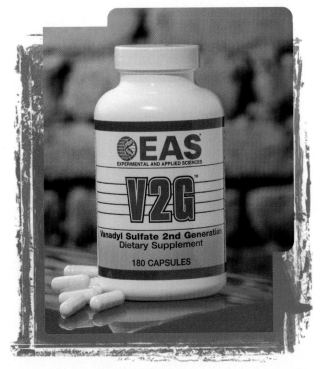

continued →

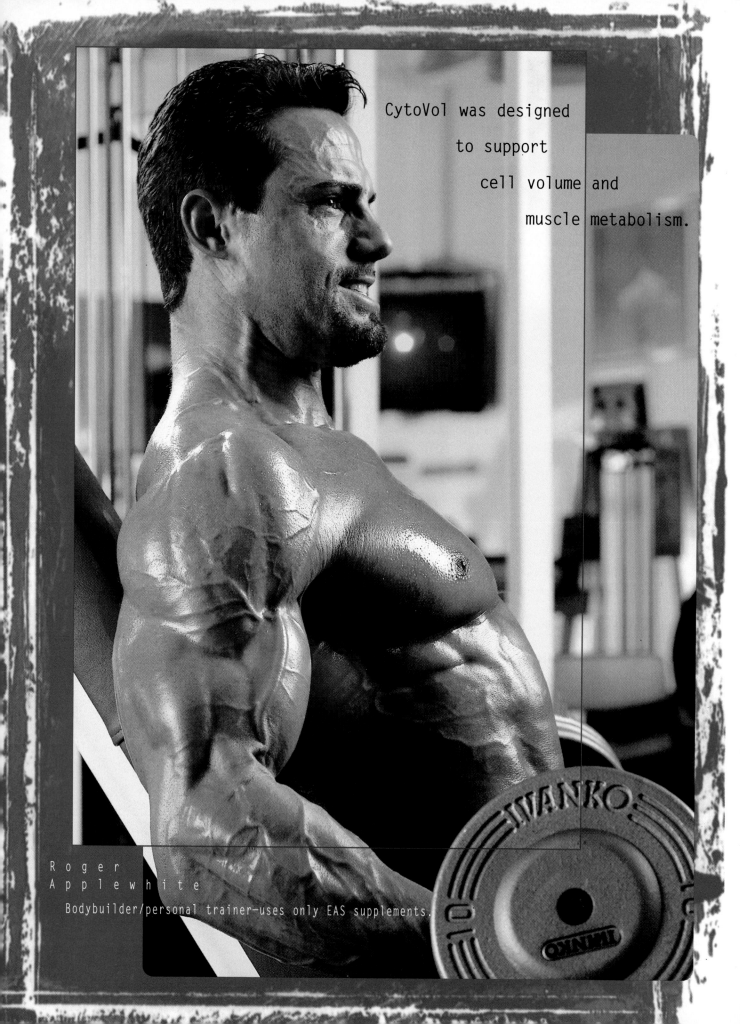

CytoVol was designed
to support
cell volume and
muscle metabolism.

Roger
Applewhite
Bodybuilder/personal trainer—uses only EAS supplements.

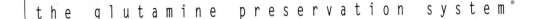

GKG®

the glutamine preservation system®

With the introduction

of GKG capsules in 1993, EAS introduced a new concept to sports nutrition—*cell volumizing.* By focusing on the vitally important nutrient glutamine (the most abundant free amino acid in muscle tissue), GKG offers a unique approach to supporting muscle metabolism. GKG not only provides the free amino acid glutamine but also the glutamine precursors alpha-ketoglutarate (AKG) and taurine, the second most abundant free amino acid in muscle, which also promotes cell volumizing.

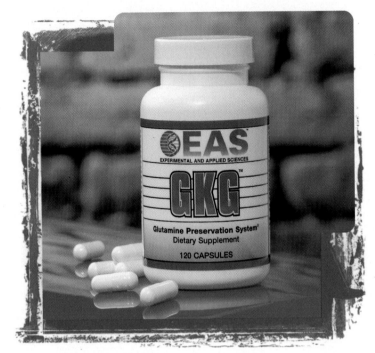

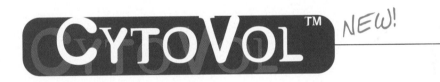

CYTOVOL™ NEW!

the new cell volumizer

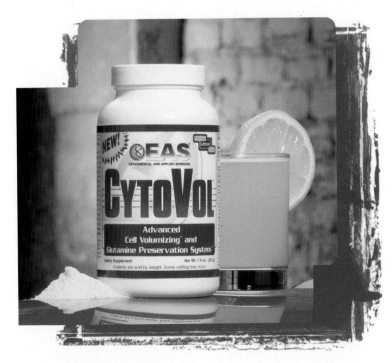

CytoVol reopens the door

to cell volumizing, incorporating a precise selection of novel cell-volumizing components along with the glutamine preservation system of GKG into a superb-tasting, convenient, lemon-flavored drink mix. CytoVol broadens the cell-volumizing focus beyond glutamine and taurine through the addition of L-alanine, glycine, and inositol—nutrients that may further potentiate cell volumizing and produce an optimal cellular environment for new muscle growth.[11] CytoVol also contains the essential glutamine synthesis cofactor manganese as well as yeast RNA to support the resistance system, which is activated by high-intensity training.

CytoVol is convenient and easy to use—it can be mixed with water, a protein drink, yogurt, or a milk shake.

continued →

Myoplex Plus Deluxe
helps take
the
guesswork out
of optimal
nutrition and
supplementation.

Eric
Hoult

A product of proper training, nutrition,
and EAS supplementation.

MYOPLEX PLUS™

precision nutrition for athletes

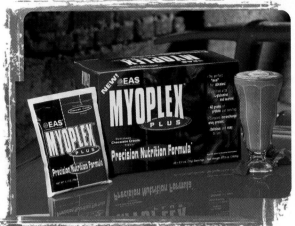

It's no secret that optimal nutrition,

combined with exercise, is essential to building a better body. And, it's also no secret that intensely training athletes and bodybuilders experience greater metabolic stress and an increased need for nutrients, including dietary protein[20] and certain micronutrients.[18]

Unfortunately, in today's busy world, it's sometimes difficult, even for the most dedicated fitness and physique enthusiasts, to find the time to shop for, prepare, and consume multiple meals, day in and day out, that contain all of the nutrients necessary to support their efforts to build better bodies.

The original Myoplex Plus formula was designed to help take the guesswork out of the complex and sometimes confusing subject of "optimal nutrition." Each serving of Myoplex Plus is fortified with 42 grams of a unique and proprietary blend of high-quality proteins, which includes ion-exchanged whey protein—perhaps the best protein available today. Ion-exchanged whey protein may also provide an additional benefit to intensely training individuals through its ability to support resistance to infection and antioxidant protection systems[2,3]—critical components on the path to a better physique. This unique formula is also enriched with 29 vitamins and minerals as well as 24 grams of energy-rich complex carbohydrates.

MYOPLEX PLUS DELUXE™

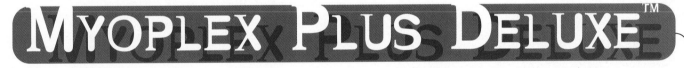

NEW! a total nutrition supplement and more

The all-new EAS supplement

Myoplex Plus Deluxe expands on the original formula by incorporating a trio of EAS' metabolic support products: V2G™ (carbohydrate metabolic support), GKG® (whole-body glutamine preservation system), and CLA (conjugated linoleic acid)—a comprehensive biochemical complement to the balanced nutrition in Myoplex Plus.

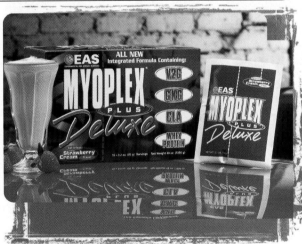

Myoplex Plus Deluxe helps take even more of the guesswork out of optimal nutrition and supplementation. This new, integrated formula offers extraordinary quality and value. And, perhaps best of all, Myoplex Plus Deluxe is absolutely delicious and super easy to use!

Myoplex Plus Deluxe is available in three delicious flavors: rich vanilla, strawberry cream, and deluxe chocolate. All make a fantastic total-nutrition shake.

MYOPLEX PLUS DELUXE BAR™   NEW!

The relentless quest for optimal nutrition can now rest upon the Myoplex Plus Deluxe precision nutrition bar. This unique formula offers the superior features of ion-exchanged whey protein, a balanced carbohydrate blend, and a fraction of the fat found in a typical candy bar. Add in the perfect metabolic complement—V2G,™ GKG,® and CLA—and you have a delicious and totally "portable" between-meal nutrition and energy support complex or post-workout nutrient repair system. The Myoplex Plus Deluxe precision nutrition bar provides satisfaction for your taste buds and optimal nutrition for your body.

Available in outrageously delicious chocolate and chocolate-peanut butter flavors.

continued →

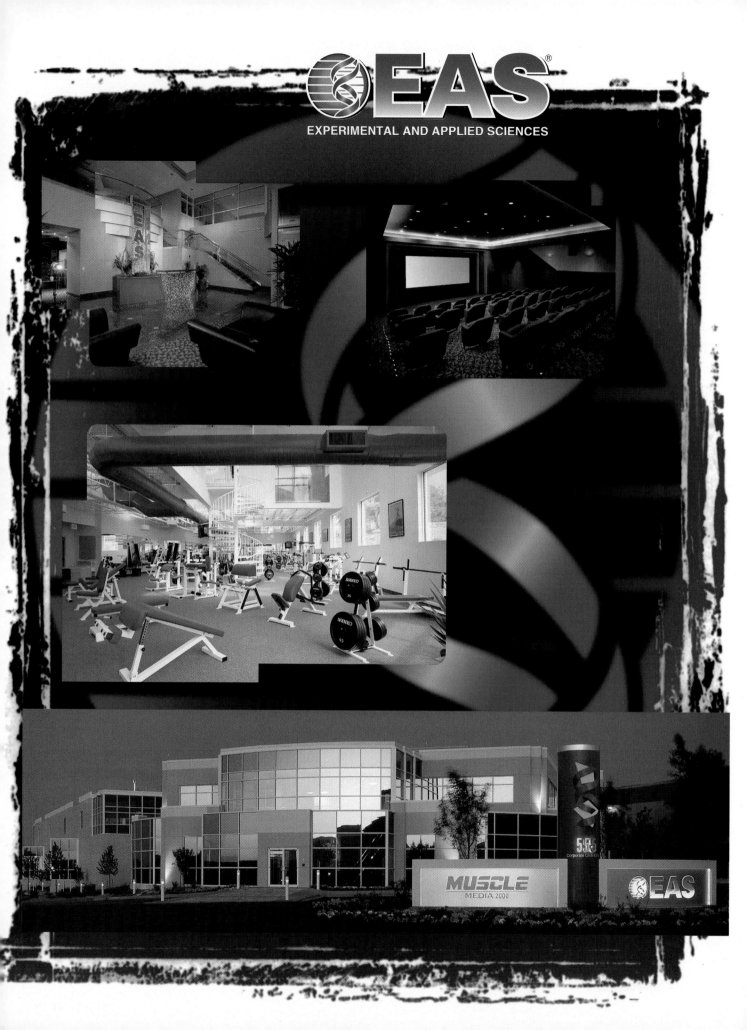

EAS Background and Philosophy

EAS is one of the nation's fastest growing privately held companies involved in research, development, and marketing of nutritional supplements for athletes and fitness enthusiasts. EAS is quickly reaching its goal to be the world's leading scientifically oriented provider of fitness-related nutritional supplements and associated educational information.

Based in Golden, Colorado, EAS internationally markets and distributes its line of nutritional supplements through direct sales and health-food retailers. The company's product line includes Phosphagen™ (creatine monohydrate). Leading sports medicine experts refer to this product as the most significant advancement in sports nutrition in recent history.

EAS was the first company to offer this supplement to athletes and to fund university research which showed Phosphagen not only helps improve sports performance but also helps increase lean body mass (one of the primary goals of weight-training athletes).

Most recently, EAS has become exclusive licensee for the distribution of pure HMB. The company collaborated in the scientific evaluation of this supplement, which caught national attention in early 1996 after university studies revealed it may significantly enhance the positive effects of intense exercise, allowing fitness buffs to boost gains in lean body mass and strength while simultaneously accelerating reductions in bodyfat.

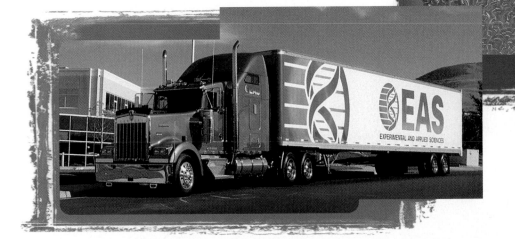

EAS Corporate Headquarters

A description of the new EAS Corporate Headquarters reads like a combination of a top-of-the-line office and warehouse complex, meshed with an entertainment center, health spa, and first-rate fitness club.

This new 60,000-square-foot facility, completed in June of 1996, juxtaposes remarkable views of the Colorado Rocky Mountains on one side and a breathtaking cityscape on the other.

Incorporated into the facility is a 3,455-square-foot corporate gym, which doubles as a research laboratory for in-house clinical studies. The fitness center is equipped with the highest quality, state-of-the-art resistance-training equipment from companies such as Strive, Flex, and Ivanko. All employees are encouraged to take advantage of the gym, which is staffed by professional, certified personal trainers, who provide motivation and instruction.

EAS employees enjoy a private game room, theater, salon, commercial-grade kitchen with spa chef, VIP locker rooms, an in-house photo studio, and spacious offices with satellite TV.

The EAS Corporate Headquarters clearly reflects a company that is dedicated to promoting fitness as well as servicing its customers. Make no mistake, EAS is not a "fly-by-night" supplement company which relies on a "get-rich-quick" philosophy or gimmicks—this is a company which builds long-term relationships with its customers and is committed to doing business the *right way*.

continued →

INVESTMENT IN SCIENCE

EAS is committed to investing in scientific research in order to benefit the company,
its consumers, and the entire nutritional supplement industry.

Unique to EAS is its partnership with the scientific community and its support of university clinical research to investigate the effectiveness of specific nutritional supplements among various population groups. This partnership has resulted in more than 20 abstract presentations at major scientific conferences throughout the world and has already resulted in the publication of three original research studies in peer-reviewed scientific and medical journals, including the prestigious *International Journal of Sport Nutrition* and *Acta Physiologica Scandinavica.*

EAS has allocated more than one million dollars to university studies to further the science of sports nutrition. In 1996 alone, we contributed grants to fund research in the areas of human performance and muscle metabolism to Kent State University, Iowa State University, Creighton University, the University of Nebraska at Omaha, the University of Memphis, State University of New York at Stonybrook, and Nottingham University in England.

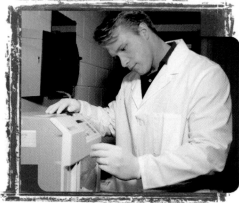

This is an unprecedented financial commitment for this industry. It not only reflects EAS' support of scientific research in the fields of human physiology and metabolism but also underscores the company's mission to apply scientific research to product development.

To assist EAS in achieving this mission, our research team collaborates with top scientists and doctors from around the world with expertise in human metabolism, physiology, and biochemistry. EAS' scientific advisors offer input on the design of clinical studies and in EAS' scientific direction—fostering discussions to advance human metabolism and performance and broaden the scope of its application.

COMMITMENT TO CUSTOMER SERVICE AND SATISFACTION

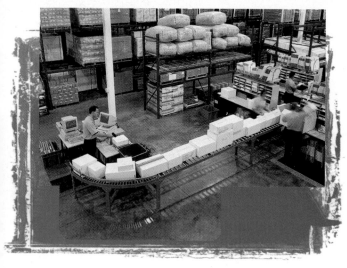

The EAS name represents the highest
caliber of people, products, ethics, and market-service philosophy.

EAS employs more than 140 individuals at its new 60,000-square-foot headquarters, which houses both office and warehouse facilities. At our headquarters, trained customer-care professionals take approximately 2,000 orders a day from customers around the world. Our warehouse personnel take great pride in the accurate, timely, and meticulous shipment of all orders. Our state-of-the-art operations allow us to process orders within 24 hours and ship them, at no premium charge, by Federal Express service.

In addition, our EAS technical-support staff is available to answer your questions. These professionals are trained experts, not only in the area of EAS product use but also in the sciences of health, exercise, and nutrition. Our experts will take time to answer all your questions, in detail, even if you're not ordering an EAS product.

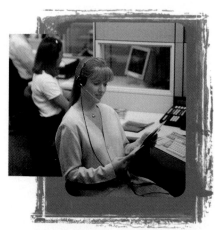

EAS also offers a guarantee that is unprecedented in this industry—a lifetime, 100% money-back guarantee. If you use any EAS product and aren't completely satisfied, you're entitled to 100% of your purchase price back. This extraordinary policy is another indicator of EAS' commitment to customer satisfaction and service.

At EAS, we confront the problems, satisfy customers' needs, and eliminate the worry. Twenty-four hours a day, seven days a week, EAS customer-care professionals are here to serve. Call us at 1-800-297-9776 (Dept. #4196).

BetaGen™

An orange-flavored drink mix, available in 30- or 90-serving containers. Nutritional information per 6.6 gram serving:

Calories	10
Carbohydrates	2 g

Vitamins and minerals: U.S. RDA%
Not a significant source of fat, saturated fat, cholesterol, dietary fiber, Vitamins A & C, calcium, and iron.

Also provides per serving:

Ca HMB Monohydrate	1,000 mg
Creatine Monohydrate	2,000 mg
Potassium Phosphate	50 mg
L-Glutamine	400 mg
Taurine	200 mg

BetaGen Ingredients:
Dextrose, Phosphagen™ (HPCE pure creatine monohydrate), calcium β-hydroxy β-methylbutyrate monohydrate, citric acid, L-glutamine, natural flavors, taurine, potassium phosphate, aspartame*, and beta-carotene for color.

***PHENYLKETONURICS:** Contains phenylalanine.

Recommended Use: Add 1 scoop to 4 oz of water or juice, and stir/mix until dissolved. Or add a serving of BetaGen to your favorite protein drink or meal-replacement powder. Use 3 servings daily. Do not exceed recommended dosage. Consult with a physician prior to use if you have any medical conditions. Do not use if pregnant or lactating.

CLA™

Available in 90-capsule containers.

Each soft gel capsule contains:
1,000 mg vegetable oil with 60% conjugated linoleic acid (CLA) and 40% other monounsaturated and saturated fatty acids. 0.02% TBHQ (antioxidant) has been added to preserve freshness.

Recommended Use:
Take 2 capsules, 3 times daily with meals.

CytoVol™

A lemon-flavored drink mix, available in 15-serving containers. Nutritional information per 15 gram serving:

Calories	45
Carbohydrates	4 g
Sodium	60 mg

Vitamins and minerals: U.S. RDA%

Calcium	30%
Phosphorus	6%

Not a significant source of fat, saturated fat, cholesterol, dietary fiber, Vitamins A & C, and iron.

Also provides per serving:

L-Glutamine	2,500 mg
Taurine	2,000 mg
Manganese	50 mcg
Calcium AKG	1,500 mg
Inositol	500 mg
Glycine	500 mg
RNA	250 mg
L-Alanine	2,000 mg

CytoVol Ingredients:
Dextrose, L-glutamine, taurine, L-alanine, calcium alpha-ketoglutarate (AKG), citric acid, natural flavors, inositol, glycine, sodium ribonucleic acid (RNA), sodium phosphate, turmeric mixed with maltodextrin for color, aspartame*, and manganese glycinate.

***PHENYLKETONURICS:** Contains phenylalanine.

Recommended Use: As a dietary supplement, mix/stir 4 tsp in 6-8 oz of cold water or juice and consume after training or before going to sleep.

GKG™

Available in 120-capsule containers.

Each capsule contains:

α-Ketoglutaric acid (Calcium alpha-ketoglutarate)	250 mg
L-Glutamine	275 mg
Taurine	150 mg
Calcium (Calcium alpha-ketoglutarate)	63 mg
Potassium (Potassium chloride and phosphate)	25 mg
Magnesium (Magnesium phosphate and oxide)	25 mg
RNA (Sodium RNA/less than 1 mg of sodium)	9.5 mg
Manganese (Albion® glycinate)	400 mcg

Recommended Use: As a dietary supplement, take 3-6 capsules after training and at bedtime. On non-training days, take 6-12 capsules at bedtime.

HMB

Available in 120- or 360-capsule containers.

Each 4-capsule serving supplies:

HMB (Calcium β-hydroxy β-methylbutyrate monohydrate)	1,000 mg
Potassium Phosphate	200 mg

Recommended Use: As a dietary supplement, take 4 capsules 3 times per day with meals. Do not exceed recommended dose. Consult with a physician prior to use if you have any medical conditions. Do not use if pregnant or lactating.

Myoplex Plus™

Vanilla, chocolate, and strawberry flavors available in boxes of 20 or 42 packets. Nutritional information per 76 gram vanilla serving:

Calories	280
Protein	42 g
Carbohydrates	24 g
Fat	2 g
Cholesterol	15 mg
Sodium	330 mg
Potassium	550 mg
Fiber	<1 g

Vitamins and minerals:	U.S. RDA%
Vitamin A (20% as beta-carotene)	40%
Vitamin C	50%
Calcium	50%
Iron	50%
Vitamin D	50%
Vitamin E	100%
Thiamin	50%
Riboflavin	50%
Niacin	50%
Vitamin B_6	50%
Folic Acid	50%
Vitamin B_{12}	50%
Biotin	50%
Pantothenic Acid	50%
Phosphorus	50%
Iodine	50%
Magnesium	50%
Zinc	50%
Copper	50%

Recommended Use: For a rich, creamy shake, combine the contents of each packet with 15 oz of cold water, juice, or skim milk and thoroughly mix in a blender or shaker for 45 seconds. Use 2-4 servings daily.

Vanilla Cream Myoplex Plus Ingredients:
MyoPro™ (unique blend of whey protein isolate from specially filtered and ion-exchanged whey protein, calcium caseinate, milk protein isolate, taurine, L-glutamine, sodium caseinate, egg albumin, and calcium alpha-ketoglutarate [AKG]), maltodextrin, corn syrup solids, vitamin and mineral blend (potassium chloride, disodium phosphate, calcium phosphate, magnesium oxide, potassium citrate, potassium phosphate, choline bitartrate, beta-carotene, ascorbic acid, dl-alpha tocopheryl acetate, ferrous fumarate, molybdenum amino acid chelate, boron proteinate, manganese gluconate, selenium amino acid chelate, niacinamide, zinc oxide, calcium pantothenate, chromium citrate, copper sulfate, Vitamin A palmitate, pyridoxine hydrochloride, riboflavin, thiamin hydrochloride, Vitamin D_3, folic acid, biotin, potassium iodide, and cyanocobalamin), natural and artificial flavor, partially hydrogenated canola oil, aspartame*, Citrimax™ (garcinia cambogia), salt, medium-chain triglycerides, xanthan gum, soy lecithin, cellulose gum, mono and diglycerides, and borage oil.

***PHENYLKETONURICS:** Contains phenylalanine.

Myoplex Plus Deluxe™

Vanilla, chocolate, and strawberry flavors available in boxes of 20 packets. Nutritional information per 83 gram vanilla serving:

Calories	300
Protein	42 g
Carbohydrates	25 g
Fat	2 g
Cholesterol	5 mg
Sodium	450 mg
Potassium	550 mg
Fiber	1 g

Vitamins and minerals:	U.S. RDA%
Vitamin A (20% as beta-carotene)	40%
Vitamin C	50%
Calcium	70%
Iron	50%
Vitamin D	50%
Vitamin E	100%
Thiamin	50%
Riboflavin	50%
Niacin	50%
Vitamin B_6	50%
Folic Acid	50%
Vitamin B_{12}	50%
Biotin	50%
Pantothenic Acid	50%
Phosphorus	50%
Iodine	50%
Magnesium	50%
Zinc	50%
Copper	50%

Also provides per serving:

Choline	100 mg
Molybdenum	50 mcg
Boron	1 mg
Manganese	400 mcg
Selenium	33 mcg
Chromium	100 mcg
Vanadyl Sulfate	10 mg
Conjugated Linoleic Acid	1,000 mg
Sodium RNA	9.5 mg

Recommended Use: For a rich, creamy shake, combine contents of packet with 16 oz of cold water, juice, or skim milk and thoroughly mix in a blender or shaker for 45 seconds. Use 2–3 servings daily.

Rich Vanilla Myoplex Plus Deluxe Ingredients:
MyoPro™ (proprietary protein blend containing whey protein isolate from ion-exchanged whey, milk protein isolate, calcium caseinate, sodium caseinate, and egg albumin), maltodextrin, GKG® (proprietary blend containing L-glutamine, calcium alpha-ketoglutarate [AKG], taurine, potassium chloride, potassium phosphate, magnesium phosphate, magnesium oxide, sodium RNA, and manganese glycinate), CLA™ (calcium conjugated linoleic acid from sunflower oil), natural and artificial flavors, partially hydrogenated canola oil, xanthan gum, V2G™ (proprietary blend containing taurine, vanadyl sulfate, and sodium selenate), vitamin and mineral blend (choline bitartrate, beta-carotene, ascorbic acid, dl-alpha tocopheryl acetate, ferrous fumarate, molybdenum amino acid chelate, boron proteinate, niacinamide, zinc oxide, calcium pantothenate, chromium citrate, copper sulfate, Vitamin A palmitate, pyridoxine hydrochloride, riboflavin, thiamin hydrochloride, Vitamin D_3, folic acid, biotin, potassium iodide, and cyanocobalamin), corn syrup solids, salt, soy lecithin, aspartame*, cellulose gum, carrageenan, Citrimax™ (garcinia cambogia), medium-chain triglycerides, mono and diglycerides, and borage oil.

***PHENYLKETONURICS:** Contains phenylalanine.

Myoplex Plus Deluxe™ Bar

Chocolate and chocolate-peanut butter flavors available in boxes of 12 bars. Nutritional information per 90 gram chocolate bar:

Calories	340
Protein	24 g
Carbohydrates	44 g
Fat	7 g
Cholesterol	<5 mg
Sodium	150 mg
Potassium	350 mg
Fiber	2 g

Vitamins and minerals:	U.S. RDA%
Vitamin A	50%
Vitamin C	50%
Calcium	25%
Iron	50%
Vitamin D	50%
Vitamin E	50%
Vitamin K	30%
Thiamin	50%
Riboflavin	50%
Niacin	50%
Vitamin B_6	50%
Folate	50%
Vitamin B_{12}	50%
Biotin	50%
Pantothenic Acid	50%
Phosphorus	25%
Iodine	50%

continued →

Magnesium	50%
Zinc	50%
Selenium	50%
Copper	50%
Manganese	50%
Chromium	80%
Molybdenum	100%

Also provides per serving:

Sodium RNA	9.5 mg
Vanadyl Sulfate	7.5 mg

Chocolate Myoplex Plus Deluxe Bar Ingredients:
MyoPro™ (proprietary protein blend containing whey protein isolate from ion-exchanged whey, calcium caseinate, and milk protein isolate), high-fructose corn syrup, sucrose, low-fat cocoa (processed with alkali), partially hydrogenated vegetable oil (cottonseed, soybean), rice flour, natural and artificial flavors, nonfat milk, milk, cocoa, unsweetened chocolate, GKG® (proprietary blend containing L-glutamine, calcium alpha-ketoglutarate [AKG], taurine, potassium chloride, potassium phosphate, magnesium oxide, magnesium phosphate, sodium RNA, and manganese glycinate), V2G™ (proprietary blend containing taurine, vanadyl sulfate, and sodium selenate), vitamin and mineral blend (dicalcium phosphate, sodium ascorbate, ferric orthophosphate, dl-alpha tocopherol acetate, niacinamide, zinc oxide, copper gluconate, calcium pantothenate, chromium citrate, Vitamin A palmitate, pyridoxine hydrochloride, riboflavin, thiamine mononitrate, folic acid, chromium chloride, sodium molybdate, biotin, potassium iodide, phylloquinone, cholecalciferol, and cyanocobalamin), CLA™ (calcium conjugated linoleic acid from sunflower oil), and lecithin.

Phosphagain 2™

Vanilla, chocolate, and strawberry flavors
available in 20-serving containers.
Nutritional information per 59 gram vanilla serving:

Calories	180
Protein	25 g
Carbohydrates	13 g
Fat	1.5 g
Cholesterol	10 mg
Sodium	380 mg
Potassium	730 mg

Vitamins and minerals:	**U.S. RDA%**
Vitamin A (10% as beta-carotene)	40%
Vitamin C	50%
Calcium	50%
Iron	20%
Vitamin D	50%
Vitamin E	50%
Thiamin	50%
Riboflavin	50%
Niacin	50%
Vitamin B_6	50%
Folic Acid	50%
Vitamin B_{12}	50%
Biotin	50%
Pantothenic Acid	50%
Phosphorus	50%
Iodine	50%
Magnesium	50%
Zinc	50%
Copper	50%

Also provides per serving:

Chromium	50 mcg
Selenium	30 mcg
Manganese	1 mg
Vitamin K	40 mcg
Molybdenum	60 mcg
Choline	80 mg

Recommended Use: Add 2 level scoops (1 serving) of Phosphagain 2™ to 14 oz of cold water, juice, or skim milk. Mix thoroughly in a blender or shaker. Drink 3 servings daily for 5 days, and then maintain at 1–2 servings daily.

Vanilla Phosphagain 2 Ingredients:
Nitrogenin 2™ proprietary protein/nitrogen reinforcing matrix (milk protein isolate, calcium caseinate, L-glutamine, taurine, calcium alpha-ketoglutarate [AKG], and egg albumin), Phosphagen™ (HPCE pure creatine monohydrate), maltodextrin, dextrose, vitamin and mineral blend (potassium phosphate, potassium citrate, salt, magnesium oxide, choline bitartrate, disodium phosphate, beta-carotene, ascorbic acid, dl-alpha tocopheryl acetate, ferrous fumarate, niacin, zinc oxide, d-calcium pantothenate, copper sulfate, Vitamin A palmitate, manganese sulfate, chromium citrate, pyridoxine hydrochloride, riboflavin, thiamin hydrochloride, sodium molybdate, Vitamin D_3, folic acid, biotin, potassium iodide, sodium selenate, Vitamin K, and cyanocobalamin), corn syrup solids, partially hydrogenated canola oil, xanthan gum, natural and artificial flavors, sodium RNA, soy lecithin, aspartame*, and carrageenan.

***PHENYLKETONURICS:** Contains phenylalanine.

PhosphaGems™

Available in 30-serving boxes.
Nutritional information per 42 gram serving:

Calories	135
Carbohydrates	35 g
Sodium	100 mg

Vitamins and minerals: ................U.S. RDA%
Not a significant source of fat, saturated fat, cholesterol, dietary fiber, Vitamins A & C, calcium, and iron.

Also provides per serving:

Phosphagen (HPCE pure creatine monohydrate)	5.2 g

Recommended Use: (One serving equals 6 "Gems.") For creatine loading, consume 4 servings daily for 5 days, then maintain at 1–2 servings daily. For best results, take one serving within 30 minutes following your workout.

PhosphaGems Ingredients:
TriCarb Complex™ (sucrose, high-dextrose corn syrup, and dextrose), Phosphagen (HPCE pure creatine monohydrate), modified starch, natural and artificial flavor, disodium phosphate, malic acid, and colored with cochineal extracts.

Phosphagen™

Available in 100, 210, 325, 500,
or 1,000 gram containers

Each 5 gram serving supplies:

Phosphagen (HPCE pure creatine monohydrate)	5 g

Recommended Use: As a dietary supplement of creatine, take 1 heaping teaspoon (5 grams), mixed into juice or water, 4 times daily for 5 days (loading dose). Thereafter, take 1 heaping teaspoon 1-2 times daily (maintenance dose). For individuals with bodyweights greater than 225 lbs, take 1 heaping teaspoon 5-6 times daily for the loading dose and 2 times daily for the maintenance dose.

Phosphagen HP™

Lemon-lime, grape, and fruit punch flavors
available in 1, 21, or 42-serving containers.
Nutritional information per 43 gram fruit punch serving:

Calories	140
Carbohydrates	34 g
Sodium	95 mg
Potassium	80 mg

Vitamins and minerals:	**U.S. RDA%**
Phosphorus	20%
Magnesium	15%

Not a significant source of fat, saturated fat, cholesterol, dietary fiber, Vitamins A & C, calcium, and iron.

Also provides per serving:

Phosphagen (HPCE pure creatine monohydrate)	5.25 g
Taurine	1,000 mg

Fruit Punch Phosphagen HP Ingredients:
Dextrose, Phosphagen (HPCE pure creatine monohydrate), taurine, natural and artificial flavor, citric acid, beet powder for color, magnesium phosphate, disodium phosphate, and potassium phosphate.

Recommended Use: Mix with 6–8 oz of cold water or juice. Drink 4 servings daily for 5 days, then maintain at 1–2 servings daily.

V2G™

Available in 180-capsule containers.

Each capsule contains:

Vanadyl Sulfate (supplying 1.5 mg of elemental vanadium [IV])	7.5 mg
Taurine	800 mg
Selenium (Sodium Selenate) (providing less than 1 mg of sodium)	33 mcg

Recommended Use: Take 2 capsules with a meal, 3 times daily. Two capsules can be taken with a protein and carbohydrate-rich meal within 1 hour following a high-intensity workout.

These statements have not been evaluated by the Food and Drug Administration. These products are not intended to diagnose, treat, cure, or prevent any disease.

Nutritional uses of HMB are licensed to Experimental and Applied Sciences, Inc. under U.S. Patent #5,348,979.

References Cited

[1] P.D. Balsom, et al., "Creatine in Humans with Special Reference to Creatine Supplementation," *Sports Medicine* 18.4 (1994) : 268-280.

[2] G. Bounous, et al., "Whey Proteins as a Food Supplement in HIV-Seropositive Individuals," *Clin. Invest. Med.* 16.3 (1993) : 204-209.

[3] G. Bounous and P. Gold, "The Biological Activity of Undenatured Whey Proteins—Role of Glutathione," *Clin. Invest. Med.* 14.4 (1991) : 296-309.

[4] C.P. Earnest, et al., "The Effect of Creatine Monohydrate Ingestion on Anaerobic Power Indices, Muscular Strength, and Body Composition," *Acta. Physiol. Scand.* 153 (1995) : 207-209.

[5] A.L. Green, et al., "Creatine Ingestion Augments Creatine Muscle Uptake and Glycogen Synthesis During Carbohydrate Feeding in Man," *J. Physiol* 491 (1996) : 63P.

[6] A.L. Green, et al., "Carbohydrate Ingestion Augments Creatine Retention During Creatine Feeding in Humans," *Acta. Physiol. Scand.* 158 (1996) : 195-202.

[7] P.L. Greenhaff, et al., "The Influence of Oral Creatine Supplementation on Muscle Phosphocreatine Resynthesis Following Intense Contraction in Man," *J. Physiol* 467 (1993) : 75P.

[8] P.L. Greenhaff, et al., "Influence of Oral Creatine Supplementation on Muscle Torque During Repeated Bouts of Maximal Voluntary Exercise in Man," *Clinical Science* 84 (1993) : 565-571.

[9] B.F. Haumann, "Conjugated Linoleic Acid Offers Research Promise," *Inform* 7.2 (1996) : 152-159.

[10] D. Häussinger, et al., "Cellular Hydration State: an Important Determinant of Protein Catabolism in Health and Disease," *Lancet* 341 (1993) : 1330-1332.

[11] D. Häussinger, et al., "Amino Acid Transport, Cell Volume and Regulation of Cell Growth," *Mammalian Amino Acid Transport* (New York: Plenum Press, 1992) 113.

[12] R.B. Kreider, et al., "Effects of Ingesting Supplements Designed to Promote Lean Tissue Accretion on Body Composition During Resistance Training," *Int. J. Sport Nutr. 6* (1996) : 234-246.

[13] R. Kreider, et al., "Effects of Ingesting a Lean Mass Promoting Supplement During Resistance Training on Isokinetic Performance," *Med. Sci. Sports Exerc.* 28 (1996) : S36.

[14] S.L. Nissen, et al., "Effect of Beta-Hydroxy-Beta-Methylbutyrate (HMB) Supplementation on Strength and Body Composition of Trained and Untrained Males Undergoing Intense Resistance Training," *FASEB J.* 10.3 (1996) : A287.

[15] S.L. Nissen, et al., "The Effect of the Leucine Metabolite β-Hydroxy β-Methylbutyrate on Muscle Metabolism During Resistance-Exercise Training," *J. Appl. Physiol.* 81.5 (1996) : 2095-2104.

[16] M. Pariza, et al., "Conjugated Linoleic Acid (CLA) Reduces Bodyfat," *Lipids*, in review (1997).

[17] M. Pariza, et al., "Mechanism of Body Fat Reduction by Conjugated Linoleic Acid," *FASEB J.* 11.3 (1997) : A139.

[18] M.J. Soares, et al., "The Effect of Exercise on the Riboflavin Status of Adult Men," *Br. J. Nutr. 69.2* (1993) : 541-551.

[19] J. Stout, et al., "The Effects of a Supplement Designed to Augment Creatine Uptake on Exercise Performance and Fat-Free Mass in Football Players," *Med. Sci. Sports Exer.*, in press (1997).

[20] M.A. Tarnopolsky, et al., "Evaluation of Protein Requirements of Trained Strength Athletes," *J. Appl. Physiol.* 73.5 (1992) : 1986-1995.

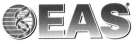

EAS supplements are available at fine health food retailers everywhere, including **GNC** GENERAL NUTRITION CENTERS LIVE WELL

To order direct **CALL 1-800-297-9776** (Dept. # 4077).

Or, use this priority NO-RISK order form to order by mail.

YES! I want to order the following EAS supplements—I understand you not only guarantee the quality and potency of every EAS product, but you also offer a lifetime money-back guarantee on all first-time purchases. In other words, if I try any EAS product and I'm not satisfied with the results, I can get my entire purchase price back, anytime!

ON THAT BASIS, SEND MY ORDER TODAY!

	Unit Price	Qty	Total
PHOSPHAGEN™			
100 g, powder	$20.95		
210 g, powder	$35.95		
325 g, powder	$52.95		
510 g, powder	$71.95		
1,000 g (kilo), powder	$121.95		
PHOSPHAGEN HP™			
21 servings, 43 g each			
Fruit Punch	$29.95		
Lemon Lime	$29.95		
Grape	$29.95		
42 servings, 43 g each			
Fruit Punch	$56.95		
Lemon Lime	$56.95		
Grape	$56.95		
Single-serving case (24 per case)			
Fruit Punch	$59.75		
Lemon Lime	$59.75		
Grape	$59.75		
PHOSPHAGEMS™			
30 servings			
Tangy Fruit Punch	$44.95		
PHOSPHAGAIN 2®			
20 servings			
Rich Vanilla	$58.00		
Deluxe Chocolate	$58.00		
Strawberry Cream	$58.00		
HMB™			
120 capsules, 250 mg HMB each	$34.95		
360 capsules, 250 mg HMB each	$89.95		
BETAGEN™ 30 servings, 6.6 g each			
Orange	$37.95		
90 servings, 6.6 g each			
Orange	$97.95		

NEW!

NEW!

NEW!

continued →

Product		Unit Price	Qty	Total
V2G™ 180 capsules, 7.5 mg vanadyl sulfate each		$34.95		
CLA™ 90 capsules, 600 mg CLA each		$29.95		
GKG® 120 capsules, 890 mg each		$29.95		
CYTOVOL™ 15 servings, 15 g each				
NEW! Lemon		$29.97		
MYOPLEX PLUS™ 20 servings, 76 g each				
Rich Vanilla		$54.95		
Deluxe Chocolate		$54.95		
Strawberry Cream		$54.95		
MYOPLEX PLUS DELUXE™ 20 servings, 83 g each				
NEW! Rich Vanilla		$63.95		
Deluxe Chocolate		$63.95		
Strawberry Cream		$63.95		
MYOPLEX PLUS DELUXE BAR™ 12 bars, 90 g each				
Chocolate		$32.95		
NEW! Chocolate Peanut Butter		$32.95		

*EAS, Inc. orders ship within 48 hours of receiving them. Shipping policy is guaranteed two-day air delivery by Federal Express. Includes packaging, handling, and insurance charges within the continental U.S. Shipping Charges: Add only $6.50 for shipping and handling on orders up to $100. Add $8.50 S&H on orders over $100 up to $200. Include $10.50 S&H on orders over $200. These rates are for orders within the continental U.S. **Colorado Residents, add 4.3% sales tax, and Golden, CO, residents add 7.3% sales tax. Check with our operators for rates on next-day air delivery by Federal Express by calling 303-279-3077. APO's and FPO's add an additional 10% of total order plus $6.50 to cover shipping charges. Alaska, Hawaii, and Canada add an additional 25% of total order plus $6.50 to cover shipping. Outside U.S. and Canada add 50% of total order plus $6.50 for shipping charges. Credit card orders are charged to EAS, Inc.

Subtotal _____

Less Coupons/Discounts _____

*Shipping and Handling _____

**CO Sales Tax _____

Grand Total _____

At EAS you can get free, expert advice from our champion bodybuilders and supplement specialists! Just call 1-800-615-8500 and ask for "technical support."

Enclosed is my ❑ Check ❑ Money Order in the amount of $ _____
(For faster service, use a money order; checks are held for 14 days. Make checks and money orders payable to EAS, Inc.)

Charge my credit card:

❑ MasterCard ❑ Visa ❑ American Express ❑ Discover Card

Credit Card Number: _____ Exp. Date: _____

Signature: _____

Telephone #: (_____) _____

Rush My Order to:

Name: _____

Address: _____

City: _____ State: _____ Zip: _____

Orders shipped **FedEx**

For Fastest Service, Use Your Credit Card And Call NOW!

1-800-297-9776

(ask for Dept. #4077)
Orders taken 24 hours a day—365 days a year!
Outside the U.S. call (303) 279-3077

Send to: EAS, Inc. (Dept. #4077), 555 Corporate Circle, Golden, CO 80401
Copyright © 1996 by Experimental and Applied Sciences, Inc.

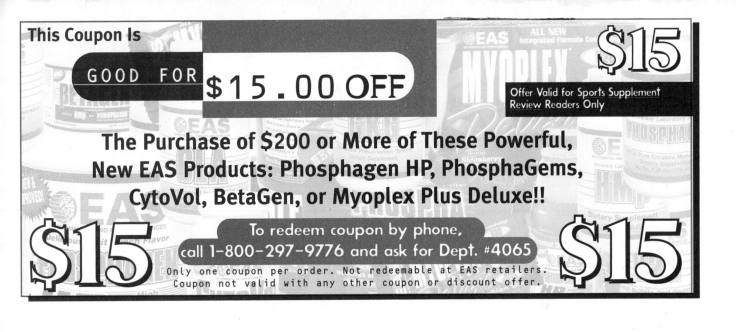

This Coupon Is

GOOD FOR **$15.00 OFF**

$15

Offer Valid for Sports Supplement Review Readers Only

The Purchase of $200 or More of These Powerful, New EAS Products: Phosphagen HP, PhosphaGems, CytoVol, BetaGen, or Myoplex Plus Deluxe!!

$15

To redeem coupon by phone, call 1-800-297-9776 and ask for Dept. #4065

$15

Only one coupon per order. Not redeemable at EAS retailers. Coupon not valid with any other coupon or discount offer.

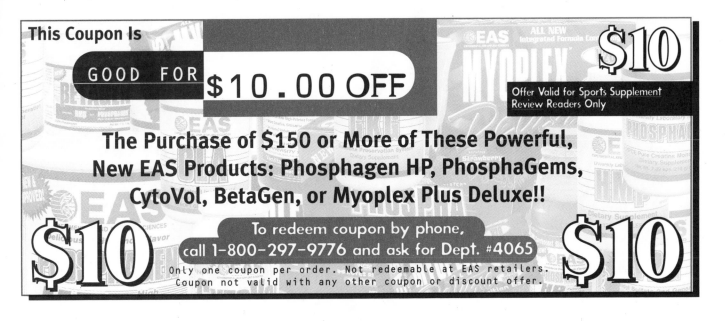

This Coupon Is

GOOD FOR **$10.00 OFF**

$10

Offer Valid for Sports Supplement Review Readers Only

The Purchase of $150 or More of These Powerful, New EAS Products: Phosphagen HP, PhosphaGems, CytoVol, BetaGen, or Myoplex Plus Deluxe!!

$10

To redeem coupon by phone, call 1-800-297-9776 and ask for Dept. #4065

$10

Only one coupon per order. Not redeemable at EAS retailers. Coupon not valid with any other coupon or discount offer.

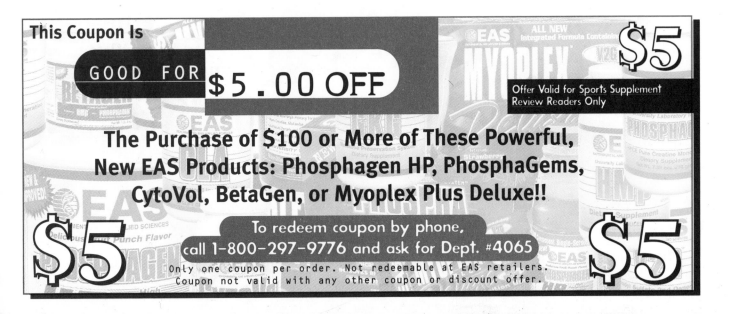

This Coupon Is

GOOD FOR **$5.00 OFF**

$5

Offer Valid for Sports Supplement Review Readers Only

The Purchase of $100 or More of These Powerful, New EAS Products: Phosphagen HP, PhosphaGems, CytoVol, BetaGen, or Myoplex Plus Deluxe!!

$5

To redeem coupon by phone, call 1-800-297-9776 and ask for Dept. #4065

$5

Only one coupon per order. Not redeemable at EAS retailers. Coupon not valid with any other coupon or discount offer.

cribe

Get This

Free!

Yours free! (a $21 value) A 100-gram bottle of the most amazing bodybuilding supplement in history—**Phosphagen.** Those of you who are already using **Phosphagen** (or another brand of creatine monohydrate) know how incredible this supplement is. **Phosphagen's** powerful effects are backed by reams of scientific data which show it **increases gains in size and muscle strength**—some users have gained up to 10 rock-hard pounds in only 10 days! Although not everyone who uses **Phosphagen** makes such extraordinary gains, it's certainly possible you could!

For those who use **Phosphagen** regularly, you'll certainly appreciate the value of receiving a free supply of this amazing supplement—those who have never tried this super bodybuilding supplement before should get ready for a big and pleasant surprise!

Phosphagen is the original creatine monohydrate supplement, introduced by Experimental and Applied Sciences—**it's the one that works!**

EAS
EXPERIMENTAL AND APPLIED SCIENCES

PHOSPHAGEN

HPLC Pure Creatine Monohydrate
Dietary Supplement

Notes

NOTES•

•SPORTS SUPPLEMENT REVIEW, 3RD ISSUE•SPORTS SUPPLEMENT REVIEW, 3RD ISSUE•SPORTS SUPPLEMENT REVIEW, 3RD ISSUE•SPORTS SUPPLEMENT REVIEW, 3RD ISSUE•SPORTS SUPPLEMENT REVIEW, 3RD ISSUE•SPORTS SUPPLEMENT REVIEW, 3RD ISSUE•SPORTS SUPPLEMENT REVIEW, 3RD ISSUE•SPORTS SUPPLEMENT REVIEW, 3RD ISSUE•SPORTS SUPPLEMENT

REVIEW•SPORTS SUPPLEMENT REVIEW, 3RD ISSUE•SPORTS SUPPLEMENT REVIEW, 3RD ISSUE•SPORTS SUPPLEMENT REVIEW, 3RD ISSUE•SPORTS SUPPLEMENT

NOTES

NOTES

NOTES•

UitalAbs, Inc.   multi vitamin

monster MATRIX - PACK

K-2 PuTE CreAtiNE

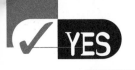

YES

You bet I want to be "updated" on the newest and "hottest" supplement breakthroughs, so I can continue my quest for the ultimate body! I understand these will be sent to me on a "semi-regular" basis...

ABSOLUTELY FREE
Sports Supplement Review
"Update"

APPLICATION FORM

Please rush my **FREE** Supplement Updates, as soon as they are published, to:

Name: _____

Address: _____

City: _____ State: _____ Zip: _____

Fill out and mail to: Mile High Publishing, Dept. #4050, P.O. Box 277, Golden, CO 80402-0277.

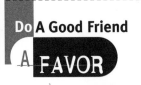

Do A Good Friend
A FAVOR

Want to make a good friend an even better friend? No problem... just tear out this card and give it to him or her, and I'll **RUSH** out a **FREE** copy of the

Sports Supplement Review! 3**RD** ISSUE

Give Him or Her This Voucher... and I'll Immediately RUSH Out a FREE Copy of the
Sports **Supplement** Review, 3**RD** ISSUE !

Bill, a good friend of mine gave me this voucher... would you please rush me a **FREE** copy of the *Sports Supplement Review, 3rd Issue* (a $29.95 value). Thanks a bunch.

Name: _____

Address: _____

City: _____ State: _____ Zip: _____

Fill out this voucher and mail it to:
Mile High Publishing, Dept. #4060, P.O. Box 277, Golden, CO 80402-0277.

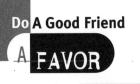

Do A Good Friend
A FAVOR

Want to make a good friend an even better friend? No problem... just tear out this card and give it to him or her, and I'll **RUSH** out a **FREE** copy of the

Sports Supplement Review! 3**RD** ISSUE

Give Him or Her This Voucher... and I'll Immediately RUSH Out a FREE Copy of the
Sports **Supplement** Review, 3**RD** ISSUE !

Bill, a good friend of mine gave me this voucher... would you please rush me a **FREE** copy of the *Sports Supplement Review, 3rd Issue* (a $29.95 value). Thanks a bunch.

Name: _____

Address: _____

City: _____ State: _____ Zip: _____

Fill out this voucher and mail it to:
Mile High Publishing, Dept. #4060, P.O. Box 277, Golden, CO 80402-0277.